T0140600

Intelligent Systems Reference Library

Volume 229

Series Editors

Janusz Kacprzyk, Polish Academy of Sciences, Warsaw, Poland

Lakhmi C. Jain, KES International, Shoreham-by-Sea, UK

The aim of this series is to publish a Reference Library, including novel advances and developments in all aspects of Intelligent Systems in an easily accessible and well structured form. The series includes reference works, handbooks, compendia, textbooks, well-structured monographs, dictionaries, and encyclopedias. It contains well integrated knowledge and current information in the field of Intelligent Systems. The series covers the theory, applications, and design methods of Intelligent Systems. Virtually all disciplines such as engineering, computer science, avionics, business, e-commerce, environment, healthcare, physics and life science are included. The list of topics spans all the areas of modern intelligent systems such as: Ambient intelligence, Computational intelligence, Social intelligence, Computational neuroscience, Artificial life, Virtual society, Cognitive systems, DNA and immunity-based systems, e-Learning and teaching, Human-centred computing and Machine ethics, Intelligent control, Intelligent data analysis, Knowledge-based paradigms, Knowledge management, Intelligent agents, Intelligent decision making, Intelligent network security, Interactive entertainment, Learning paradigms, Recommender systems, Robotics and Mechatronics including human-machine teaming, Self-organizing and adaptive systems, Soft computing including Neural systems, Fuzzy systems, Evolutionary computing and the Fusion of these paradigms, Perception and Vision, Web intelligence and Multimedia.

Indexed by SCOPUS, DBLP, zbMATH, SCImago.

All books published in the series are submitted for consideration in Web of Science.

Chee Peng Lim · Ashlesha Vaidya · Yen-Wei Chen ·
Vaishnavi Jain · Lakhmi C. Jain
Editors

Artificial Intelligence and Machine Learning for Healthcare

Vol. 2: Emerging Methodologies and Trends

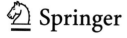

Springer

Editors
Chee Peng Lim
Deakin University
Victoria, VIC, Australia

Ashlesha Vaidya
Royal Adelaide Hospital
Adelaide, SA, Australia

Yen-Wei Chen
College of Information Science
and Engineering
Ritsumeikan University
Kusuatsu, Shiga, Japan

Vaishnavi Jain
ASF Insignia
Kyndryl Solutions Pvt Ltd.
Gurugram, Haryana, India

Lakhmi C. Jain
Liverpool Hope University
Liverpool, UK

KES International
Shoreham-by-Sea, UK

ISSN 1868-4394   ISSN 1868-4408 (electronic)
Intelligent Systems Reference Library
ISBN 978-3-031-11172-3   ISBN 978-3-031-11170-9 (eBook)
https://doi.org/10.1007/978-3-031-11170-9

© The Editor(s) (if applicable) and The Author(s), under exclusive license to Springer Nature
Switzerland AG 2023
This work is subject to copyright. All rights are solely and exclusively licensed by the Publisher, whether
the whole or part of the material is concerned, specifically the rights of translation, reprinting, reuse
of illustrations, recitation, broadcasting, reproduction on microfilms or in any other physical way, and
transmission or information storage and retrieval, electronic adaptation, computer software, or by similar
or dissimilar methodology now known or hereafter developed.
The use of general descriptive names, registered names, trademarks, service marks, etc. in this publication
does not imply, even in the absence of a specific statement, that such names are exempt from the relevant
protective laws and regulations and therefore free for general use.
The publisher, the authors, and the editors are safe to assume that the advice and information in this book
are believed to be true and accurate at the date of publication. Neither the publisher nor the authors or
the editors give a warranty, expressed or implied, with respect to the material contained herein or for any
errors or omissions that may have been made. The publisher remains neutral with regard to jurisdictional
claims in published maps and institutional affiliations.

This Springer imprint is published by the registered company Springer Nature Switzerland AG
The registered company address is: Gewerbestrasse 11, 6330 Cham, Switzerland

Preface

This volume is a sequel of the edition on *Artificial Intelligence and Machine Learning for Healthcare*. A number of artificial intelligence/machine learning (AL/ML)-based image and data analytics solutions for addressing medical and healthcare problems are presented in the first volume. In this second volume, a total of ten chapters dedicated to emerging methodologies and future trends of AL/ML in the medical and healthcare domains are covered. A description of each contribution is as follows.

Ruiz and Velasquez analysed new paradigms to develop preventive, participatory, predictive, and personalised medicine (4P medicine). The foundation and potential for AI and ML to solicit knowledge through intelligent image and data processing are explained. Considering health-related databases only grow in complexity and size, AI and ML play a critical role to establish automated tools for processing and extraction of healthcare information and knowledge. The formation of multi-disciplinary teams to design and develop new intelligent solutions for supporting decision-making is vital, contributing towards the advancement of 4P medicine in the future.

Belciug provided a guide on survival analysis and practical examples in oncology. Several methodologies, which include Kaplan–Meier survival curves, logrank test, hazard ratio, and Cox regression, are introduced to determine the best course of medical treatment. A step-by-step guide for performing survival analysis and interpreting the obtained results is provided.

Kapoteli et al. devised a general approach to sentiment analysis pertaining to COVID-19 vaccination and reviewed several use cases. Based on a Twitter dataset on COVID-19 vaccination, both supervised and unsupervised models for sentiment analysis are explored. The developed methodology is useful for mining information on public attitudes, forecasting opinions and reactions related to vaccine update in near real time, which is critical in dealing with health emergency situations.

Michailidis et al. utilised data mining techniques for incident prediction and general medical knowledge acquisition. ML methodologies that are useful for healthcare support are explained, which include classification, regression, clustering, and association rules. A study on stroke prediction is used to illustrate the effectiveness of ML models, while issues and challenges of data mining in stroke prediction and general healthcare support are also discussed.

Ageing is a real concern nowadays in many countries. Within the European ageing population, hearing loss, cardiovascular diseases, cognitive impairments, mental health, and balance disorders are prevalent medical conditions that cause tremendous social and financial issues. Bellandi et al. conducted a study on preventing, slowing the development of, or dealing effectively with the effects of these medical conditions and related issues. An eHealth platform leveraging AI and ML models is devised. Personalised notifications and alerts can be generated by collecting and analysing daily activity data of the elderly through the integration of heterogeneous smart devices, e.g. wearables and environment sensors. This allows an affordable, secure, and privacy-preserving living environment to be established for promoting healthy and independent living for the ageing population.

Game-based virtual reality (VR) rehabilitation protocols offer a promising therapeutic alternative for activating neuro-motor functions as well as sustaining motivation and achieving rehabilitation goals of patients. Jeyakumar et al. studied a wide range of VR-based applications for rehabilitation treatments and discussed the role of virtual games for rapid recovery during post-therapy. Case studies on sports rehabilitation exercises for athletes suffering from musculoskeletal injuries and guidelines for them to return to play are also presented.

Learning and playing games are useful for children to develop social skills. Mihova et al. reviewed on the use of serious games to improve the communication skills of youngsters with Autism Spectrum Disorder (ASD). Specialised games are useful tools to help the development of a child's skills based on certain parameters. The review and findings assist stakeholders in understanding the impacts of using smartphones, mobile apps, and computer games as a therapeutic approach to enhancing social skills of ASD children.

Ovalle-Magallanes et al. presented an overview and future trend on deep learning-based coronary stenosis detection in X-ray angiography images. The basic methodologies of convolutional neural networks, attention modules, vision transformers, and quantum computing are explained. The use of hybrid methods for enhancing the effectiveness of deep learning models is described. Challenges and future directions on stenosis detection methods are also discussed.

Hoppe et al. conducted a systematic literature review on the potential benefit of AI in the healthcare sector. The main factors concerning AI in health care are analysed, which include management tasks, medical diagnostics, medical treatment, and drug discovery. Utilising structural equation modelling, medical diagnostics, and drug discovery is identified as positive and significant influencing factors with respect to the potential benefit of AI in health care. Various recommendations to further exploit the potential of AI in health care are provided.

Beltempo et al. analysed the barriers associated with AI in the healthcare sector. Based on a systematic literature review, several key barriers concerning AI in health care are identified and examined, namely disagreement in data protection, lack of compatibility with ethical aspects, quality of training data, knowledge, and trust of physicians in AI-supported systems. Opinions solicited from interviews with medical professionals and AI developers are compared and discussed. Potential resolutions to undertake the identified barriers are derived, contributing towards advancing AI for the healthcare sector in future.

The editors are grateful to all authors for their contributions and to Springer editorial team for their support throughout the compilation of both volumes of this edition. We sincerely hope that the selected chapters in both volumes offer new knowledge and ideas for readers to design, develop, and implement AI/ML systems for delivering better healthcare services and realising 4P medicine for the betterment of our society.

Victoria, Australia	Chee Peng Lim
Adelaide, Australia	Ashlesha Vaidya
Kusuatsu, Japan	Yen-Wei Chen
Gurugram, India	Vaishnavi Jain
Liverpool/Shoreham-by-Sea, UK	Lakhmi C. Jain
May 2022	

Contents

10 Barriers of Artificial Intelligence in the Health Sector 251
Laura Beltempo, Jasmin Zerrer, Ralf-Christian Härting,
and Nathalie Hoppe

Chapter 1
Artificial Intelligence for the Future of Medicine

Rocío B. Ruiz and Juan D. Velásquez

Abstract Since its origins, medicine has been more linked to the cure of diseases than to their prevention. This is due to multiple factors, training of health professionals aimed at curing diseases, lack of quality data, processing capacity, poor multidisciplinary approach, etc. However, this paradigm is changing, focusing on maintaining the health of individuals to avoid diseases, improving social welfare. To achieve this, the new approach proposes that medicine must be Preventive, Participatory, Predictive, and Personalized (P4 Medicine). In this chapter, we will analyze how artificial intelligence can convincingly contribute to the construction of P4 Medicine, through the processing of key data such as DNA, electronic medical records and environmental variables to which people have been exposed. Here we can find complex data such as Computed Tomography images, electroencephalograms, free text in electronic medical records, pharmacological data, etc. These data have grown exponentially and efforts to improve their quality are already paying off. However, it is no longer possible for a health professional to analyze them to provide a better diagnosis or carry out preventive work on diseases, requiring the formation of multidisciplinary teams to find new solutions to ancient problems, such as healthcare, where data processing, knowledge extraction and its subsequent parameterization in support systems for medical decision-making are vital to save lives. In this sense, artificial intelligence, together with new methods for processing complex data and computational resources to process massive data, will be key to improving the humanity health.

Keywords Artificial intelligence · Machine learning · Healthcare · P4 medicine

R. B. Ruiz · J. D. Velásquez (✉)
Department of Industrial Engineering, Web Intelligence Consortium, Chile Research Centre, University of Chile, Av. Beauchef 851, East Tower, Office 619, 8370456 Santiago, Chile
e-mail: jvelasqu@dii.uchile.cl

R. B. Ruiz
e-mail: rocio.ruiz@wic.uchile.cl

Instituto Sistemas Complejos de Ingeniería (ISCI), Santiago, Chile

© The Author(s), under exclusive license to Springer Nature Switzerland AG 2023
C. P. Lim et al. (eds.), *Artificial Intelligence and Machine Learning for Healthcare*,
Intelligent Systems Reference Library 229,
https://doi.org/10.1007/978-3-031-11170-9_1

1

1.1   Introduction

Artificial Intelligence (AI) is perhaps the greatest technological revolution of the 21st century. Its beginnings can be placed in the late 50s, when the famous English mathematician Alan Turing began to wonder what conditions are needed to consider a machine as intelligent. His ideas were reflected in his seminal article *"Computing Machinery and Intelligence"* [1]. However, the main concept was coined in 1956 by John McCarthy in the Dartmouth Summer Research Project on Artificial Intelligence [2], defining AI as *"the science and engineering of making intelligent machines, especially intelligent computer programs"*. Currently, practically no technological development escapes the use or influence of AI. We can find it in everyday situations such as the coffee machine that prepares us a cappuccino or sophisticated ones such as those that allow us to calculate the most optimal path so that an emergency vehicle (ambulance, fire truck, etc.) finds the optimal route to save lives or even very complex ones like a robot performing a complex surgery on a patient with a critical heart condition. In that sense, the IA has two main branches: virtual and physical. The first one is related with the informatics approaches where the algorithms are used for creating complex computer systems. The second one is close to robotics, where the algorithms are used to give the correct movement to the physic parts of a devices to perform an specific task.

But, what is intelligence? A very simple question with a no simple answer. In fact, we don't have a general agreement on the definition of intelligence, but some good approaches have been presented during the last century, such as the capacity to give good answers from the point of view of truth or facts [3], the ability to continue an abstract thinking [4], the combination of abilities necessaries to survive in a particular culture [5], the ability to solve problems, to create products valued based on cultural settings [6] and from Random House Unabridged Dictionary (2006), the *"capacity for learning, reasoning, understanding, and similar forms of mental activity; aptitude in grasping truths, relationships, facts, meanings, etc."*. It seems the learning capacity is an important issue when we try to explain what intelligence is.

Can a machine be intelligent as a human being? For now and hopefully for the future, the answer is no. But a very good approach is to give the machines the capacity of learning from data originated in a source, for example environmental data for a good prediction about future conditions. In that sense, if during the learning process the machine gets enough capacity to predict future scenarios, and making good predictions for taking correct decisions, we will be in front of an intelligent machine. But the reasoning and understanding capacities are not present in that machine.

For creating an intelligent machine, the learning process is essential because it is where the machine can identify patterns from the data and define rules on how to use them to make its best prediction regarding a future situation. However, data is not always required to make a machine perform tasks as an intelligent being would. Who has not ever played chess with the computer? Normally chess programming is based on rules of piece movements, being unnecessary data regarding the moves of other players. But these rules intrinsically contain a series of patterns that the programmer has programmed into algorithms. Clearly, the algorithm that represents the cybernetic player can be improved by finding new patterns that the programmer never imagined. This is where once again the massive processing of data from other players' plays becomes extremely relevant. Indeed, the algorithm that represents the cybernetic player can be continuously improved until it reaches the point where it learns from patterns of so many plays that it practically covers a large part of the universe of possibilities that a human player would have, making the machine beat the man, which has already happened, but it has not been a process of reasoning, but rather of processing capacity.

There is no doubt that the applications developed and to be developed based on AI are beyond any prediction that we can make at the moment. However, it is practically an assumed fact that the world we know is undergoing dizzying changes where AI in many cases has taken a leading role. This is how in healthcare and in medicine in general, the next step in its development cannot be taken without the support of AI.

Since immemorial time, medicine has been focused on the cure of diseases and ailments of all kinds of patients [7], who have in common that symptoms have first manifested before decisions can be made, which in many cases may arrive late. However, the focus is changing, where the maintenance of healthy begins to to be relevant. Indeed, medicine is moving from a reactive to a proactive discipline being participatory, predictive, personalized and preventive P4 medicine [8]. The foregoing will be possible to the extent that we can obtain information and knowledge of the data related to the health of patients, in particular their DNA, electronic medical records and the environment in which they have lived, among other data. This is a huge challenge, starting with the maintenance and consolidation of data that ensures secure access for study purposes and of course to help patients with their ailments. Followed by the data storage and processing capacity for the extraction of patterns that help all health personnel in tasks such as diagnosis, treatment, medication, etc. And finally, to provide adequate help to both the patient and the health personnel to achieve the primary objective that goes beyond the cure of the disease, we refer to the maintenance of good health in the population. Given this scenario, artificial intelligence is playing a key role in massive data processing that allows the creation of countless applications, which cover practically all branches of medicine, such as radiology, nephrology, nutrition, psychiatry, neurology, etc. [9].

This chapter is organized as follow. Section 1.2 introduces the process about how the machines learn. In Sect. 1.3, the possible applications of artificial intelligence in medicine is shown. A short review about papers related with P4 medicine is developed in Sect. 1.4. And finally, as chapter's summary, some reflections on the current and future potential of the application of artificial intelligence in medicine are shown.

1.2 How Do Machines Learn?

How do we human beings learn? through examples which are reflected in our neural network that then allow us to analyze sounds, images, movements, structures, tastes, etc. In this sense, the automatic learning of a machine is very similar, that is, many examples are needed so that the machine can extract patterns from the data that then allows it to extrapolate a future decision. When they receive data that did not belong to the set of examples as input and for which you are looking for an output, it will give you the best prediction based on what it had learnt before [10].

According to [11] an algorithm is capable to learn when given a task, training experience, and a performance measure, so its achievement on the task improves with experience. Based on experiences learned, the algorithms can take decisions, make predictions, classify objects, predict cancer in a patient, give directions to the robots, recognize the human voice, and a huge set the possible uses and applications. In this context, the data play a central role in achieving a correct training of the algorithms. In other words, if the data are not clean and consolidated, the training of the algorithm will be affected and its learning capacity will be reduced, which will affect all the uses described above, making it impossible to create applications.

Machine learning is the concept that groups the set of algorithms that are capable of learning from the data. It was defined by Arthur L. Samuel as a *"field of study that gives computers the ability to learn without being explicitly programmed"* [12]. Depending of type of data and the algorithm to use, the learning process can be classified in supervised, unsupervised, reinforcement [13], and deep learning [14].

In **supervised learning**, a set of training data is created where the input and output vector are known. Then the algorithm learns the associations between inputs and outputs to create a mathematical model, which is validated and tested with real data before it can be used. A different situation happens in **unsupervised learning** where the algorithm learns the associations in the training data but the output is unknown, identifying undiscovered patterns. In **reinforcement learning** the algorithm learns a behaviour through trial-and-error to maximize a defined reward. Finally, **deep learning** allow to process big amount of raw data to extract patterns for detection or classification of issues.

1.2.1 Machine Learning Process

Giving a collection of data we are trying to extract patterns and rules about how to use them. The basic assumption is that the data was not created randomly, i.e., there are intrinsic relationships among them, for example regularities, which can then be detected and represented as patterns that allow a machine learning algorithm to be trained. In other words, if the data are dirty, their dispersion is high or there are no possible relationships among them, then there will be no machine learning algorithm able to create an analysis, predict, classify, or model the phenomenon under study. In that sense, statistical techniques are used to analyze the quality of the data and make prospects of its possible uses in a training process of a machine learning algorithm [15].

Figure 1.1 shows a conceptual diagram about the machine learning algorithms, where the deep learning one is part of the artificial neural network family. Depending on the kind of data to be processed and the phenomenon under study to be modeled, is the machine learning algorithms to use.

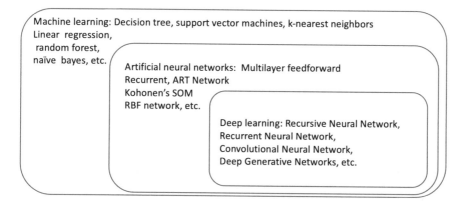

Fig. 1.1 Machine learning algorithms, concepts and classes, based on [14]

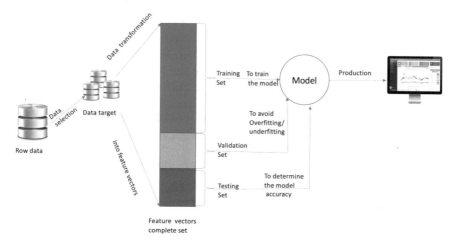

Fig. 1.2 Machine learning general training process workflow

Figure 1.2 shows the general learning process for machine learning algorithms focused in supervised learning. From a set of row data, the target data, i.e. the data to be considered to analyze the phenomenon under study, are selected. Next, a feature vector transformation process is developed. The feature vectors set is divided in three parts: training, validation, and testing. The training data are used to train the model by applying a selected machine learning algorithm. Then the model is validated to check if there are problems of overfitting/underfitting. And finally, testing is applied to get some effectiveness measure such as accuracy. After the whole process, the model is put into production, being useful for taking decisions.

1.2.2   Machine Learning in Medicine

Considering the current amount of data related to people's health, and that its future growth will be exponential, it is no longer possible by using traditional methods of extracting information and knowledge, fundamentally manual, can obtain any benefit from these data [16]. In this way that machine learning algorithms have become the new way of processing large volumes of data, in many cases complex and multivariable, and in particular medical data [17].

Machine learning algorithms and a subset of them, like deep learning, allow to create a computational model to process medical data for getting novel patterns from raw data, for instance, digitized X-ray images of a human chest to detect if the patient has pneumonia or COVID-19 [18]. The learning model is trained by using a set of learning techniques, in this case an object detection technique to predict if a new chest X-ray image is classify as normal, pneumonia, or COVID-19.

Medical data are available in an enormous variety of types and sources, which include diseases, public health data, prognosis, diagnosis, images, time series, etc., and everything indicates that its growth will continue to be exponential, as more and better sensor devices are added to medical exams [19]. Almost by construction, medical data are complex to analyze, even when there are very few records to analyze a disease, the mere fact that these records have high dimentionality makes them a challenge in machine learning. Additionally, in many cases it is not entirely clear what methods have been used to ensure the quality of medical data, which directly influences the predictive quality of the model to be trained [20].

There is no doubt that the applications of machine learning, and deep learning in particular, in medicine are enormous and will continue to expand in the incoming years. In [17] presents a study on the use of machine learning in medical research in recent years. From there it follows that the most used algorithms have been Random Forrest, Decision Tree, Support Vector Machine, Naïve Bayes, Artificial Neural Networks, and clustering techniques. Especial attention with Deep Learning algorithms, used in an important set of papers, in particular Convolutional neural network (CNN) for medical imagine processing [21].

1.3   Artificial Intelligence in Medicine

During the last decade, Artificial Intelligence research has grown exponentially in projects related to medicine. Indeed only in 2016, AI projects related to medicine attracted much more investment than AI projects related to other sectors of the global economy [22, 23]. What factors explain this heightened growth and interest?, among the reasons we can find is the great capacity of AI to improve the efficiency and effectiveness of healthcare delivery. AI in medicine aims to optimize clinical decision-making by using data related with health to provide information and patterns for improving the healthcare of the individuals.

Then, what AI algorithms can do for the future of medicine? It is an inescapable fact that in the developed world, the amount of data related to each person's health is growing by leaps and bounds. Also that the reality of the quality and consolidation of these data in many countries is doubtful. However, steps are being taken in the right direction to achieve the digitalization of computer systems related to electronic medical data, continuous improvement in data quality, interoperability of systems, and security protocols that guarantee that the access, processing, and use of the data will be carried out in accordance with the law [24]. In this context, there is only one question: what do we do with medical data? This is where AI plays a central role. With the avalanche of data that health information systems are producing day by day, the number of exams that patients must perform, DNA analyzes that are less expensive every day, and the data provided by the patients themselves through applications for Smartphones or other devices, the possibility of a human being able to analyze all this is simply impossible, which is why advanced mechanisms are required in data processing and in the presentation of information and patterns for making relevant clinical decisions.

Consider the following situation. A person suffers from a severe headache and tells a friend about his ailment. Immediately the friend takes out a medicine that he carries in his backpack that a doctor diagnosed him with years ago and that has always helped him with his headaches. Immediately afterwards, he gives a pill to his friend so that he can make the strong pain that he is suffering disappear. Several questions immediately arise: (1) if they are different persons, why give them the same drug? (2) does the friend know the person's medical history?; (3) The dose delivered is correct?; (4) Will there be any contraindications? And we could continue asking questions, but the fact is that the advisable thing would be that if they are different persons, the treatment at least would not have to be the same. This is the essence of precision medicine that is the basis of the medicine of the future. Precision medicine, sometimes called personalized medicine is defined by the National Institute of Health (NIH) precision medicine as *"refers to a new treatment and prevention method based on understanding of individual gene, environment and life-style"* [25]. And to achieve this, information and knowledge extracted from quality data per individual are required, considering their medical history, DNA, environment, and lifestyle.

Figure 1.3 shows the integration of several data sources related with the patients, and the respective data processing by using artificial intelligence tools, machine learning algorithms and deep learning algorithms. The outcome aims to provide information, patterns, knowledge, etc, to improve the decision-making for different users, such as healthcare professionals and patients.

In Fig. 1.3, the collection of data presented is only a part of the data that are related to the life and healthcare of people. Among these data we also find those from online social networks [26] and those provided by people through smartphone applications related to healthcare [27]. Clearly, the more quality data that can be collected from an individual, the better the diagnosis to cure a disease or the advice to maintain their health, making the patient central in their healthcare. However, such amount of data cannot be processed directly by human beings, so a large data processing capacity is

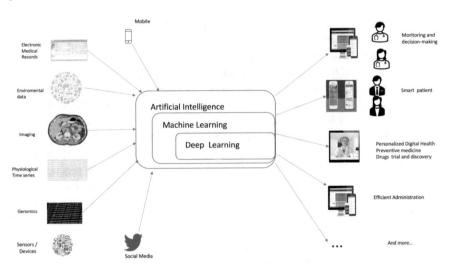

Fig. 1.3 Artificial intelligence as enable factor for future medicine

needed together with advanced algorithms for the extraction of information, patterns, and knowledge. The final result points to multiple users, starting with the patient, being able to make correct use of this new knowledge, which is key in healthcare.

There is no doubt that AI is causing a great positive revolution in terms of people's healthcare. However, not everything is a rose garden. As it is sensitive personal data, its processing must be carried out under strict security measures and ethical considerations [28]. Indeed, what would happen when analyzing the DNA data of an individual, it is detected that she/he has a high probability of developing diabetes in the future, will this be a prevalence? will health insurance cover this disease? will the individual suffer some kind of discrimination? We must not forget that the use of AI in healthcare is to help people in an ethical and responsible manner [29], taking care that their personal data is not used for purposes other than to support health maintenance or cure the disease that affects an individual. In no way can they be used for other purposes that violate the fundamental human rights [30].

1.4 AI Applications in Medicine

As mentioned above, the development of high-throughput, data-intensive research assays, and technologies in medicine has created a need for researchers to develop strategies to analyze, integrate, and interpret the massive amounts of data they generate. Traditional approaches do not allow working with 'big data', which presents the opportunity to improve people's health, so the use of AI techniques suggest that they could be particularly appropriate. In addition, the results of the application of medical exams reveal a great heterogeneity in the pathophysiological factors and processes that contribute to a disease, suggesting that there is a need to adapt or 'customize' the medicines to the nuanced characteristics and, often, unique to individual patients [31].

P4 Medicine represents the foundations of a model of clinical medicine, which offers the opportunity to modify the healthcare paradigm: the participation of the individual is essential to put into practice the other three aspects of P4 Medicine with each patient [32].

In Fig. 1.4 a summary about the P4 Medicine is shown. The future of health services focuses on giving people a complete picture of the many factors that affect their health. Personalized medicine proposes the integration of numerous biological data points, including molecular, cellular, and phenotypic longitudinal measurements, as well as individual genome sequences, to better define the health or well-being of each person, predict transitions to disease and guide medical interventions [33–35]. The implementation of the P4 from the clinical point of view will create predictive and personalized models that represent the well-being of each patient or of a disease, which will allow the design of new pharmacological tests that take into account the heterogeneity of responses to therapies and disease stratification [36].

1.4.1 Predictive Medicine

Predictive medicine is a branch of medicine that aims to identify patients at risk of developing a disease, allowing for early prevention or treatment of that disease. Single or more commonly multiple assays are used to identify markers of future disease disposition [38].

The goal of predictive medicine is to obtain and catalog the characteristics of individual patients, analyze that data to predict an individual patient's risk for an outcome of interest, predict which treatment in which individual will be most effective, and then intervene before the event occurs. However, previously limited to the realm of genetics, genetics-based risk prediction has been of limited benefit because whole genome sequencing is still relatively expensive, and most diseases affecting today's population depend on different variables [39]. These are not only influenced by genetics but also by demographic, psychosocial data, eating habits, stress levels, etc. Therefore, the need arises to collect and organize different types of data to perform a more complete analysis of people.

In recent years, machine learning algorithms such as deep learning that can account for complex interactions among features is shown to be promising in predictive modeling in healthcare [40]. Artificial intelligence can help doctors make better clinical decisions. Algorithms can unlock clinically relevant information hidden in the vast volume of healthcare data guided by clinically relevant questions asked by healthcare professionals. In clinical trials of most medical studies, specific hypotheses or questions are clearly defined, and algorithms are trained to predict

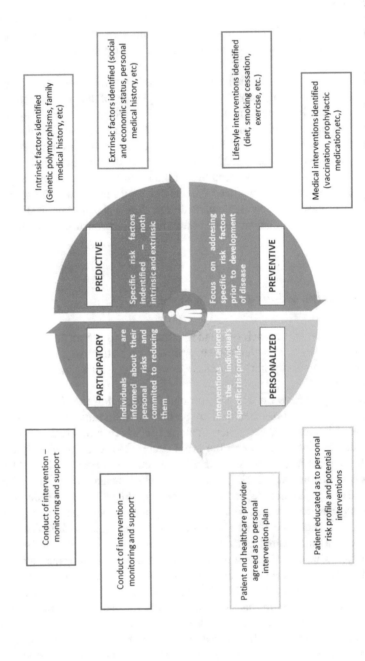

Fig. 1.4 Summary scheme of the definitions and components of the 4Ps of medicine: predictive, preventive, personalized, and participatory. Own elaboration based on [37]

certain outcomes, given that a set of features and insights can be developed through prediction [41].

Artificial intelligence is used in many different health conditions and healthcare applications, for example, to assess the readmission of patients to hospitals [42], to detect patients who will suffer adverse effects when taking medications [43], in chronic diseases such as diabetes [44] and hypertension [45]; just to name a few. Table 1.1 presents some research that has applied artificial intelligence in predictive medicine.

1.4.2 Participatory Medicine

Participatory medicine focuses on the patient, in order to empower people to make more informed decisions related to their health, where the individual/patient is at the center of any related health care initiative [61]. In recent times, the role of patients in managing their own health has been changing [62]. People have gone from being mere observers to more active, committed and empowered actors in the decision-making process shared with the health team [63, 64]. For example, vaccination is strictly participatory since the individual is responsible for administering it, including that of children. This issue has become highly relevant due to the pandemic, and the multiple recently developed COVID-19 vaccines, given their differences in composition, timing of administration, effectiveness, and potential adverse events [65].

AI applied to participatory health involves individuals and their representatives, who would be the main beneficiaries of this technology [66, 67]. People can collect, record, and track indicators to quantify their health, providing insights into their overall health status [68], giving AI the opportunity to further understand their health.Continuing with the example in the pandemic context, thanks to AI, surveillance, monitoring of close contacts, compliance with quarantines, and the reduction of workload for health teams have been facilitated. Along with this, mobile technology has been harnessed to collect data on the symptoms reported by individuals combined with other data from different sources to obtain information on the disease and the spread of infection, contributing to knowledge about the prevalence and transmission of asymptomatic COVID-19 [69]. Images from security cameras, facial recognition, bank card records, and GPS data from vehicles and mobile phones have also been used to closely monitor possible contacts between infected people. In this way, data on the location and movements of people were collected to alert neighbors/patients to new cases.

AI applications within participatory health have been evaluated in the context of a wide variety of health conditions, health promotion activities, and healthcare settings through: social media, mobile apps, chatbots, health records, questionnaires, and open collaborative health studies [64, 67]. Each allows for the generation, production, or collection of various types of data, reflecting various facets of health, including psychological, physical, social, physiological, or cognitive indicators.

Table 1.1 Summary of research focusing on predictive medicine

Author, year	Area	Description	Data	AI tasks
Goh et al. [46]	Sepsis	An artificial intelligence algorithm was developed, which uses structured data and unstructured clinical notes to predict and diagnose sepsis	Singapore government-based hospital	NLP— Voting ensemble
Dhaese et al. [47]	COVID-19	Predict the onset of symptoms consistent with a viral illness three days before symptoms	Data from portable devices	The set of probabilistic rules comprises a Markov network
Elujide et al. [48]	Psychotic disorders	Early classification of five psychotic disorders: bipolar disorder, vascular dementia, attention deficit/hyperactivity disorder, insomnia and schizophrenia	Yaba Psychiatric Hospital, Yaba, Lagos State, Nigeria	Deep learning— Multilayer perceptron—Support vector machine—Random forest—Decision tree
Noor et al. [49]	Depression	This article presents a model to predict depression risk based on electrocardiogram (ECG) and classification of normal, abnormal heartbeats and PVC (Premature Ventricular Contraction)	Electrocardiograms with heart rates from UEA and UCR Time Series Classification Repository	Autoencoder LSTM
Vijayalaxmi et al. [50]	Multi-disease/Diabetes	This work aims to develop a portable and affordable diagnostic system to measure basic health parameters such as Body mass index (BMI), temperature, pulse rate, blood oxygen saturation level, blood pressure, and blood glucose content to predict the future health complications that could be used to take preventive measures	Dataset of Pima Indians Diabetes, which is taken from the national institute of diabetes and digestive and kidney diseases	Decision tree—Naive Bayes—K-neighbors classifiers
Lauritsen et al. [51]	Sepsis, AKI, and ALI, respectively	Presents an alert scoring system for the early detection of chronic diseases	Secondary health care data for all residents of four Danish municipalities (Odder, Hedensted, Skanderborg and Horsens)	Convolutional neural network
Jiang et al. [52]	COVID-19	Develop a model that predicts which COVID-19 patients are at increased risk of worsening and complications	Patient data from two hospitals in Wenzhou, Zhejiang, China	Support Vector Machine—K-neighbors classifier—Logistic Regression—Decision Tree—Random Forest
Kanegae et al. [53]	Hypertension	This study used machine learning techniques to develop and validate a new hypertension risk prediction model	Annual health checks that companies perform on their employees in Japan	XGBoost - Logistic Regression

(continued)

Table 1.1 (continued)

Author, year	Area	Description	Data	AI tasks
Rebane et al. [54]	Adverse Drug Events	A System for Detecting Medications, Adverse Drug Events, and Their Relations from Clinical Notes	Clinical notes provided by the University of Massachusetts Medical School through the MADE1.0 challenge	Recurrent Neural Networks LSTM—NLP—Support Vector Machine—Random Forest
Kalmady et al. [55]	Schizophrenia	Early diagnosis of schizophrenia in patients without prior treatment with antipsychotic drugs	Data from functional magnetic resonance imaging (fMRI) and alterations in resting-state (RS) from patients attending the clinical services of the National Institute of Mental Health and Neurosciences (NIMHANS, India)	Principal Components Analysis - Logistic Regression
Schmidt et al. [56]	Vision	Individual prediction of the progression of macular degeneration (disease that affects a person's central vision)	Monthly standardized optical coherence tomography (OCT) images, demographic and genetic characteristics of patients with muscle degeneration who participated in the HARBOR clinical trial	Sparse Cox proportional hazards (CPH) model
Choi et al. [57]	Multiple diseases	Build a general temporal predictive model to predict (all) diagnoses and medication categories for a visit (for all medical conditions); as well as forecasting the time to the next doctor visit	EHR from primary care patients from Sutter Health Palo Alto Medical Foundation	Recurrent Neural Network GRU - Continuous-time Markov chains—Latent space models—Logistic Regression—Multilayer Perceptron
Esteban et al. [58]	Kidney transplant	The objective is to predict, based on the information obtained from the electronic medical record of each patient, if any post-kidney transplant event (death, rejection or transplant loss) will occur within the next six or twelve months after each clinic visit	Database collected at Charité Hospital in Berlin with patients who have undergone or are awaiting a kidney transplant	Recurrent Neural Networks (GRU and LSTM)—Logistic Regression—Artificial Neural Networks
Francis et al. [59]	Colorectal cancer	Predict delayed discharge and readmission in enhanced recovery following laparoscopic colorectal cancer surgery	Colorectal cancer patients undergoing laparoscopic surgery within the enhanced recovery after surgery (ERAS) program	Artificial Neural Networks—Logistic Regression
Ng et al. [60]	Breast Cancer	Research using thermography and artificial intelligence for breast cancer diagnosis	Patient data from Singapore General Hospital	Artificial Neural Networks

Tables 1.2 and 1.3 present the tools that have been used to apply AI in participatory medicine: papers that work with social networks and research where different devices and applications are used.

1.4.3   Personalized Medicine

Personalized medicine is the tailoring of therapies to defined subsets of patients based on their likelihood to respond to therapy or their risk of adverse events [85]. It uses an individual's genetic profile to guide decisions about disease prevention, diagnosis, and treatment. Knowing a patient's genetic profile can help clinicians select the appropriate drug or treatment and administer it at the appropriate dose or regimen [86].

Personalized medicine has the potential to tailor therapy with the best response and the largest safety margin to ensure better patient care. By enabling every patient to receive early diagnosis, risk assessment and optimal treatment, it promises to improve care while lowering costs [87].

The focus of personalized medicine is on identifying which approaches will be effective for which patients based on genetic, environmental, and lifestyle factors. If information is collected from different sources for the same individual, a specific profile of the subject can be established, in which the sensitivity to certain risk factors can be accurately determined, and with this, appropriate measures can be taken to reduce the risk of developing the disease. Furthermore, risk assessment can benefit from precision medicine by generating estimates that lead to evidence-based recommendations for different outcomes [88], including historical data [89]. In addition, precision medicine's focus on the individual will lead to accumulating evidence of multiple exposures and thus characterizing the body's short- and long-term response to changes that occur, exposures to environmental factors, and occupational agents [88].

The use of Artificial Intelligence techniques applied to personalized medicine can contribute to the detection or prediction of diseases, achievement of accurate diagnosis, and optimal treatment. Some examples are based on personalized diagnosis and treatment based on Cardiac Imaging [90], applications of artificial intelligence in early detection of cancer [91] (such as automatic classification of cancer based on images [92] and on genes [33]), computer-aided detection and computer-aided diagnosis of colorectal polyps [93], and automatic health-record heart failure with preserved ejection fraction patient phenotyping [33]. Finally, it is highlighted that in recent times, the pandemic prompted the execution of research in personalized medicine applied in the timely diagnosis of COVID-19, in order to be able to deal with the disease, from containing the spread of the virus to the correct treatment of patients [34].

Table 1.4 presents some studies that focus on the use of artificial intelligence to support personalized medicine.

Table 1.2 Summary of some outstanding papers that apply artificial intelligence in social networks associated with participatory medicine

Author, year	Area	Description	Platform	AI Tasks
Adikari et al. [70]	COVID-19	This research aims to investigate the human emotions related to the COVID-19 pandemic expressed on social media over time in Australia	Twitter	NLP—Word embeddings—Markov models—The growing self-organizing map algorithm
Amin et al. [71]	Dengue	Detection of dengue disease based on posts on social networks, differentiating whether it is a general discussion or whether people are actually infected	Twitter	Logistic Regression - Support Vector Machine—Naive Bayes—ANN/DNN—RNN/LSTM
Mann et al. [72]	Depression	It focuses on detecting the severity of depression symptoms in higher education students	Instagram	Deep learning—Resnet—LSTM and NLP
Tao Wang et al. [73]	Eating disorders	Social interactions in online eating disorder communities	Twitter	Sentiment Analysis—K-means
Nguyen et al. [74]	Mental Health	Identify adverse drug reactions (ADR) of psychiatric medications mentioned in social media	Social media: Twitter, Reddit, and LiveJournal	Deep Learning
Adams et al. [75]	Joint and muscle pain relief	Seeks to uncover safety and efficacy issues in Amazon reviews of joint and muscle pain relief products	Amazon's online product reviews	Sentiment analysis
Yang et al. [76]	Breast Cancer	Extract medical terms (conditions, symptoms, treatments, effectiveness and side effects) for each question in an online health forum	Medlinehelp.org	Sentiment analysis—Clustering—Latent Dirichlet Allocation
Rastegar-Mojarad et al. [77]	Patient experience	Create a corpus of patient experience at healthcare facilities (e.g. hospitals, urgent care facilities, and medical centers	Yelp Reviews	NLP—Sentiment analysis

Table 1.3 Summary of some outstanding papers that apply artificial intelligence with different devices/applications, associated with participatory medicine.

Author, year	Health Domain	Purpose	Description	Technology/AI Tasks
Lin et al. [78]	Heart diseases	Device/Diagnosis	Electrocardiogram (ECG) analysis for the detection of heart disease	The front-end IoT-based hardware, a wearable ECG patch that includes an analog front-end circuit and a Bluetooth module, which can detect ECG signals. Use of convolutional neural networks
Mathew et al. [79]	Diagnosis of diseases	Supportive care/Diagnosis	The proposed system seeks to create an alternative for an individual to request an appointment with a doctor for a diagnosis	People can interact with the chatbot, and through a series of queries, the chatbot will identify the user's symptoms and therefore diagnose the disease and recommend treatment. One of NLP and other techniques of deep learning
Sullivan et al. [80]	Smoking cessation	Treatment	Messaging program intervention to confirm that patients with drug dependence take the medications	Conversational agent—NLP—Other Deep Learning Techniques
Wall et al. [81]	Autism Spectrum Disorder	Treatment	To study the effects of a new automatic facial expression recognition tool to analyze the behavior of children with autism during social interactions	Autism glass / Google glass
Stein et al. [82]	Obesity	Supportive care	Evaluate weight loss, changes in meal quality, and app acceptability among Lark Weight Loss Health Coach AI (HCAI) users, to increase access to healthcare through mobile health	Application/Automatic detection through the data delivered by the user's mobile phone.
Fitzpatrick et al. [83]	Anxiety and Depression	Supportive care	Provide a tool to monitor symptoms and manage episodes of anxiety and depression	Chatbot mobile apps
Paasche-Orlow et al. [84]	Cancer	Supportive care	Palliative care in cancer patients at home and counseling in hospitalized patients	Embodied conversational agent

Table 1.4 Summary of research where personalized medicine is applied to deal with different problems in the field of health

Author, year	Area	Description	Data	AI Tasks
Patel et al. [94]	COVID-19	They developed a classifier to predict the need for intensive care and mechanical ventilation (ICU admission), in low-resource clinical settings or community hospitals where radio imaging might not be readily accessible. Using sociodemographic, clinical, and blood panel profile data that are collected at admission	Positive patients seen at the Keck Medical Center of USC, Verdugo Hills Hospital, and Los Angeles County + USC Medical Center	Random Forest
Murugan et al. [95]	COVID-19/ Neumonia	Perform a differential diagnosis between COVID-19, pneumonia and normal, using X-ray images	Chest X-ray images of COVID-19, normal, and pneumonia collected from the publicly available repositories	Deep Learning: Convolutonial (CNN) Neural Networks— CNN-ResNet50 based Extreme Learning Machine classifier (ELM)
Bibi et al. [96]	Leukemia	IoMT-based automated leukemia detection and classification usirg deep learning	Two publicly available datasets for leukemia, i.e., ALL-IDB and ASH image bank	Clinical gadgets—Deep Learning: Convolutional Neural Network densa (DCNN) y Convolutional Neural Network residual (RCNN)
Nanmaran et. al [97]	Brain Tumor	This research work analyzes the role of image fusion in an improved brain tumor classification model	The images are collected from http://kaggle.com	Support vector machine—KNN classifier—Decision tree
Mckinney et al. [98]	Breast cancer	Artificial intelligence system to improve the correct interpretat on of mammograms and thus predict breast cancer	Two datasets from the UK and the USA. The UK dataset was collected from three breast screening sites in the UK National Health Service Breast Screening Programme (NHSBSP). The US dataset was collected from Northwestern Memorial Hospital (Chicago)	Deep Learning
Franzmeier [99]	Alzheimer	Use of cerebrospinal fluid-derived Alzheimer's disease biomarkers, magnetic resonance imaging (MRI), arnyloid-PET, and fluorodeoxyglucose positron emission tomography (FDG-PET), to predict rates of Cognitive Impairment	Autosomal Dominant Alzheimer's Disease (ADAD) Data	Support Vector Regression
Zhou et al. [100],2019	Alzhaimer	In this article, the authors aim to make maximum use of multimodal neuroimaging and genetic data to identify Alzheimer's disease (AD) and its prodromal state, Mild Cognitive Impairment (MCI), in normally aging subjects	The Alzheimer's Disease Neuroimaging Public Initiative (ADNI) Database	Deep Learning

(continued)

Table 1.4 (continued)

Author, year	Area	Description	Data	AI Tasks
Long et al. [101]	Eye Diseases	AI agent for diagnosis, risk stratification and treatment suggestions, accurately diagnoses and provides treatment decisions for congenital cataracts in an in silico test, in a website-based study, in a 'find a needle in a haystack' and in a multi-hospital clinical trial	All cases used in the in silico test were collected from the Children's Cataract Program of the Chinese Ministry of Health, China	Deep learning—Convolutional neural networks
Tan et al. [102],2017	Spine Care	Comparison of NLP ML and Rule-Based Systems to Identify Lower Back Pain-Related Imaging Findings of the Lumbar Spine	Cohort consisted of patients enrolled in four integrated health systems (Kaiser Permanente of Washington, Kaiser Permanente of Northern California, Henry Ford Health System, Mayo Clinic Health System)	NLP
Frunza [103]	Disease—Treatment	Construction of an application that is capable of classifying disease-treatment relationships in short texts. Also to identify disease names and symptoms or signs are the data used in that diagnosis. Also to extract the sentence containing those details of an article	The data used for this research was a 'live' template	Naïve Bayesian
Khan et al. [104]	Nephritis/Heart disease	Medically diagnosed disease such as acute nephritis disease and heart disease symptoms, images or signs are the data used in medical diagnosis	The data set is obtained from the UCI Machine Learning Repository	Artificial Neural Networks
Kumar [105]	Kidney Stones	The objective of this article is to diagnose kidney stone disease by using three different neural network algorithms that have different architecture and characteristics	The data set used in this work is collected from different medical laboratories that test kidney stone patients	Radial basis function (RBF)—Learning vector quantization (LVQ)—Multilayer perceptron (MLP)
Douali et al. [31]	Disease Detection	Genomic and Personalized Medicine for classification as a means of detecting diseases in the Decision support system	Use of a database of patients with cardiovascular diseases	Fuzzy rules
Yang et al. [106]	Heart Disease	This paper presents support vector machine (SVM)-based two-dimensional reduction methodologies for diagnosing heart disease	University of California Irvine (UCI) Repository	Support Vector Machine and Radial Basis Function (RBF) type of Artificial Neural Networks
Orunesu [107], 2004	Grave Disease	Research studied the clinical outcome of Graves' disease after antithyroid therapy by defining a set of achievable variables capable of predicting, as soon as possible, the progression of the disease	Patients with a diagnosis of hyperthyroidism caused by GD, treated with MMI therapy for 18 months at the Department of Internal Medicine of the University of Genoa and at the Endocrinology Division of the Galliera Hospital of Genoa	Artificial Neural Networks

1.4.4 Preventive Medicine

Due to rising health care costs, early disease prevention has never been more important than it is today. Given the above, the concept of preventive medicine is strengthened, which is based on Medical practices that are designed to avert and avoid disease[108].

Digital health announces that thanks to technological progress embodied in applications, wearable technology, remote monitoring, telemedicine, and communication tools, among other diagnostic devices; the quality of patient care will be optimized, as well as a more timely response to any situation. This occurs because these tools make data available, which are extracted and used for the detection, prediction, and support for diagnosis/decision making of anomalies [109].

AI-driven health interventions fall into four categories relevant to global health researchers: (1) diagnosis, (2) patient morbidity or mortality risk assessment, (3) disease outbreak prediction and surveillance, and (4) health policy and planning [110]. Through the use of AI, huge amounts of data derived from different sources can be interpreted to facilitate diagnosis and increase the ability to execute early initiatives and prevent diseases to reduce the burden on both the patient and caregivers. Then executing successful interventions depends on the knowledge of the causes of the disease, the transmission dynamics, the identification of risk factors and groups, the methods of early detection and treatment, the implementation of these methods and the continuous evaluation and development of the methods. prevention methods and treatment. The identification of the determinants of a disease at the population level is a prerequisite, to prevent its appearance in a single individual, providing the basis for targeted and specific treatment [109].

The application of AI in disease prevention has been carried out in the evaluation of breast cancer risk [111], heart disease diagnosis [112], early prognosis in patients with liver disorders [113], prediction of admissions, complications and mortality in ICUs [114], and the prognosis of severity and outcome of cerebrovascular accidents [115], among others.

Table 1.5 shows a summary of some research that applies Machine Learning and Deep Learning algorithms in the field of preventive medicine.

1.5 Summary

People's healthcare is changing, going from being a task focused on curing diseases to one based on preserving health, through various methods that anticipate possible illnesses, treatments to maintain indicators of internal biology of the human body within certain margins and of course, considering that people are the center of any initiative regarding healthcare. Hence, the adequate collection of quality data related to people's lives and health is very important. For several years, enormous efforts have been made to improve the processes of capturing and storing data related to

Table 1.5 Summary of research works that seek the prevention of diseases/events in the field of health.

Author, year	Area	Description	Data	AI Tasks
Ravaut et al. [116]	Diabetes	Develop a model to predict 3 years in advance whether a patient diagnosed with diabetes will visit a doctor due to adverse outcomes from complications of the disease within 3 months	Health system administrative data in Ontario, Canada	Decision Tree
Nejra et al. [117]	Smoking	Application of Artificial Intelligence Techniques to Predict Effects of Cigarette Smoking on Hematological Parameters and Attributable Diseases	A dataset was created which consisted of healthy adult male subjects, including smokers and non-smokers in the age range from 18 to 55 years	Artificial Neural Networks
Mora et al. [118]	ICU	Proposes various artificial intelligence approaches to obtain information on risk factors for multidrug resistance during the first 48 h after ICU admission	Data from Hospital Universitario de Fuenlabrada (UHF) in Madrid, Spain	Logistic Regression—Decision trees—XGBoost— Artificial neural networks
Yang et al. [119]	Heart Disease	Artificial Intelligence-Assisted Identification of Genetic Factors Predisposing High-Risk Individuals to Asymptomatic Heart Failure	Northeast Taiwan Community Medicine Research Cohort Participants enrolled and screened at Chang Gung Memorial Cardiology Outpatient Clinic Hospital, Keelung	Random forest—support vector machine (SVM)—Least absolute shrinkage—Selection operator (LASSO) methods
2020	COVID-19	COVID-19 Forced Cough Record Pre-Screening Tool, AI-based	Built COVID-19 cough record data collection channel via website (opensigma.mit.edu)	CNN ResNet50s
Lu et al. [120]	Diet	An Artificial Intelligence System for Dietary Assessment that requires an input of two meal images or a short video	Databases: MADiMa database that compiles images from different data sources and a new database named "Fast food" database, which contains images of food from the "McDonald's" fast food chain	Deep Learning
Kanegae [53]	Hypertension	This study used machine learning techniques to develop and validate a new risk prediction model for new-onset hypertension in Japan	Included individuals who underwent health checkups at the Japan Health Promotion Foundation	XGBoost—Ensemble—Logistic Regression

(continued)

Table 1.4 (continued)

Author, year	Area	Description	Data	AI Tasks
Regalia et al. [121]	Epilepsia	The objective of this research is to provide updated evidence of the effectiveness of the detection and monitoring of generalized tonic-clonic seizures (GTCS) based on the combination of sensors with motion (accelerometers, ACC) and electrodermal activity (EDA) sensors	The detection algorithm has been trained on E4 epilepsy data patients experiencing GTCS in Epilepsy Monitoring Units (EMUs), labeled by at least 2 qualified epileptologists using gold standard v-EEG in Level IV Epilepsy Centers	Wearable
Rebane et al. [54]	Adverse events	Predicting Adverse Drug Events (ADEs) at a patient's last visit, based on medical record data from all previous visits	The medical database consists of information on patient diagnoses and medications obtained from the Stockholm University HealthBank	Recurrent Neural Network RETAIN and Timeline
Zellweger et al. [35]	Heart Disease	This study aims to evaluate the diagnostic power of AI to predict the risk of the presence/absence of coronary artery disease	Ludwigshafen Risk and Cardiovascular Health Study (LURIC)	Memetic pattern-based algorithm (MPA); Ensemble tree methods based on classification and Regression tree—Logistic regression—Ensemble Logistic Regression methods—Voting Algorithms—Self-organizing maps
Christiansen et al. [122]	Glucose Measurement	Accuracy and performance of a fourth-generation subcutaneous glucose sensor (Guardian Sensor 3) was evaluated in the abdomen and arm	This study was conducted at six research centers in the United States and enrolled subjects diagnosed with type 1 or type 2 diabetes	Sensor
Liu et al. [123]	Bone Fracture	This study sought to predict key risk factors of hip bone fracture for the elderly	Patients aged over 60 years and admitted for first-time low-trauma hip fracture to National Taiwan University Hospital	Artificial Neural Networks
Spasic et al. [124]	Mental Health	Automatically classify sentences in suicide notes using a scheme of 15 topics, mostly emotions	Dataset consisting of suicide notes from Challenge on Sentiment Classification (2011)	NLP—Sentiment analysis—Topic classification—Naïve Bayes classifier
Jang et al. [125],2011	Heart Disease	Detection of atrial fibrillation through cardiac monitoring devices	Using patient recordings from the MIT-BIH AF database	Support Vector Machine
Zhang et al. [126], 2008	Critical Care	The study develops real-time alarm algorithms specific to each patient to detect adverse effects of clinical and medical conditions	This research was conducted in the Pediatric Multidisciplinary ICU (P-MICU) at Boston Children's Hospital, where patient data was collected	Decision Tree—Artificial Neural Network

health, its subsequent maintenance, transmission, and exploitation. However, despite all these efforts, in many places there is still no unified electronic medical record, which is essential to apply the concepts behind 4P medicine. But it is a matter of time before the situation gradually improves. For now, efforts have been focused on using the data related to people's health in the best possible way to create various applications and systems that are aimed at gradually improving population's health. Considering this scenario and the inescapable fact that health-related data only grows in complexity and size, it is essential to have automated tools for its processing to extract information and knowledge to support decision-making in the field of healthcare. This is where artificial intelligence plays an essential role, enabling massive data processing, process automation, timely delivery of information and knowledge and, of course, support for diagnosis. We are at the gates of a new medicine, much more participatory, predictive, preventive and personalized, where the joint work between health personnel and artificial intelligence is bearing increasingly significant fruits. But remember, with all this tremendous technological power comes great responsibility. The processing of data related to people's health must be carried out in a safe, responsible and, above all, ethical manner, taking care to safeguard the human rights of individuals above all else. Only in this way can the benefits of AI be accessed in the field of healthcare.

Acknowledgements The authors gratefully acknowledge financial support from ANID PIA/APOYO AFB180003. This work was supported by projects ANID (National Research and Development Agency of Chile) Doctorado Nacional #2116137

References

1. Turing, A. Computing machinery and intelligence. Mind (1950)
2. McCarthy, J., Minsky, M.L., Rochester, N., Shannon, C.E.: A proposal for the Dartmouth summer research project on artificial intelligence, 31 Aug 1955. AI Mag. **27**(4), 12–12 (2006)
3. Thorndike, E.I.: Intelligence and its measurement: a symposium–i. J. Educ. Psychol. **12**(3), 124 (1921)
4. Terman, L.M.: Intelligence and its measurement: a symposium–ii. J. Educ. Psychol. **12**(3), 127 (1921)
5. Anastasi, A.: What counselors should know about the use and interpretation of psychological tests. J. Counsel. Dev. **70**(5), 610–615 (1992)
6. Gardner, H.: Frames of mind: theory of multiple intelligences. Fontana Press (1993)
7. Subbarayappa, B.V.: The roots of ancient medicine: an historical outline. J. Biosci. Bangalore **26**(2), 135–143 (2001)
8. Hood, L., Friend, S.H.: Predictive, personalized, preventive, participatory (p4) cancer medicine. Nat. Rev. Clin. Oncol. **8**(3), 184–187 (2011)
9. Koteluk, O., Wartecki, A., Mazurek, S., Kołodziejczak, I., Mackiewicz, A.: How do machines learn? artificial intelligence as a new era in medicine. J. Person. Med. **11**(1), 32 (2021)
10. Thrun, S., Pratt, L. Learning to Learn. Springer (2012)
11. Mitchell, T.: Learning to Learn. McGraw-Hill (1997)
12. Samuel, A.L.: Machine learning. Technol. Rev. **62**(1), 42–45 (1959)

13. Ray, S.: A quick review of machine learning algorithms. In 2019 International Conference on Machine Learning, Big Data, Cloud and Parallel Computing (COMITCon), pp. 35–39. IEEE (2019)
14. Janiesch, C., Zschech, P., Heinrich, K.: Machine learning and deep learning. Electron. Markets **31**(3), 685–695 (2021)
15. Gudivada, V., Apon, A., Ding, J.: Data quality considerations for big data and machine learning: going beyond data cleaning and transformations. Int. J. Adv. Softw. **10**(1), 1–20 (2017)
16. Awaysheh, A., Wilcke, J., Elvinger, F., Rees, L., Fan, W., Zimmerman, K.I.: Review of medical decision support and machine-learning methods. Veterinary Pathol. **56**(4), 512–525 (2019)
17. Garg, A., Mago, V.: Role of machine learning in medical research: a survey. Comput. Sci. Rev. **40**, 100370 (2021)
18. Das, S., Roy, S.D., Malakar, S., Velásquez, J.D., Sarkar, R.: Bi-level prediction model for screening covid-19 patients using chest X-ray images. Big Data Res. **25**, 100233 (2021)
19. Tao, X., Velásquez, J.D.: Multi-source information fusion for smart health with artificial intelligence. Inf. Fusion **83–84**, 93–95 (2022)
20. Lee, C.H., Yoon, H.-J.: Medical big data: promise and challenges. Kidney Res. Clin. Practice **36**(1), 3 (2017)
21. Garain, A., Basu, A., Giampaolo, F., Velasquez, J.D., Sarkar, R.: Detection of covid-19 from CT scan images: a spiking neural network-based approach. Neural Comput. Appl. **33**(19), 12591–12604 (2021)
22. Buch, V.H., Ahmed, I., Maruthappu, M.: Artificial intelligence in medicine: current trends and future possibilities. Bri. J. General Practice **68**(668), 143–144 (2018)
23. CB Insights Research: Healthcare remains the hottest AIcategory for deals (2017)
24. Chan, K.S., Fowles, J.B., Weiner, J.P.: Electronic health records and the reliability and validity of quality measures: a review of the literature. Med. Care Res. Rev. **67**(5), 503–527 (2010)
25. Wang, Z.-G., Zhang, L., Zhao, W.-J.: Definition and application of precision medicine. Chin. J. Traumatol. **19**(05), 249–250 (2016)
26. Flavia Guinazu, M., Cortes, V., Ibanez, C.F., Velasquez, J.D.: Employing online social networks in precision-medicine approach using information fusion predictive model to improve substance use surveillance: a lesson from twitter and marijuana consumption. Inf. Fusion **55**, 150–163 (2020)
27. González, F., Vera, F., González, F., Velásquez, J.D.: Kefuri: a novel technological tool for increasing organ donation in Chile. In: 2020 IEEE/WIC/ACM International Joint Conference on Web Intelligence and Intelligent Agent Technology (WI-IAT), pp. 470–475. IEEE (2020)
28. Knoppers, B.M., Thorogood, A.M.: Ethics and big data in health. Curr. Opin. Syst. Biol**4**, 53–57 (2017)
29. Morley, J., Machado, C.C.V., Burr, C., Cowls, J., Joshi, I., Taddeo, M., Floridi, L.: The ethics of AI in health care: a mapping review. Soc. Sci. Med. **260**, 113172 (2020)
30. Mann, J.M., Gostin, L.O., Gruskin, S., Brennan, T., Lazzarini, Z., Fineberg, H.V.: Health and human rights. In: Health and Human Rights in a Changing World, pp. 16–31. Routledge (2013)
31. Douali, N., Jaulent, M.-C.: Genomic and personalized medicine decision support system. In: 2012 IEEE International Conference on Complex Systems (ICCS), pp. 1–4 (2012)
32. Hood, L., Flores, M.: A personal view on systems medicine and the emergence of proactive p4 medicine: predictive, preventive, personalized and participatory. New Biotechnol. **29**(6), 613–624 (2012)
33. Gifari, M.W., Samodro, P., Kurniawan, D.W.: Artificial intelligence toward personalized medicine. Pharmaceut. Sci. Res. **8**(2), 1 (2021)
34. Lin B., Wu, S.: Digital transformation in personalized medicine with artificial intelligence and the internet of medical things. Omics: J. Integr. Biol. **26**(2), 77–81 (2022)
35. Zellweger, M.J., Tsirkin, A., Vasilchenko, V., Failer, M., Dressel, A., Kleber, M.E., Ruff, P., März, W.: A new non-invasive diagnostic tool in coronary artery disease: artificial intelligence as an essential element of predictive, preventive, and personalized medicine. EPMA J. **9**(3), 235–247 (2018)

36. Flores, M., Glusman, G., Brogaard, K., Price, N.D., Hood, L.: P4 medicine: how systems medicine will transform the healthcare sector and society. Pers. Med. **10**(6), 565–576 (2013)
37. Doherty, T.M., Di Pasquale, A., Michel, J.-P., Del Giudice, G.: Precision medicine and vaccination of older adults: from reactive to proactive (a mini-review). Gerontology **66**(3), 238–248
38. Taylor, C.A., Draney, M.T., Ku, J.P., Parker, D., Steele, B.N., Wang, K., Zarins, C.K.: Predictive medicine: computational techniques in therapeutic decision-making. Comput. Aided Surgery: Off. J. Int. Soc. Comput. Aided Surgery (ISCAS) **4**(5), 231–247 (1999)
39. Jen, M.Y., Shahrokhi, M., Varacallo, M.: Predictive medicine. In: StatPearls. StatPearls Publishing, Treasure Island (FL) (2022)
40. Deo, R.C.: Machine learning in medicine. Circulation **132**(20), 1920–1930 (2015)
41. Yang, Christopher C.: Explainable artificial intelligence for predictive modeling in healthcare. J. Healthcare Inform. Res. **6**(2), 228–239 (2022)
42. Xue, Y., Klabjan, D., Luo, Y.: Predicting ICU readmission using grouped physiological and medication trends. Artif. Intell. Med. **95**, 27–37 (2019)
43. Yang, H., Yang, C.C.: Using health-consumer-contributed data to detect adverse drug reactions by association mining with temporal analysis. ACM Trans. Intell. Syst. Technol. **6**(4), 1–55 (2015)
44. Krieg, S.J., Robertson, D.H., Pradhan, M.P., Chawla, N.V.: Higher-order networks of diabetes comorbidities: disease trajectories that matter. In: 2020 IEEE International Conference on Healthcare Informatics (ICHI), pp. 1–11 (2020)
45. Martinez-Ríos, E., Montesinos, L., Alfaro-Ponce, M., Pecchia, L.: A review of machine learning in hypertension detection and blood pressure estimation based on clinical and physiological data. Biomed. Signal Process. Control **68**, 102813 (2021)
46. Goh, K.H., Wang, L., Kwang Yeow, A.Y., Poh, H., Li, K., Lin Yeow, J.J., Heng Tan, G.Y.: Artificial intelligence in sepsis early prediction and diagnosis using unstructured data in healthcare. Nature Commun. **12**(1), 1–10 (2021)
47. D'Haese, P.-F., Finomore, V., Lesnik, D., Kornhauser, L., Schaefer, T., Konrad, P.E., Hodder, S., Marsh, C., Rezai, A.R.: Prediction of viral symptoms using wearable technology and artificial intelligence: a pilot study in healthcare workers. PLOS ONE **16**(10), e0257997 (2021) (Public Library of Science)
48. Elujide, I., Fashoto, S.G., Fashoto, B., Mbunge, E., Folorunso, S.O., Olamijuwon, J.O.: Application of deep and machine learning techniques for multi-label classification performance on psychotic disorder diseases. Inf. Med. Unlocked **23**, 100545 (2021)
49. Noor, S.T., Asad, S.T., Khan, M.M., Gaba, G.S., Al-Amri, J.F., Masud, M.: Predicting the risk of depression based on ECG using RNN. Comput. Intell. Neurosci. (2021)
50. Vijayalaxmi, A., Sridevi, S., Sridhar, N., Ambesange, S.: Multi-disease prediction with artificial intelligence from core health parameters measured through non-invasive technique. In: 2020 4th International Conference on Intelligent Computing and Control Systems (ICICCS), pp. 1252–1258. IEEE (2020)
51. Lauritsen, S.M., Kristensen, M., Olsen, M.V., Larsen, M.S., Lauritsen, K.M., Jørgensen, M.J., Lange, J., Thiesson, B.: Explainable artificial intelligence model to predict acute critical illness from electronic health records. Nat. Commun. **11**(1), 3852 (2020) (Nature Publishing Group)
52. Jiang, X., Coffee, M., Bari, A., Wang, J., Jiang, X., Huang, J., Shi, J., Dai, J., Cai, J., Zhang, T., Zhengxing, W., He, G., Huang, Y.: Towards an artificial intelligence framework for data-driven prediction of coronavirus clinical severity. Comput. Mater. Continua **62**, 537–551 (2020)
53. Kanegae, H., Suzuki, K., Fukatani, K., Ito, T., Harada, N., Kario, K.: Highly precise risk prediction model for new-onset hypertension using artificial intelligence techniques. J. Clin. Hypertension **22**(3), 445–450 (2020)
54. Rebane, J., Karlsson, I., Papapetrou, P.: An investigation of interpretable deep learning for adverse drug event prediction. In: 2019 IEEE 32nd International Symposium on Computer-Based Medical Systems (CBMS), pp. 337–342. IEEE (2019)
55. Kalmady, S.V., Greiner, R., Agrawal, R., Shivakumar, V., Narayanaswamy, J.C., Brown, M.R.G., Greenshaw, A.J., Dursun, S.M., Venkatasubramanian, G.: Towards artificial

intelligence in mental health by improving schizophrenia prediction with multiple brain parcellation ensemble-learning. NPJ Schizophrenia **5**(1), 1–11 (2019)

56. Schmidt-Erfurth, U., Waldstein, S.M., Klimscha, S., Sadeghipour, A., Hu, X., Gerendas, B.S., Osborne, A., Bogunović, H.: Prediction of individual disease conversion in early amd using artificial intelligence. Invest. Ophthalmol. Vis. Sci. **59**(8), 3199–3208 (2018)

57. Choi, E., Bahadori, M.T., Schuetz, A., Stewart, W.F., Sun, J.: Doctor AI: Predicting clinical events via recurrent neural networks. In: Machine Learning for Healthcare Conference, pp. 301–318. PMLR (2016)

58. Esteban, C., Staeck, O., Baier, S., Yang, Y., Tresp, V.: Predicting clinical events by combining static and dynamic information using recurrent neural networks. In: 2016 IEEE International Conference on Healthcare Informatics (ICHI), pp. 93–101. IEEE (2016)

59. Francis, N.K., Luther, A., Salib, E., Allanby, L., Messenger, D., Allison, A.S., Smart, N.J., Ockrim, J.B.: The use of artificial neural networks to predict delayed discharge and readmission in enhanced recovery following laparoscopic colorectal cancer surgery. Tech. Coloproctol. **19**(7), 419–428 (2015)

60. Ng, E.Y.-K., Fok, S.C., Peh, Y.C., Ng, F.C., Sim, L.S.J.: Computerized detection of breast cancer with artificial intelligence and thermograms. J. Med. Eng. Technol. **26**(4), 152–157 (2002)

61. Swan, M.: Health 2050: The realization of personalized medicine through crowdsourcing, the quantified self, and the participatory biocitizen. J. Pers. Med. **2**(3), 93–118 (2012)

62. DeBronkart, D.: From patient centred to people powered: autonomy on the rise. BMJ 350 (2015)

63. Millenson, M.L.: When "patient centred" is no longer enough: the challenge of collaborative health: an essay by Michael L Millenson. BMJ 358 (2017)

64. Coughlin, S., Roberts, D., O'Neill, K., Brooks, P.: Looking to tomorrow's healthcare today: a participatory health perspective. Internal Med. J. **48**(1), 92–96 (2018)

65. Gonzalez-Hernandez, G., Sarker, A., O'Connor, K., Savova, G.: Capturing the patient's perspective: a review of advances in natural language processing of health-related text. Yearbook Med. inform. **26**(01), 214–227 (2017)

66. Wright, M.T., Springett, J., Kongats, K.: What is participatory health research? In Participatory Health Research, pp. 3–15. Springer (2018)

67. Denecke, K., Gabarron, E., Grainger, R., Th Konstantinidis, S., Lau, A., Rivera-Romero, O., Miron-Shatz, T., Merolli, M.: Artificial intelligence for participatory health: applications, impact, and future implications. Yearbook Med. Inform. **28**(01), 165–173 (2019)

68. Almalki, M., Gray, K., Sanchez, K.M.: The use of self-quantification systems for personal health information: big data management activities and prospects. Health Inf. Sci. Syst. **3**(1), 1–11 (2015)

69. Staccini, P., Fernandez-Luque, L., et al.: Secondary use of recorded or self-expressed personal data: consumer health informatics and education in the era of social media and health apps. Yearbook Med. Inform. **26**(01), 172–177 (2017)

70. Adikari, A., Nawaratne, R., De Silva, D., Ranasinghe, S., Alahakoon, O., Alahakoon, D., et al.: Emotions of covid-19: content analysis of self-reported information using artificial intelligence. J. Med. Internet Res. **23**(4), e27341 (2021)

71. Amin, S., Irfan Uddin, M., Hassan, S., Khan, A., Nasser, N., Alharbi, A., Alyami, H.: Recurrent neural networks with TF-IDF embedding technique for detection and classification in tweets of dengue disease. IEEE Access **8**, 131522–131533 (2020)

72. Mann, P., Paes, A., Matsushima, E.H.: See and read: detecting depression symptoms in higher education students using multimodal social media data. In: Proceedings of the International AAAI Conference on Web and Social Media, vol. 14, pp. 440–451 (2020)

73. Wang, T., Brede, M., Ianni, A., Mentzakis, E.: Social interactions in online eating disorder communities: A network perspective. PloS One **13**(7), e0200800 (2018)

74. Nguyen, T., Larsen, M.E., O'Dea, B., Phung, D., Venkatesh, S., Christensen, H.: Estimation of the prevalence of adverse drug reactions from social media. In. J. Med. Informa. **102**, 130–137 (2017)

75. Adams, D.Z., Gruss, R., Abrahams, A.S.: Automated discovery of safety and efficacy concerns for joint & muscle pain relief treatments from online reviews. Int. J. Med. Inform. **100**, 108–120 2017

76. Yang, F.C., Lee, A.J.T., Kuo, S.-C.: Mining health social media with sentiment analysis. J. Med. Syst. **40**(11), 1–8 (2016)

77. Rastegar-Mojarad, M., Ye, Z., Wall, D., Murali, N., Lin, S., et al.: Collecting and analyzing patient experiences of health care from social media. JMIR Res. Protocols **4**(3), e3433 (2015)

78. Lin, Y.J., Chuang, C.-W., Yen, C.-Y., Huang, S.-H., Huang, P.-W., Chen, J.-Y., Lee, S.-Y.: Artificial intelligence of things wearable system for cardiac disease detection. In: 2019 IEEE International Conference on Artificial Intelligence Circuits and Systems (AICAS), pp. 67–70 (2019)

79. Mathew, R.B., Varghese, S., Joy, S.E. Alex, S.S.: Chatbot for disease prediction and treatment recommendation using machine learning. In: 2019 3rd International Conference on Trends in Electronics and Informatics (ICOEI), pp. 851–856 (2019)

80. Sullivan B.: Pilot trial of the first conversational agent for smoking cessation (QuitBot). In: Clinical Research Trial Listing (Smoking Cessation) (NCT03585231)

81. Wall, D.P.: Superpower glass project: a mobile at-home intervention for children with autism. Clinical Trial Registration NCT03569176, clinicaltrials.gov, July 2018. Submitted: 14 June 2018

82. Stein, N., Brooks, K., et al.: A fully automated conversational artificial intelligence for weight loss: longitudinal observational study among overweight and obese adults. JMIR Diabetes **2**(2), e8590 (2017)

83. Fitzpatrick, K.K., Darcy, A., Vierhile, M.: Delivering cognitive behavior therapy to young adults with symptoms of depression and anxiety using a fully automated conversational agent (Woebot): a randomized controlled trial. JMIR Mental Health **4**(2), e7785

84. Boston Medical Center: Conversational agents to improve quality of life in palliative care. Clinical Trial Registration NCT02750865, clinicaltrials.gov, December 2021. submitted: March 30, 2016

85. Bates, S.: Progress towards personalized medicine. Drug Discovery Today **15**(3–4), 115–120 (2010)

86. Schork, N.J.: Personalized medicine: time for one-person trials. Nature **520**(7549):609–611 (2015)

87. Vogenberg, F.R.,, Barash, C.I., Pursel, M.: Personalized medicine. Pharm. Therapeut. **35**(10):560–576 (2010)

88. Bollati, V., Ferrari, L., Leso, V., Iavicoli, I.: Personalised medicine: implication and perspectives in the field of occupational health. La Medicina del Lavoro **111**(6), 425 (2020)

89. Orlando, L.A., Ryanne Wu, R., Myers, R.A., Neuner, J., McCarty, C., Haller, I.V., Harry, M., Fulda, K.G., Dimmock, D., Rakhra-Burris, T., et al.: At the intersection of precision medicine and population health: an implementation-effectiveness study of family health history based systematic risk assessment in primary care. BMC Health Services Res. **20**(1), 1–10 (2020)

90. Dilsizian, S.E., Siegel, E.L.: Artificial intelligence in medicine and cardiac imaging: harnessing big data and advanced computing to provide personalized medical diagnosis and treatment. Curr. Cardiol. Rep. **16**(1), 1–8 (2014)

91. Ullah, M., Akbar, A., Yannarelli, G.G.: Applications of artificial intelligence in early detection of cancer, clinical diagnosis and personalized medicine (2020)

92. Sollini, M., Bartoli, F., Marciano, A., Zanca, R., Slart, R.H.J.A., Erba, P. A.: Artificial intelligence and hybrid imaging: the best match for personalized medicine in oncology. Eur. J. Hybrid Imaging **4**(1), 1–22 (2020)

93. Alagappan, M., Glissen Brown, J.R., Mori, Y., Berzin, T.M.: Artificial intelligence in gastrointestinal endoscopy: the future is almost here. World J. Gastrointest. Endosc. **10**(10), 239 (2018)

94. Patel, D., Kher, V., Desai, B., Lei, X., Cen, S., Nanda, N., Gholamrezanezhad, A., Duddalwar, V., Varghese, B., Oberai, A.A.: Machine learning based predictors for covid-19 disease severity. Sci. Rep. **11**(1), 1–7 (2021)

95. Murugan, R., Goel, T.: E-diconet: extreme learning machine based classifier for diagnosis of covid-19 using deep convolutional network. J. Ambient Intell. Hum. Comput. **12**(9), 8887–8898 (2021)
96. Bibi, N., Sikandar, M., Ud Din, I., Almogren, A., Ali, S.: IoMT-based automated detection and classification of leukemia using deep learning. J. Healthcare Eng. (2020)
97. Nanmaran, R., Srimathi, S., Yamuna, G., Thanigaivel, S., Vickram, A.S., Priya, A.K., Karthick, A., Karpagam, J., Mohanavel, V., Muhibbullah, M.: Investigating the role of image fusion in brain tumor classification models based on machine learning algorithm for personalized medicine. Comput. Math. Methods Med. (2022)
98. McKinney, S.M., Sieniek, M., Godbole, V., Godwin, J., Antropova, N., Ashrafian, H., Back, T., Chesus, M., Corrado, G.S., Darzi, A., et al.: International evaluation of an AI system for breast cancer screening. Nature **577**(7788), 89–94 (2020)
99. Franzmeier, N., Koutsouleris, N., Benzinger, T., Goate, A., Karch, C.M., Fagan, A.M., McDade, E., Duering, M., Dichgans, M., Levin, J., et al.: Predicting sporadic Alzheimer's disease progression via inherited Alzheimer's disease-informed machine-learning. Alzheimer's Dementia **16**(3), 501–511 (2020)
100. Zhou, T., Thung, K.-H., Zhu, X., Shen, D.: Effective feature learning and fusion of multimodality data using stage-wise deep neural network for dementia diagnosis. Hum. Brain Map. **40**(3), 1001–1016 (2019)
101. Long, E., Lin, H., Liu, Z., Xiaohang, W., Wang, L., Jiang, J., An, Y., Lin, Z., Li, X., Chen, J., et al.: An artificial intelligence platform for the multihospital collaborative management of congenital cataracts. Nat. Biomed. Eng. **1**(2), 1–8 (2017)
102. Tan, W.K., Hassanpour, S., Heagerty, P.J., Rundell, S.D., Suri, P., Huhdanpaa, H.T., James, K., Carrell, D.S., Langlotz, C.P., Organ, N.L., et al.: Comparison of natural language processing rules-based and machine-learning systems to identify lumbar spine imaging findings related to low back pain. Acad. Radiol. **25**(11), 1422–1432
103. Frunza, O., Inkpen, D., Tran, T.: A machine learning approach for identifying disease-treatment relations in short texts. IEEE Tran. Knowl. Data Eng. **23**(6), 801–814 (2011)
104. Khan, I.Y., Zope, P., Suralkar, S.R.: Importance of artificial neural network in medical diagnosis disease like acute nephritis disease and heart disease. Int. J. Eng. Sci. Innovat. Technol. **2**, 210–217 (2013)
105. Kumar, K., Abhishek, B.: Artificial Neural Networks for Diagnosis of Kidney Stones Disease, vol. 10. GRIN Verlag Germany (2012)
106. Yang, C., An, B., Yin, S.: Heart-disease diagnosis via support vector machine-based approaches. In: 2018 IEEE International Conference on Systems, Man, and Cybernetics (SMC), pp. 3153–3158 (2018)
107. Orunesu, E., Bagnasco, M., Salmaso, C., Altrinetti, V., Bernasconi, D., Del Monte, P., Pesce, G., Marugo, M., Mela, G.S.: Use of an artificial neural network to predict graves' disease outcome within 2 years of drug withdrawal. Eur. J. Clin. Invest. **34**(3), 210–217 (2004)
108. Clarke, E.A.: What is preventive medicine? Can. Fam.Phys. **20**(11), 65 (1974)
109. Chang, A.: The role of artificial intelligence in digital health. In: Digital Health Entrepreneurship, pp. 71–81. Springer (2020)
110. Schwalbe, N., Wahl, B.: Artificial intelligence and the future of global health. Lancet **395**(10236), 1579–1586 (2020)
111. Gastounioti, A., Desai, S., Ahluwalia, V.S., Conant, E.F., Kontos, D.: Artificial intelligence in mammographic phenotyping of breast cancer risk: a narrative review. Breast Cancer Res. **24**(1), 1–12 (2022)
112. Johnson, K.W., Soto J.T., Glicksberg, B.S., Shameer, K., Miotto, R., Ali, M., Ashley, E., Dudley, J.T.: Artificial intelligence in cardiology. J. Am. Col. Cardiol. **71**(23), 2668–2679 (2018)
113. Ahn, J.C., Connell, A., Simonetto, D., Hughes, C., Shah, V.H.: Application of artificial intelligence for the diagnosis and treatment of liver diseases. Hepatology **73**(6), 2546–2563 (2021)

114. Greco, M., Caruso, P.F., Cecconi, M.: Artificial intelligence in the intensive care unit. Seminars Respirat. Crit. Care Med. **42**(1) (2021) (Thieme Medical Publishers, Inc.)
115. Damen, J.A.A.G., Hooft, L., Schuit, E., Debray, T.P.A., Collins, G.S., Tzoulaki, I., Lassale, C.M., Siontis, G.C.M., Chiocchia, V., Roberts, C.: et al.: Prediction models for cardiovascular disease risk in the general population: systematic review (2016)
116. Ravaut, M., Sadeghi, H., Leung, K.K., Volkovs, M., Kornas, K., Harish, V., Watson, T., Lewis, G.F., Weisman, A., Poutanen, T., et al.: Predicting adverse outcomes due to diabetes complications with machine learning using administrative health data. NPJ Digit. Med. **4**(1), 1–12 (2021)
117. Nejra, K., Lejla, K., Nermana, K., Amina, K., Božana, L., Amina, L., Almir, B.: Application of artificial intelligence techniques to predict effects of cigarette smoking on hematological parameters and attributable diseases. In: International Conference on Medical and Biological Engineering, pp. 313–318. Springer (2021)
118. Mora-Jiménez, I., Tarancón-Rey, J., Álvarez-Rodríguez, J., Soguero-Ruiz, C.: Artificial intelligence to get insights of multi-drug resistance risk factors during the first 48 hours from ICU admission. Antibiotics **10**(3), 239 (2021)
119. Yang, N.I., Yeh, C.-H., Tsai, T.-H., Chou, Y.-J., Hsu, P.W.-C., Li, C.-H., Chan, Y.-H., Kuo, L.-T., Mao, C.-T., Shyu, Y.-C., et al.: Artificial intelligence-assisted identification of genetic factors predisposing high-risk individuals to asymptomatic heart failure. Cells **10**(9), 2430 (2021)
120. Lu, Y., Stathopoulou, T., Vasiloglou, M.F., Pinault, L.F., Kiley, C., Spanakis, E.K., Mougiakakou, S.: goFOODTM: an artificial intelligence system for dietary assessment. Sensors **20**(15), 4283 (2020)
121. Regalia, G., Onorati, F., Lai, M., Caborni, C., Picard, R.W.: Multimodal Wristworn devices for seizure detection and advancing research: focus on the Empatica wristbands. Epilepsy Res. **153**, 79–82 (2019)
122. Christiansen, M.P., Garg, S.K., Brazg, R., Bode, B.W., Bailey, T.S., Slover, R.H., Sullivan, A., Huang, S., Shin, J., Lee, S.W., et al.: Accuracy of a fourth-generation subcutaneous continuous glucose sensor. Diabetes Technol. Therapeut. **19**(8), 446–456 (2017)
123. Liu, Q., Cui, X., Chou, Y.-C., Abbod, M.F., Lin, J., Shieh, J.-S.: Ensemble artificial neural networks applied to predict the key risk factors of hip bone fracture for elders. Biomed. Signal Process. Control, **21**, 146–156 (2015)
124. Irena Spasić, Pete Burnap, Mark Greenwood, and Michael Arribas-Ayllon. A naïve bayes approach to classifying topics in suicide notes. *Biomedical informatics insights*, 5:BII–S8945, 2012
125. Jang, K.J., Balakrishnan, G., Syed, Z., Verma, N.: Scalable customization of atrial fibrillation detection in cardiac monitoring devices: Increasing detection accuracy through personalized monitoring in large patient populations. In: 2011 Annual International Conference of the IEEE Engineering in Medicine and Biology Society, pp. 2184–2187. IEEE (2011)
126. Zhang, Y., Szolovits, P.: Patient-specific learning in real time for adaptive monitoring in critical care. J. Biomed. Inform. **41**(3), 452–460 (2008)

Chapter 2
A Survival Analysis Guide in Oncology

Smaranda Belciug

Abstract Survival analysis has a crucial role in oncology. These statistical methods are ubiquitous in oncology, helping physicians determine the death risk, the best course of treatment, and even help in discovering new therapies. The aim of this chapter it to provide a guide on some survival analysis statistical methods as well as practical examples on how to apply them in oncology. We begin with some theory regarding survival analysis in general, followed by Kaplan–Meier survival curves, logrank test and hazard ration to determine the best course of treatment. The chapter ends with the Cox regression. This chapter is a step-by-step guide in performing survival analysis and in interpreting the obtained results.

Keywords Survival analysis · Kaplan–Meier curve · Logrank test · Hazard ratio · Cox regression

2.1 Introduction

Cancer remains the main health challenge we are facing nowadays. Seems like every day you find out that another person you know has been diagnosed with cancer. After the shock wave, you feel sad for that person, and guilty because you are somehow happy that this did not happen to you or your loved ones. Even if heart diseases still remain the first cause of death worldwide, the death rate caused by them is rapidly falling. Why is that? Because we found out what causes heart diseases: high blood pressure, high weight, high glucose levels, smoking, drinking, etc. Knowing the cause, we have the means to prevent them. Unfortunately, this is not the case for cancer. We still do not know what causes cancer.

Sadly enough, nowadays most people Google first the symptoms, before speaking to a physician. No matter what we are Googling, cancer will appear on the result page. So, we are alarmed, and while waiting for the doctor's appointment we start Googling for that type of cancer. The most searched questions are: what is the 5-year

S. Belciug (✉)
Department of Computer Science, Faculty of Sciences, University of Craiova, Craiova, Romania
e-mail: sbelciug@inf.ucv.ro

© The Author(s), under exclusive license to Springer Nature Switzerland AG 2023
C. P. Lim et al. (eds.), *Artificial Intelligence and Machine Learning for Healthcare*,
Intelligent Systems Reference Library 229,
https://doi.org/10.1007/978-3-031-11170-9_2

survival rate? What is the overall survival? If there is need for surgery, what is the morbidity? What about the mortality rate? So, the number one outcome of interest is survival—overall, disease-free, recurrent, surgery survival.

The Global cancer prevalence rose from 0.54 to 0.64% since 1990. For instance for prostate cancer the rates rose from 67.8% to 98.6%, due to better AI prediction, [1]. Even if the cancer rates are rising, the death rates are falling. This can only mean one thing: early diagnosis and/or better novel treatments, hence people have better and longer survival rates. The 5-year survival rates for all cancers have increased from 50.3% to 67% [2–4]. Table 2.1 and Fig. 2.1 present how the 5-year survival rates for different types of cancers have changed from 1970–1977 to 2007–2013 in the USA.

WHO's global target (25×25) is a 25% reduction in deaths from cancer in people aged 30–69 years by 2025 [5]. Cancer survival research is crucial for developing cancer control strategies [6], control measures [7], so that the effectiveness and costs of them to be assessed [8, 9].

Survival analysis concerns the time until a certain event takes place: i.e. the time that passes from the start of chemotherapy until the tumor stops shrinking (the patient stops responding to treatment), the time elapsed from when a cancer surgery is over

Cancer type	1990–1997 (%)	2007–2013 (%)
All-cancers	50.3	67
Prostate	67.8	98.6
Thyroid	92.1	98.2
Melanoma	81.9	91.7
Breast (female)	74.8	89.7
Uterus	82.3	86.9
Bladder	72.3	77.3
Kidney	50.1	74.1
Non-hodgkin lymphoma	46.5	71
Cervix uteri	67.1	69.1
Mouth/throat	52.5	64.5
Colon	49.8	64.1
Leukemia	34.3	60.65
Myeloma	24.6	49.6
Ovary	36	46.5
Stomach	15.2	30.6
Brain	22.4	30.5
Esophagus	5	18.8
Lung	12.2	18.1
Liver	3.4	17.6
Pancreas	2.5	8.2

Table 2.1 5-year cancer survival rates in the USA comparison

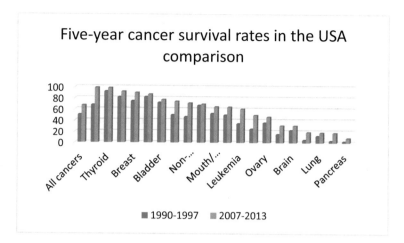

Fig. 2.1 5-year cancer survival rates comparison

until the patients gets out of the ICU (Intensive Care Unit), or the time that passed from the moment the patient started radiotherapy, till she/he passed away.

In this chapter, we are going to present statistical models that are used in survival analysis, along with examples and explanations regarding the obtained results.

2.2   Survival Analysis

Survival analysis deals with survival times. In order for you to start such an analysis you need two variables: a numeric metric of time (i.e. number of days, weeks, or months), and a categorical variable that identifies the event (i.e. irresponsive to treatment, death). The merged variables give us a lot of information about whether a subject has entered or left the study, and if and when the subject has met a certain criterion or not.

Unfortunately, in practice things are never that simple, and we might find ourselves in two situations:

- The *start time* cannot be specified. For example, we cannot establish exactly when was the exact onset of the disease. Some cancers progress at a faster pace than others, being more aggressive, but there is no precise method to determine the debut of cancer.
- The *end time* is difficult to be determined. If the end time is given by the time of death, then there is no problem in establishing it, but if a person decides to leave the study, or she/he survives more than the time that was set to be recorded (i.e. 5-year survival rate), things change. This is the case of the *censored survival time*.

In Fig. 2.2 we present an example of how we can record the survival times. The figure is converted into a table, Table 2.2.

The dotted line from Fig. 2.2 gives us information about the study: the patients were recruited the first 5 months of the study. The timeline from month 5 till month 9 represents the follow-up part of the study. The black square signifies that the patient has died, whereas the grey circle means that the patient did not die. To be more specific: patient 1 was recruited at the beginning of the study and stayed in the study till month 3, time of which she/he died. The second patient enrolled in the study from month 0, and did not have any event (i.e. died) during the whole observation period, so she/he represents a censored data. Patient 3 also started from the beginning of the study, but died five months later. The fourth patient enrolled on month 1 and stayed

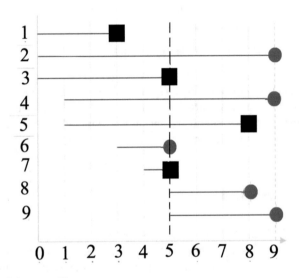

Fig. 2.2 Survival time recordings

Table 2.2 Tabulated survival time recordings

Patient	Start time	Time of death/censored	Death/censored	Survival time
1	0	3	D	3
2	0	9	C	9*
3	0	5	D	5
4	1	9	C	9*
5	1	8	D	7
6	3	5	C	2*
7	4	5	D	1
8	5	8	C	3*
9	5	9	C	4*

Fig. 2.3 Survival analysis tree structure diagram

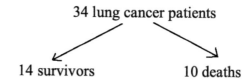

until the end of it. The fifth patient enrolled on month 1, and had an event (i.e. death) on month 8. The sixth patient enrolled on month 3, but left the study on month 5. Patient 7 joined the study on month 4 and passed away on month 6. Both patients 8 and 9 joined on month 5, the first leaving the study on month 8 (censored data), while the latter on month 9 (censored).

You can see in Table 2.2 that the censored data are marked with (*).

In general, we use survival analysis in oncology to review the outcomes of clinical trials, cohort studies, etc. For instance, if we have a cohort of 30 patients who have been diagnosed with lung cancer between 2017 and 2019, they have started chemotherapy and/or immunotherapy and were observed until the end of 2021, we wish to review their *survival time*. So far, we have seen that survival analysis contains a *starting period*, in which the patients are enrolled, followed by the *observation period* or *follow-up*, when the patients are observed. Besides these two stages, there exists another one named the *final period*. In this stage the collected data is analyzed, and conclusions are drawn.

Let us presume that from the 30 lung cancer patients, 6 of them left the study during the observation period. The 6 patients will be excluded from the statistical analysis process. From the remaining 24 patients, 14 survived and 10 passed away. This observation is depicted in a tree structure diagram, as the one presented in Fig. 2.3.

A more thorough tree diagram will include even the patients that left the study. See Fig. 2.4.

We can compute the *death rate* or the *death risk* using the following formula:

$$deathrate = \frac{number\,of\,deaths}{number\,of\,subjects}.$$

In our example the death rate is 0.41, that is 41%.
The *death probability* is computed as:

$$Deathprobability = \frac{D}{N - 0.5 \times L}$$

Fig. 2.4 Survival analysis tree diagram 2

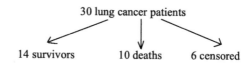

where N is the cohort size, D is the number of deaths, and L is the number of patients that left the study during the observation period. The death probability in our case is 0.37, that is 37%.

Having computed the death risk, we can compute the *survival probability* as 1—*death probability for that interval*. By plotting the cumulative survival probability, we obtain the *survival curve*. The curve starts at 1 meaning that all patients are alive and approaches 0 as patients start to die. In the following sections we shall discuss more about survival curves, starting with the *Kaplan–Meier survival curves*.

2.3 Kaplan–Meier Survival Curve

Kaplan–Meier curves were invented in 1958 by Edward L. Kaplan and Paul Meier, and they can be used if the data is incomplete [10]. They represent the standard for reporting the survival rate of patients, being used in over 70% of the oncology papers [11].

Kaplan–Meier curves use three types of data regarding the patient: the date the patient entered the study, the last date of observation (i.e. the last time the patient was seen alive), and whether the last observation was due to the death of the patient, or because the patient left the study. We can use Kaplan–Meier curves to determine the survival probability of a patient given certain conditions. For example, by recording the survival times of patients that undergo chemotherapy, we can compute the probability of a new patient to survive a certain period of time if she/he undergoes the same protocol.

We denote the survival time with a random variable X. P_n is the probability of a patient to survive the nth day after the last chemotherapy session, conditioned by the fact that she/he survived all the other $n-1$ days before that. $\overline{P_n}$ is the total probability of surviving all the n days, and we compute it as follows:

$$\overline{P_n} = P_1 \cdot P_2 \cdot \ldots \cdot P_n$$

We compute the intermediate survival probabilities using:

$$p_k = p_{k-1} \times \frac{r_k - f_k}{r_k},$$

where p_k is the probability of surviving k units of time, r_k is the number of patients with a death risk at the k moment, that survived k units of time, and f_k the number of deaths reported at the k moment. If no patient has died the survival rate is 100%. We compute the standard error of the probability of surviving using:

$$SE_{pk} = p_k \cdot \sqrt{\frac{(1 - p_k)}{r_k}}.$$

If we presume that p_k is governed by the Normal distribution, than we can compute the 95% interval as follows:

$$\left(p_k - 1.96 \times SE_{p_k}, \, p_k + 1.96 \times SE_{p_k}\right)$$

The standard error does not always give accurate approximations if there are extreme values in the data sample. If this is the case, the Greenwood formula is preferred:

$$SE_{p_k} = p_k \cdot \sqrt{\sum_{j=1}^{k} \frac{f_j}{r_j \cdot \left(r_j - f_j\right)}}.$$

Let us presume that we have a sample data that contains 16 patients that have been diagnosed with stage IV lung cancer. All the patients have undergone chemotherapy treatment with a certain type of drug, drug A. The patients are monitored 14 months. We start the survival analysis from day 0 (Table 2.3).

Using the survival probability formula, we compute the survival probability at a given time. Table 2.4 presents these calculations.

The corresponding Kaplan–Meier curve is plotted in Fig. 2.5.

Kaplan–Meier survival curves have a drawback: if we wish to compare two or multiple sample data, we can obtain only a comparison at a certain moment in time, not a global one. To resolve this issue, we can use the logrank test, or hazard ratio.

Table 2.3 Life table for lung cancer patients that underwent chemotherapy with drug A

No. of subjects	Survival time (months)	Event/Censored
1	2	1
2	3	1
3	5	1
4	5	1
5	5	1
6	5	0
7	7	1
8	7	1
9	7	1
10	9	0
11	10	0
12	10	0
13	11	1
14	11	1
15	12	1
16	12	1

Table 2.4 Survival probabilities, standard error and confidence interval

Time	Events	Survival rate	p_k	*SE*	Confidence interval
0	0	1	0	0	(1, 1)
2	1	0.9375	0.9375	0.0605	(0.6323, 0.991)
3	1	0.875	0.9333	0.0826	(0.586, 0.9672)
5	3	0.6875	0.7857	0.1159	(0.4046, 0.8563)
7	3	0.4812	0.7	0.1285	(0.2241, 0.6993)
9	0	0.4812	1	0.1285	(0.2241,0.6993)
10	0	0.4812	1	0.1285	(0.2241, 0.6993)
11	2	0.2406	0.5	0.1364	(0.04473, 0.5204)
12	2	0	0	0	(0, 0)

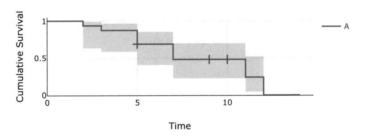

Fig. 2.5 Kaplan–Meier survival curve

2.4 The Logrank Test

The logrank test is a non-parametric test that uses the null hypothesis H_0: "there is no difference between the two groups". We perform this test by dividing the time scale according to observed events (i.e. deaths), while ignoring the censored data. For each interval we compute the observed number of deaths and the expected one, summing them up.

If we have two groups of patients, each group receives a certain chemotherapy drug. We will divide the survival time in time periods. Each period ends with one or multiple deaths. For each death unit, and each patient group, we compute the number of patients that are at death risk. Let us denote with r_1 the number of patients with death risk for sample group 1, and with r_2 the number of patients with death risk for sample group 2. Next, we compute the number of observed deaths for each group, f_1 and f_2. With this information we proceed on building the following table, Table 2.5.

The expected number of deaths for each group is computed using the following formula:

Table 2.5 Death and survival data regarding the two sample groups of patients

	Group 1	Group 2
Deaths	f_1	f_2
Survivals	$r_1 - f_1$	$r_2 - f_2$
Total	r_1	r_2

$$e_i = \frac{r_i \cdot f}{r}, i = 1, 2.$$

Next, we must sum up the observed values, O_i, as well as the expected values, E_i:

$$O_i = \sum_j f_{ji}, \quad i = 1, 2,$$

$$E_i = \sum_j e_{ji}, \quad i = 1, 2.$$

The logrank statistics is computed as follows:

$$X^2 = \frac{(O_1 - E_1)^2}{E_1} + \frac{(O_2 - E_2)^2}{E_2}.$$

For multiple groups we will use:

$$T = \sum_{j=1}^{n} \sum_{i=1}^{m} \frac{\left(O_{ij} - E_{ij}\right)^2}{E_{ij}}.$$

To verify whether we accept or reject the null hypothesis, we will use the $O_1 + O_2 = F_1 + E_2$ as control equality. The statistic value is compared with a χ^2 distribution with $(n-1)(m-1)$ degrees of freedom. n represents the number of groups, whereas m represents the number of time intervals [12, 13].

Let us exemplify how the logrank test works. Let us presume that we are conducting a clinical trial, with two types of immunotherapy drugs, A and B. For 14 months we have monitored the two groups of patients diagnosed with IV grade lung cancer. The first group contains the 16 patients from the Kaplan–Meier section, whereas the second group contains 12 patients. Table 2.6 presents the data regarding the two sample groups.

Using the survival probability formula, we compute the survival probability at a given time. Table 2.7 presents these calculations.

The corresponding Kaplan–Meier curve is plotted in Fig. 2.6.

For a better comparison we shall plot both curves in the same plot. Figure 2.7 present this plot.

Using the logrank equations we can build the following table, Table 2.8:

Table 2.6 Life table for lung cancer patients that underwent chemotherapy with drug *B*

No. of subjects	Survival time (months)	Event/Censored
1	14	1
2	14	0
3	5	1
4	5	0
5	10	1
6	10	1
7	10	0
8	11	0
9	11	0
10	14	0
11	14	0
12	14	0

Table 2.7 Survival probabilities, standard error and confidence interval

Time	Events	Survival rate	p_k	SE	Confidence interval
0	0	1	0	0	(1,1)
5	1	0.9167	0.9167	0.0605	(0.6323, 0.991)
10	2	0.7333	0.8	0.0826	(0.586, 0.9672)
11	0	0.7333	1	0.1159	(0.4046, 0.8563)
14	1	0.5867	0.8	0.1285	(0.2241, 0.6993)

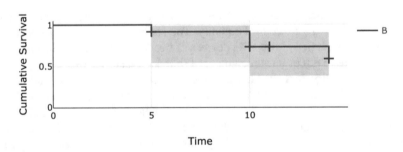

B - Survival Function (S_t) - with confidence interval

Fig. 2.6 Kaplan–Meier survival curve second group

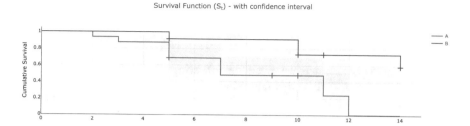

Fig. 2.7 Kaplan–Meier curves for both sample patients

Table 2.8 Goodness of fit table

Group	Observed frequency	Expected frequencies
Group 1	12	6.829
Group 2	4	9.170

Fig. 2.8 Goodness of fit histogram

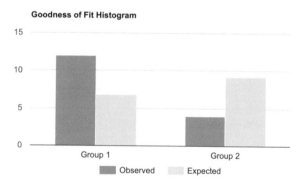

The Goodness of Fit histogram is presented in Fig. 2.8.

The test statistic χ^2 equals 6.829, while the p-level equals 0.0089. This means that we will reject the null hypothesis, implying that there are significant differences between the survival rates of the patients that use drug A, versus drug B.

2.5   The Hazard Ratio

Besides the information regarding the difference between two groups of observations, we might be interested in seeing how truly different the two groups are. In this matter, we cannot use the logrank test, but we can apply the hazard ratio. Technically, we will measure the relative survival between the two groups by comparing the observed and expected numbers [14–19]. The hazard ratio is computed using the following formula:

$$R = \frac{O_1 / E_1}{O_2 / E_2}.$$

Returning to our example, we obtain the following results (Fig. 2.9; Table 2.9).

The obtained results show that the estimated relative risk of dying when undergoing imunotherapy with drug A is 3.1839 of the estimated relative risk of dying when undergoing chemotherapy with drug B. More specifically, if the hazard ratio equals 1, it means that there is no difference in survival rates / event rate over time between the two sample groups. If the hazard ratio is greater than 1, just like in our example, then the risk of having an event is greater in the group that uses drug A versus the group that uses drug B. Please note that the hazard ratio indicates an increase of hazard when using drug A, which is an increase in the rate of the event, not the chances of it happening.

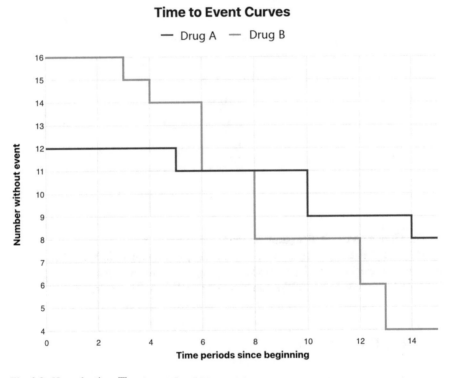

Fig. 2.9 Hazard ratio—Time to event curves

Table 2.9 Hazard ratio results	Hazard	95% Confidence interval	χ^2	p-value
	3.1839	(1.194, 8.487)	4.494	0.034

2.5.1   Cox Regression Model

The chapter ends with the *Cox's proportional hazard regression model* or *Cox regression*, which creates a *survival function* that gives us a certain event's probability (i.e. death, irresponsive to treatment) to happen at a particular time t. Having previously observed and recorded data, we can build the model, and afterwards use it to make predictions on new patients. Cox regression can analyze multiple factors. Some may think that instead of using the Cox regression, we might be able to use the multilinear regression. This is not possible due to the following:

- in general, samples that contain survival times have exponential or Weibull distributions, and multiple linear regression cannot be applied unless the sample data is governed by the Gaussian distribution.
- Survival times contain censored data.

When using the Cox proportional hazard regression method, we need to compute the *survival function* and the *hazard function*. We compute the survival function as it follows:

$$S(t) = \{T > t\},$$

where t is the time, and T is the time remaining till the patient's death. Hence, we can write the *lifetime* distribution as:

$$F(t) = 1 - S(t).$$

We compute the number of deaths per time unit as: $f(t) = \frac{d}{dt}F(t)$. The *hazard function* is:

$$\lambda(t) = P\{t < T < t + dt\} = \frac{f(t)dt}{S(t)} = -\frac{S'(t)dt}{S(t)}.$$

Practically, by computing the hazard function we find the patient's death risk within the timeframe dt, when previously given T time left to live. The Cox regression model presumes that variables within the hazard function are independent and have a constant effect over the time of the survival, and each of them can be a predictor or covariance:

$$h(t; Z_1, Z_2, \ldots, Z_k) = h_0(t) \cdot \exp(b_1 Z_1 + b_2 Z_2 + \cdots + b_k Z_k).$$

The function can be afterwards transformed into:

$$ln\left[\frac{h(t; Z_1, Z_2, \ldots, Z_k)}{h_0(t)}\right] = b_1 Z_1 + b_2 Z_2 + \cdots + b_k Z_k.$$

The $h_0(t)$ is the *underlying hazard function* and represents the hazard when all the variables equal 0. Two assumptions must be fulfilled [20–22]:

- The hazard and the independent variables have a log-linear relationship;
- The *hypothesis of proportionality*: the relationship between the underlying hazard function and log-linear function of covariates exists.

Let us see how the Cox regression works on another fictional example. Our sample data contains 17 patients diagnosed with lung cancer. The dataset contains four attributes, four predictor variables (time, age, number of affected lymph nodes, number of months that have passed since the surgery), and the categorical variable (survival). The data is presented in Table 2.10.

First, we were interested in plotting the Kaplan–Meier curve to see the survival after the oncological lung surgery. Figure 2.10 show the curve together with 95% confidence interval.

Next, we built two cohorts of patients. The first had no cancerous lymph node detected, the other had more than one. We have plotted the survival curve for both groups using Kaplan–Meier (Fig. 2.11).

We have applied the Cox regression model having as event the Survival attribute, and as duration the Time attribute. The obtained results are in Table 2.11. The summary statistic table indicates the significance of the covariates in predicting the Survival risk. The large confidence interval indicates that the sample data is small.

Table 2.10 Fictional lung cancer patient dataset

# Patient	Time	Age	No lymph nodes	Months from surgery	Survival
0	12	57	1	6	1
1	18	65	3	7	1
2	24	63	0	12	1
3	24	56	2	16	1
4	11	62	4	10	0
5	26	75	0	23	1
6	16	48	0	11	1
7	19	51	0	9	1
8	5	66	1	5	0
9	6	63	2	4	1
10	4	68	4	2	0
11	15	66	5	10	0
12	20	65	0	18	1
13	28	59	1	25	1
14	12	70	1	11	0
15	12	72	2	10	1
16	28	65	0	26	1

Fig. 2.10 Kaplan–Meier curve and 95% confidence interval for survival after oncological lung surgery

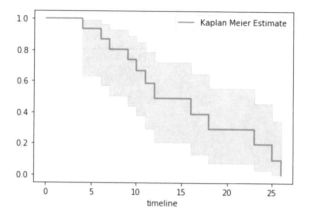

Fig. 2.11 Kaplan–Meier curve and 95% confidence interval for two lung patient cohorts

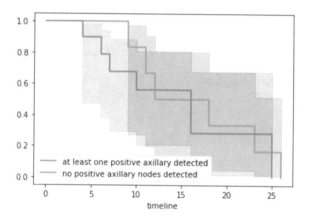

The p-level shows us that the number of months that have passed since the oncological surgery is significant, while the others are not. The hazard ratio for this attribute is 0.71 showing a strong relationship between the number of months that have passed since the surgery and decreased risk of death. Notice that the hazard ration for Age is 1.01, which suggests only a 1% increase for the higher age group. Technically:

- Hazard ratio = 1: no effect
- Hazard ratio < 1: reduction in the hazard
- Hazard ratio > 1: increase in hazard.

Let us see now which attributes affect the most from the following plot (Fig. 2.12):

From Fig. 2.12, we can clearly see that the number of months that have passed since the surgery is indeed significant, while the others are not. As a final note, we have plotted the survival probabilities for different persons in our dataset. From the graph (Fig. 2.13), we can see that patient 13 has the highest chances of survival, whereas patient 8 has the lowest.

Table 2.11 Results of Cox hazard regression

	Age	Number of lymph nodes	Months from surgery
Coef.	0.01	−0.05	−0.34
Exp(coef.)	1.01	0.95	0.71
SE(coef.)	0.06	0.30	0.12
Coef. lower 95%	−0.10	−0.63	−0.58
Coef. upper 95%	0.13	0.53	−0.10
Exp. (coef.) lower 95%	0.91	0.53	0.56
Exp. (coef.) upper 95%	1.13	1.71	0.90
Z	0.26	−0.16	−2.82
p-level	0.80	0.87	<0.005
$-\log 2(p)$	0.33	0.20	7.70

Fig. 2.12 Significant attributes

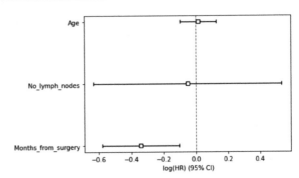

Fig. 2.13 Survival probabilities for patients: 0, 4, 8, and 13

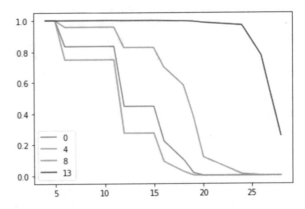

2.6   Conclusions

This chapter provides a survival analysis guide with applications in oncology. Survival analysis represents an important part of cancer research. It can be applied to determine the survival rate of patients, to determine which treatment protocol is more efficient, or to establish whether new therapies are indeed better than the old ones. Using survival analysis in clinical trials we can move forward in providing the best care for cancer patients.

In this chapter we have discussed the theory behind Kaplan–Meier survival curves, logrank test, hazard ration, and Cox regression, as well as practical examples. We hope that this chapter will provide data scientists and oncologists a better understanding of the survival analysis process.

Acknowledgements   The author would like to thank the reviewers for taking their time to review this chapter, and for their important comments that led to a better version of this work.

References

1. Wulczyn, E., et al.: Predicting prostate cancer specific mortality with artificial intelligence-based Gleason Grading. Commun. Med. **1**(10). https://doi.org/10.1038/s43856021-00005-3
2. https://ourworldindata.org/cancer
3. Jemal, A., Ward, E.M., Johnson, C.J., Cronin, K.A., Ma, J., Ryerson, A.B., Mariotto, A., Lake, A.J., Wilson, R., Sherman, R.L., Anderson, R.N., Hensley, S.J., Kohler, B.A., Penberthy, L., Feuer, E.J., Weir, H.K.: Annual report to the nation of the status of cancer, 1975–2014, feature survival, JNCI: J. Natl. Cancer Inst. **109**, 9 (2017). https://doi.org/10.1093/jnci/djx030
4. Allemani, C., Weirm H.K., Carreira, H., Harewood, R., Spika, D., Wang, X.S., Bannon, F., Ahn, J.V., Johnson, C.J., Bonaventure, A., Gragera, R.M., Stiller, C., Azevedo e Silva, G., Chen, W.Q., Ogunbiyi, O., Rachet, B., Soeberg, M., You, H., Coleman, M.P.: Global surveillance of cancer survival 1995–2009: analysis of individual data for 25 676 887 patients from 279 population-based registries in 67 countries (CONCORD-2). Lancet **385**(9972), 977–1010 (2015)
5. WHO (2012). Decisions and list of resolutions of the 65th World Health Assembly: prevention and control of noncommunicable diseases: follow-up to the high-level meeting of the United Nations General Assembly on the prevention and control of non-communicable diseases (A65/DIV/3). World Health Organization, Geneva
6. Coleman, M.P., Forman, D., Byrant, H., et al., The ICBP Module 1 Working Group: Cancer survival in Australia, Canada, Denmark, Norway, Sweden, and the UK, 1995–2007 (the International Cancer Benchmarking Partnership): an analysis of population-based cancer registry data. Lancet **377**, 127–138 (2011)
7. Department of Health: Improving Outcomes: a Strategy for Cancer. Department of Health, London (2011)
8. Rachet, B., Maringe, C., Nur, U., et al.: Population-based cancer survival trends in England and Wales up to 2007: an assessment of the NHS cancer plan for England. Lancet Oncol. **10**, 351–369 (2009)
9. Rachet, B., Ellis, L., Maringe, C., et al.: Socioeconomic inequalities in cancer survival in England after the NHS Cancer Plan. Br. J. Cancer **103**, 446–453 (2010)
10. Kaplan, E.L., Meier, P.: Nonparametric estimations for incomplete observations. J. Am. Stat. Assoc. **53**(282), 457–481 (1958)

11. Stalpers, L.J., Kaplan, E.L.: Edward L. Kaplan and the Kaplan-Meier survival curve. BSHM Bull. **33**, 109–135 (2018)
12. Bland, J.M., Altman, D.G.: The logrank rest. BMJ **328**(74447), 1073 (2004)
13. Gorunescu, F., Belciug, S.: Incursiune in Biostatistica, Editura Albastra – Grupul Microinformatica (2014)
14. Altman, D.G.: Practical Statistic for Medical Research. Chapman and Hall (1991)
15. Belciug, S.: Artificial Intelligence in Cancer: Diagnostic to Tailored Treatment. Elsevier (2020)
16. Georgiev, G.Z.: One-tailed versus two-tailed tests of significance in A/B testing, https://blog.analytics-toolkit.com/2017/one-tailed-two-tailed-tests-significance-ab-testing/ (2017)
17. Stare, J., Maucort-Boulch, D.: Odds ratio, hazard ratio and relative risk. Metodoloskizvezki **13**(1), 59–67 (2016)
18. Sashegyi, A., Ferry, D.: On the interpretation of the hazard ratio and communication of survival benefit. Oncologist **22**(4), 484–486 (2017)
19. Spruance, S.L., Reid, J.E., Grace, M., Samore, M.: Hazard ratio in clinical trials. Antimicrob. Agents Chemother. **48**(8), 2787–2792 (2004)
20. Cox, D.R.: Regression models and life tables. J. Roy. Stat. Soc. B **34**, 187–202 (1972)
21. Andersen, P., Gill, R.: Cox's regression model for counting processes, a large sample study. Ann. Stat. **10**, 1100–1120 (1982)
22. Harrell, F.E., Jr.: Regression Modeling Strategies: With Applications to Linear Models, Logistic Regression, and Survival Analysis. Springer (2001)

Chapter 3
Social Media Sentiment Analysis Related to COVID-19 Vaccinations

Evridiki Kapoteli, Vasiliki Chouliara, Paraskevas Koukaras⊙, and Christos Tjortjis⊙

Abstract The wake of the COVID-19 pandemic has yet again highlighted how vital immunization is for public health. Despite the dramatic spread of SARS-CoV-2 and its variants, there is a rising trend of people refusing to be vaccinated. As a result, governments and health experts must gather and understand public ideas and perceptions about vaccines to design engagement and education efforts about vaccine advantages. Sentiment analysis is a common method for acquiring a broad picture of public opinion, that enables the classification of people as those who are in favor or against vaccination, as well as the determination of the factors that influence their attitudes and beliefs. The purpose of this chapter is to describe the general approach to sentiment analysis in the context of vaccinations and review its different use cases. The chapter's experimental component integrates the utilization of a dataset retrieved from Kaggle, which contains COVID-19 vaccine-related Twitter data. When attempting to perform sentiment analysis, certain methodological steps need to be considered after data collection, including data pre-processing, technique selection and model construction, as well as model evaluation and results interpretation. Both supervised and unsupervised sentiment analysis methods are investigated in the model construction step, with the former involving the implementation of Support Vector Machines and Logistic Regression algorithms, and the latter involving the use of TextBlob and Valence Aware Dictionary and sEntiment Reasoner (VADER) sentiment analysis tools. The performance of each algorithm and tool is evaluated, as is the performance of each sentiment detection approach

E. Kapoteli · V. Chouliara · P. Koukaras · C. Tjortjis (✉)
The Data Mining and Analytics Research Group, School of Science and Technology, International Hellenic University, 570 01 Thermi, Greece
e-mail: c.tjortjis@ihu.edu.gr

E. Kapoteli
e-mail: ekapoteli@ihu.edu.gr

V. Chouliara
e-mail: vchouliara@ihu.edu.gr

P. Koukaras
e-mail: p.koukaras@ihu.edu.gr

© The Author(s), under exclusive license to Springer Nature Switzerland AG 2023
C. P. Lim et al. (eds.), *Artificial Intelligence and Machine Learning for Healthcare*, Intelligent Systems Reference Library 229,
https://doi.org/10.1007/978-3-031-11170-9_3

in order to select the best performing one. Social media platforms have become a common source of information and misinformation regarding vaccines. Our effort aims to emphasize the importance of mining such readily available public attitudes, as well as forecast opinions and reactions related to vaccine uptake in near real-time. Such insights could be critical in dealing with health emergency situations like the ongoing coronavirus pandemic.

Keywords Machine learning · Lexicon-based · Sentiment analysis · Classification · Natural language processing · Vaccination · Tweets · COVID-19

Term Definition Table

Data mining	The process used to convert raw data into useful information.
Accuracy	The total number of instances that have been correctly classified by the trained classifier when tested with unseen data.
Training Set	The input dataset of an algorithm with known correct outputs.
Feature vector	The mathematical representation of an object's numeric or symbolic characteristics known as features.
Class	The output category of the data instances.
Polarity	The expression that takes positive, negative, or neutral values and determines the sentimental aspect of an opinion

3.1 Introduction

At the time of writing, it has been two years since WHO declared SARS-CoV-2 a global pandemic on March 11, 2020 [1]. During that time, the coronavirus affected more than 220 countries, causing over 377 million infections and 6 million fatalities worldwide [2, 3]. With new variants of concern emerging and old ones continuing to leave their mark in the form of human casualties, the global community is still on high alert.

In the light of the COVID-19 pandemic, scientists made an unparalleled effort on building safe and effective vaccines to mitigate the spread. However, due to the rapid development of vaccines, as well as worries regarding their safety, efficacy, and side effects, there is a trend of people who refuse to be vaccinated. Vaccine hesitancy and a decreased likelihood of complying to health guidance measures are both associated with susceptibility to misinformation. While public belief in COVID-19 misinformation is not very widespread, a substantial portion of individuals finds this type of misinformation highly reliable, posing a potential threat to public health [4].

Low vaccination coverage, especially in areas of the developing world, is believed to be one of the factors contributing to the formation of new variants [5] highlighting, yet again, how vital immunization is for public health. As a result, governments and health experts must gather and understand public ideas and perceptions about vaccines to design engagement and education efforts about vaccine advantages.

Current sources for gathering such data and inferring insights into COVID-19 include social media sites, which serve as both information and communication channels, providing rich data for opinion mining or sentiment analysis. Researchers have already thoroughly examined what processes and steps are required when analyzing data obtained from social media [6]. During the crisis people all over the world turned to social media to remain up to date on the latest coronavirus information, often compromising their mental health causing more anxiety and depression [7]. Additionally, social media were extensively used to express opinions and concerns on covid-related news, indicating that they may be harnessed to predict events related to the global spread of the disease in real-time [8].

Throughout the pandemic, sentiment analysis and machine learning have proven to be very useful techniques in applications such as predicting COVID-19 ICU needs [9] or identifying public opinion on social distancing [10], mask usage [11], and vaccines [12]. Sentiment analysis, in particular, is a common method for acquiring a broad picture of public opinion and human emotions by observing the behaviors of people as they interact with social media tools [13]. It provides the polarity of a given text and enables the classification of people, as those who are in favor or against vaccination, as well as the determination of the factors that influence their attitudes and beliefs. The concept of sentiment analysis has also been considered in order to propose a novel method for extracting sentiment from user-generated social media opinions [14].

Sentiment analysis relies on data mining and Natural Language Processing (NLP) techniques to detect, gather, and distill information from the massive textual content available online [15]. Depending on the level it is performed, sentiment analysis can be classified as document-level, sentence-level, or aspect level [16]. Document-level sentiment analysis is carried out under the assumption that each document is a representation of its author's opinion on a single main entity. A sentence-level sentiment analysis is performed when individual sentences in a document are reviewed to determine whether the opinion, they reflect is positive, negative, or neutral. Finally, when a document covers multi-aspect entities about which different opinions are expressed, an aspect- level sentiment analysis task is performed to determine the sentiment expression for each of the aspects present [17].

There exist three types of approaches for sentiment classification: supervised machine learning, unsupervised lexicon-based and hybrid approach, which combines both. The first class of approaches requires a labeled dataset with entries of known polarity, which is divided into training and testing sets. The training set is used to train a Machine Learning (ML) algorithm of our choice to recognize the class of previously unseen entries [18]. This approach, however, is not without limitations. For starters, the model's performance is dependent on the volume of training data, which means that the greater the collection of labeled data, the better the performance.

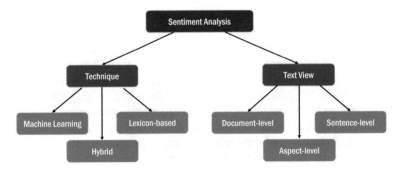

Fig. 3.1 Sentiment analysis aspects

Moreover, when a classifier is applied to a domain other than the one in which it was trained, its performance may be reduced.

The lexicon-based approach determines the overall sentiment polarity of a document based on a lexicon, a set of predefined words, each of which has a polarity score assigned to it. Although this sentiment analysis method does not require a set of training data, it is susceptible to informal language, such as that used on social media, since lexicons may be lacking context-specific terms [19]. Hybrid sentiment analysis is a combination of ML and lexicon-based methodologies often used to overcome the disadvantages of each technology when employed separately [20]. Figure 3.1 depicts a summary of the different sentiment analysis expressions based on the text-level and the technique used.

The purpose of this chapter is to describe the general approach to sentiment analysis in the context of vaccinations and review its different use cases. The literature we reviewed demonstrates that scientists have experimented with several methods to detect and understand public opinion towards vaccination not only for COVID-19 vaccines, but also for HPV and MMR vaccines.

As for the experimental part of the chapter, we utilize a dataset retrieved from Kaggle which contains COVID-19 vaccine-related data acquired from Twitter. The data were pre-processed in order to eliminate any irrelevant information to our analysis, such as mentions, links, numbers, stop-words and emojis. Following that, the pre-processed dataset is given as input to popular ML algorithms such as Support Vector Machines (SVM) and Logistic Regression (LR), as well as to well-known sentiment analysis tools such as TextBlob and Valence Aware Dictionary and sEntiment Reasoner (VADER). The goal of this comparison is to measure the performance of each model and each tool and report the efficacy of each sentiment detection approach.

The structure of the remainder of the chapter is as follows. Section 3.2 discusses recent studies that used both ML and lexicon-based techniques to perform sentiment analysis on vaccinations. Section 3.3 describes the proposed methodology in detail, while Sect. 3.4 describes the experimental setup, including information on data collection and pre-processing, model selection, and the class imbalance problem. The experimental results are then analyzed by reporting the performance metrics of the models and tools that were used. The chapter ends with conclusions, discussion, contribution and future directions overview, as well as a list of references.

3.2 Literature Review

Over the past few years, a plethora of studies on sentiment analysis regarding vaccination have been conducted. Moreover, data mining techniques have been used successfully to deal with epidemics [21]. With the ongoing pandemic, academics are relying on social media sentiment analysis more than ever before to study people's feeling. The next paragraphs provide detailed descriptions of how the research community has approached the sentiment analysis task on vaccinations thus far.

3.2.1 Machine Learning-Based Sentiment Analysis Studies

Du et al. [22], proposed a hierarchical ML based model to analyze public sentiment on HPV vaccines related tweets and classify them into 10 distinct categories. The training dataset comprised of 6000 random tweets, manually annotated and the chosen classification algorithm was SVM with RBF kernel. Based on the traits of the data set, different combinations of word n-grams, word clusters and part of speech tags were used as features, and it has been observed that the highest score is achieved when all three are used together. The authors considered parameter optimization to be critical because it has a significant impact on the performance of the system, particularly when dealing with highly imbalanced data set like the one studied. When the hierarchical classification and the baseline model employing word n-grams as the feature and default SVMs parameters were put into testing, the former outperformed the latter both on overall performance and on each category.

Following this paper, the same authors in their next study [23], evaluated the performance of the proposed system on a large-scale dataset. For that, they extracted English tweets that contained keywords regarding HPV vaccines for a 5-month long period and randomly selected 500 of them for manual annotation according to the hierarchical classification scheme. The procedure of the performance evaluation was the following: the ML model was used to classify the annotated tweets and the resulted label was then compared to the label obtained after the manual annotation. Afterwards, precision, recall, F-measure, micro-averaged and macro-averaged scores were calculated, which indicated a promising overall performance but an unsatisfactory performance on categories with limited number of instances. However, the impact of this behavior on the result was not deemed to be significant, since the ratio of those tweets compared to the whole corpus was observed to be small.

The authors were not limited to these findings, and they additionally conducted a time series analysis, aiming to reveal trends and patterns of HPV vaccines related sentiments, as well as if and how sentiment categories associate to different days of the week. The quadratic models used to investigate the trends, fitted the data quite well and they showed a weak trend for "Negative" sentiment category, first increasing and then decreasing, and exactly the opposite trend for the "Positive" group. It was also found that different sentiments are strongly associated to different days of the week. For instance, the percentage of "Negative" tweets was minimum on Wednesdays and maximum on weekends. Finally, the time series analysis indicated there is a link between mainstream events and the content on Twitter, implying that mass media can influence the public opinion on Twitter regarding the HPV vaccination.

One year later, Yuan and Crooks in their paper [24], employed supervised ML along with community detection on online social networks, opting to uncover communication patterns among pro- and anti-vaccine users on Twitter. The data collection includes MMR vaccine related tweets, published by a large number of users after a measles outbreak in California. Each user must then be classified into one of the following groups: anti-vaccination, pro-vaccination and neutral to vacci-nation. To train a supervised model that could do so, the authors hand-labeled a small portion of the tweets' corpus, to the three aforementioned classes. Afterwards, several supervised learning models with different features were trained with labeled data, to choose the one that delivers the best results and then employed the model. Logistic Regression, SVM, k-Nearest Neighbors and Naïve Bayes were some of the examined models, but SVM with a linear kernel was used due to its higher perfor-mance. The users' opinion was then determined by aggregating the resulted labeled tweets and the findings suggest that users belonging in the anti-vaccination class are as the authors say, "highly clustered and enclosed communities".

Another example of how a ML based sentiment analysis model can be combined with community detection to monitor online discussions on vaccination across different opinion groups in real time is the one referred to Kunneman et al. research [25]. According to Kunneman et al., insights gained from automatically classifying tweets containing a negative stance towards vaccinations, can be used for vaccination campaigns. The authors studied Dutch vaccine related tweets in a five-year period, with their main goal being to discover as accurately as possible messages with a negative stance towards vaccination. The authors started by annotating a collection of tweets based on their stance as "Negative", "Neutral", "Positive" or "Not clear", and some additional categories like relevance, subject and sentiment. However, the agreement on the annotation categories was poor, which made the authors discern three types of annotated data and try out different combinations of them to test if the addition of labeled data that are less reliable, could improve the performance. The different types of labeled data are the following:

- "strict": describes tweets that were given the same label by two annotators and comprise the most reliable type.
- "lax": denotes tweets that were labeled with a certain category by one of the two annotators.
- "one": denotes the portion of annotated tweets that were annotated by only one coder.

This collection of coded tweets was used to train and test different configurations for the classifier. The authors examined Multinomial Naïve Bayes and SVM for different combinations of strict, lax and one, and found that SVM outperforms Naïve Bayes when trained on strict and lax types of labeled data. This model with a F1-score of 0.36, also outperforms general purpose sentiment analysis tools, even if it was trained only on a small dataset.

D'Andrea et al. [26], proposed a system that can analyze the public stance of Italian-language tweets regarding the vaccination topic. The authors retrieved and pre-processed a collection of tweets, from which they randomly selected a subset to manually label and use during the training phase. Several experiments were then conducted to determine the optimal combination of text representation and classification approaches. Deep learning-based methods yielded the worst results, while the rest evaluated methods achieved comparable results. The bag-of-words scheme along with a SVM model achieved the best results and thus, was adopted to classify the expressed stance of each tweet as being in favor, neutral or not in favor of vaccination, with 64.84% accuracy. Following that, the dynamics of public opinion towards vaccination in Italy were tracked for a 10-month period, in relation to vaccine-related events that could trigger an opinion shift. 64% of the analyzed tweets were neutral, approximately 19% were in favor of vaccination and the remaining 17% were not in favor of vaccination.

The discovery of COVID-19 vaccines was undoubtedly one of the most significant successes in the virus's containment and mitigation. However, they have unwittingly and unintentionally became a bone of contention among mankind, necessitating in that way a regular inspection of public opinion.

Towards this end, Cotfas et al. [27], employed classical ML and deep learning algorithms to analyze the opinions regarding COVID-19 vaccination by taking into consideration the one-month period from the first vaccine announcement (from Pfizer and BioNTech), until the first vaccination took place in UK. Tweets have been gathered from November 9 until December 8, and four approaches have been investigated:

- Bag-of-Words representation followed by classical ML
- Word embeddings followed by classical machine learning
- Word embeddings followed by deep learning
- Bidirectional Encoder Representations from Transformers (BERT).

The goal was to categorize the data into 3 categories, in favor, against and neutral. For this purpose, the performance of several ML algorithms has been investigated: Multinomial Naive Bayes (MNB), Random Forest (RF), Support Vector Machine (SVM), Bidirectional Long Short-Term Memory (Bi-LSTM) and Convolutional Neural Network (CNN). Additionally, the Term Frequency-Inverse Document Frequency (TF-IDF) which is used as a weighting factor, seems to improve the classification algorithms. The insights gained from this process are that in the case of vaccine classification, classical ML algorithms have outperformed deep learning approaches. Also, the model that seems to perform best here, is BERT with an accuracy of 78.94%. The authors complete the process with the connection between the data at specific periods and the events in the media at the same periods and they conclude that "tweets reflect the hot topics in the society at large."

Supervised sentiment analysis was also conducted by Villavicencio et al. [28], to analyze Filipinos' sentiment regarding the COVID-19 vaccines. To this end, the authors collected vaccine-related Twitter posts written in English and Filipino, manually annotated them, and preprocessed them, in order to prepare them for sentiment classification. The Naïve Bayes classifier was then used to categorize the tweets as negative, neutral, or positive, achieving an accuracy of 81.77%. The findings indicate that the majority of the collected tweets had positive polarity, while neutral and negative polarities comprised the 9% and 8% of the dataset, respectively. This study, however, is hampered by the fact that only a small number of tweets (993) were used to extract the sentiment.

The study of Kwok et al. [29], employed ML techniques to uncover issues and sentiments of Australians regarding COVID-19 vaccination on the Twitter platform. For this reason, from January 2020 to October 2020, English tweets posted by Australian Twitter users were collected and analyzed by performing Latent Dirichlet Allocation and sentiment analysis. Tweets were classified into two sentiments, namely positive and negative, and into eight emotions among anger, fear, trust, joy, and more. The majority of tweets (67%) were determined to be positive, 30% were negative, and 3% were neutral. Regarding the emotions detected in tweets, trust and anticipation were the most frequently found positive emotions, whereas fear and sadness were the top two negative emotions.

3.2.2 Lexicon-Based Sentiment Analysis Studies

A small dataset of 9581 tweets was used by Raghupathi et al. [30], to study the public sentiment towards vaccination. The authors applied text analysis techniques and sentiment analysis on the collected dataset of tweets. For conducting sentiment analysis, the authors used a lexicon and rule-based sentiment analysis tool, namely Valence Aware Dictionary and Sentiment Reasoner. Next, K-means algorithm was used to cluster the document collection by topics using a bag-of-words approach. Three different clusters were derived, with the first one containing most tweets (7361) discussing about studies or innovations regarding vaccines, while tweets belonging to the second cluster focused on discussions about U.S. outbreaks. In general, it was found that negative tweets outnumbered positive ones by a small margin, particularly there were 43.3% negative and 40.4% positive. Since, the time period of this study coincided with a measles outbreak, the authors highlight how machine learning, sentiment analysis, NLP and text analysis speed up the process of public sentiment understanding, when it comes to infectious diseases.

Moving on to a more recent matter of concern, in the following we explore sentiment analysis studies during the coronavirus pandemic, with a focus on vaccines. Several studies followed a lexicon approach to sentiment analysis and employed the VADER or the TextBlob tools. For instance, Wang et al. [20], performed Twitter sentiment analysis using VADER to explore the differences in public sentiments and opinions about COVID-19 on social media between New York and California states.

Furthermore, VADER was used by Hung et al. [31], to identify whether a tweet expressed positive, neutral, or negative attitude towards COVID-19, based on tweets originating from all over the United States. Bhagat et al. [32], used TextBlob to study public attitude towards online learning from news articles on the internet. A hybrid sentiment analysis was conducted by Shofiya and Abidi [10], in which sentiment polarities of social distancing related tweet texts from Canada were extracted using SentiStrength tool and then used as labels to train an SVM algorithm.

Sattar and Arifuzzaman [33], performed sentiment analysis to detect the public sentiment regarding vaccination during the coronavirus pandemic, using English language tweets. For that purpose, two datasets are used, one containing tweets about various vaccines, and the other containing tweets about people's lifestyle following vaccination and a lexicon-based approach to sentiment analysis was followed comparing both TextBlob and VADER tools. The daily distribution of the tweets for each vaccine, depicted for both tools indicate a similar trend, with VADER tending to misclassify some neutral tweets as negative and positive ones. Therefore, the results retrieved solely using TextBlob are reported which indicate that most of the tweets (60–70%) were neutral, and in the remaining part the percentage of positive tweets outnumbered that of negative tweets, despite reports of adverse reactions caused by some of the vaccines. Additionally, the positive sentiment was equally prevalent when it came to maintaining COVID-19 safety precautions after vaccination.

Hu et al. [34], investigated the public's perception of COVID-19 vaccines in the United States. Over 300,000 tweets were analyzed using sentiment and emotion analysis techniques, as well as topic modeling and word cloud mapping, to track the progression of sentiment and emotion patterns between March 2020 and February 2021. The authors identified three periods in the pandemic timeframe that show significant shifts in public sentiment and emotion, but also 11 major events and topics as likely causes of such changes. The Valence Aware Dictionary for Sentiment Reasoning tool was used for sentiment analysis, which revealed an increase in positive sentiment alongside a decrease in negative sentiment about COVID-19 vaccinations in the majority of states. Finally, the findings of the emotion analysis indicate that the emotions of trust and anticipation were coupled with a combination of fear, sadness, and anger.

In order to analyze sentiments and opinions about the COVID-19 vaccines Yousefinaghani et al. [35], collected over 4.5 million tweets posted between January 2020 and January 2021 using Twitter as their data source. For polarity assignment, the Valence Aware Dictionary and sEntiment Reasoner (VADER) was used, classifying tweets as positive if they had a score of 0.25 or higher, negative if they had a score of 0.25 or lower, and neutral if they had a score between those values. It was found that the majority of the tweets were assigned to the neutral category (41%), while 34% of them were assigned to the positive category and 25% to the negative category. Furthermore, the authors classified vaccine-related Twitter discussions as either anti-vaccine, vaccine hesitant or pro-vaccine and contrasted the online discourse toward major vaccine makers, identified main themes and keywords and took into consideration accounts features and posts engagement metrics.

More interestingly, Marcec and Likic [36], were the first to analyze how people's sentiment toward each COVID-19 vaccine manufacturer was formed on Twitter, using a lexicon-based sentiment analysis. During a 4-month study period, the authors collected tweets written in English that mentioned AstraZeneca/Oxford, Pfizer/BioNTech, and Moderna vaccines. The AFINN lexicon was then employed to compute the daily average sentiment of tweets and events or news that could have influenced the sentiment were identified.

3.2.3 Hybrid Sentiment Analysis Studies

Other researchers studied vaccine hesitancy on Twitter employing sentiment analysis tools [37]. In particular, they performed a sentence-level sentiment analysis and applied a hybrid approach on a large collection of vaccine-related tweets written in English or Spanish and posted between June 2011 and April 2019. At the beginning, a sample of the collected tweets was randomly chosen and annotated as either positive, negative, or neutral. The tweets were then preprocessed, and the SVM classifier was trained on a random selection of 5000 tweets from each sentiment polarity category. The authors addressed any errors and repeated the process until the algorithm's accuracy was greater than 85%. The majority of the tweets were classified as neutral by the algorithm, but descriptive analysis revealed an increase on the percentage of positive and negative tweets and a decrease on neutral tweets over the study period.

The authors found that the number of tweets related to vaccines was ever-growing over time, which was in part due to the increasing number of Twitter users. When examining the sentiment of tweets on different days of the week the findings match those of Du et al., described before. Positive tweets increased on Wednesdays and declined on weekends, while the opposite holds for negative tweets.

The sentiment of tweets was also examined on different locations unveiling significant differences, which made the authors advocate that public health authorities could use Twitter sentiment analysis as an additional tool to detect regions prone to vaccine hesitancy and act accordingly. Finally, because the study covered such a long period of time, the authors were able to show that Twitter users' attitudes on vaccinations tend to remain consistent over time.

Khakharia et al. [38], used an open-source dataset comprising of COVID-19 vaccine-related tweets from all over the world and TextBlob to determine the sentiment polarity of each tweet as being positive, zero or negative. Only positive and negative tweets were kept, having their sentiment polarity converted to binary sentiment. The dataset was then pre-processed and divided into 70% training and 30% testing data before being fed into the ML algorithms under consideration, which included Multinomial Naïve Bayes, SVM and Logistic Regression. It was found that the LR classifier achieved the best results with a 97.3% accuracy score, the SVM classifier came in second with an accuracy of 96.26%, and the Multinomial Naïve Bayes classifier came in third with an accuracy of 88%.

3.3 Methodology

After reviewing a wide range of sentiment analysis applications in the existing literature, we decided to study and compare machine learning-based sentiment analysis methods using SVM and LR algorithms, lexicon-based sentiment analysis methods using VADER and a python library, commonly used for sentiment analysis, called TextBlob.

3.3.1 Methodology Outline

Our suggested methodology requires a labeled collection of domain-specific tweets, that are categorized according to the opinion they express. Depending on the sentiment detection approach followed, different additional actions may be needed. In order to determine the sentiment label of a tweet, classifiers must be trained on a dataset containing the numerical feature vector of the given tweet, whereas VADER and TextBlob must calculate the tweet text's compound score and polarity metric, respectively. The objective is to determine and inform the reader about which sentiment detection method performs best and could be used to predict the sentiment of future tweets with unknown polarity.

3.4 Experiments

3.4.1 Dataset

The chosen Twitter dataset is about different COVID-19 vaccines and was obtained from Kaggle.[1] It contains 6000 tweet instances and it is organized into three columns that report the tweet id, the tweet content, and the tweet's sentiment annotation. Based on the dataset's description, tweets with negative sentiment were labeled as "1", tweets with neutral sentiment were labeled as "2", while tweets with positive sentiment were labeled as "3". As a result, we must handle a three-way classification problem with negative, neutral, and positive classes. The negative class includes 420 tweets, the neutral class 3680 tweets and the positive class 1900 tweets. All

---

[1] https://www.kaggle.com/datasciencetool/covid19-vaccine-tweets-with-sentiment-annotation.

the experiments outlined below were carried out using the Python programming language.

3.4.2 Dataset Pre-Processing

Due to the informal nature of the Twitter platform and the length constraint it enforces, tweets are frequently written in informal language including hashtags, emoticons, slangs, abbreviations, username mentions ("@") and URLs [39]. However, the presence of these elements might harm the performance of the sentiment detection model, necessitating a cleaning process.

Following data collection, data pre-processing ensures data quality and prepares it for subsequent processes by retaining only content essential to the study. There are a variety of pre-processing approaches available; however, in our case, we started by eliminating duplicate tweets and extracting the tweet content without any hashtags, URLs, or emoticons. Next, we removed multiple whitespaces as well as special characters, including symbols, accent, and punctuation marks. The remaining words were converted to lowercase. The last step of the cleaning process involves the elimination of stopwords, which are frequently used words that neither affect the polarity of the tweet, nor give extra meaning to the analysis. To accomplish this step, we used the Natural Language Toolkit (NLTK) [40] library's stopwords list, which encompasses 179 such words. We also used preprocessor[2] and neattext[3] Python packages in order to execute the remainder pre-processing steps. The former works well with simple preprocessing, whereas the latter is a textual data cleaning and pre-processing NLP package.

3.4.3 Sentiment Analysis

Once the pre-processing procedure is finished the data can be given as input to any ML algorithm or sentiment analysis tool. As previously stated, we opted for reviewing both supervised and lexicon-based instances of the sentiment analysis task. Thus, the following sub-sections report in detail the development, as well as the performance of TextBlob, VADER, Logistic Regression, Naïve Bayes and SVM. The performance of the aforementioned approaches was evaluated using four frequently used metrics: accuracy, precision, recall, and f-score.

---

[2] https://pypi.org/project/preprocessor/.
[3] https://pypi.org/project/neattext/.

3.4.3.1   Lexicon-Based Sentiment Analysis Tools

TextBlob

TextBlob[4] constitutes one of the most well-known lexicon-based sentiment analysis tools. It is a Python library that supports sentiment analysis in addition to other NLP tasks. This tool performs a sentence-level sentiment analysis and returns the polarity and subjectivity scores for each input text. The polarity can be any float number between -1 and $+1$, with -1 representing negative sentiments and $+1$ representing positive sentiments. On the other hand, subjectivity can be any float number between 0 and 1, with 0 being the most objective and 1 being the most subjective [33, 41]. In our implementation, the input text was labeled as "Positive" when its polarity was more than zero, "Negative" when it was less than zero, and "Neutral" when it was equal to zero.

Vader

VADER (Valence Aware Dictionary and sEntiment Reasoner) [42] is an open-source lexicon and rule-based sentiment analysis tool intended to identify sentiments expressed in social media data. It combines a sentiment lexicon with a collection of lexical features that are commonly labeled as positive or negative based on their semantic orientation. This is because, in addition to reporting negativity and positivity rating, VADER also reports how negative or positive a sentiment is [41].

In order to implement VADER in Python, we used the vaderSentiment[5] package and we initialized a sentiment intensity analyzer. VADER examines each text snippet to determine whether any of its words are in the VADER lexicon. The negative, neutral, positive and compound metrics are then returned, which indicate the sentiment of the given tweet. We extracted the compound score that is said to be the most widely used and useful metric for sentiment analysis [33, 43].

The compound score is the float result of the sum of the valence scores of each word in the lexicon, which have been normalized to be between -1, which signifies the negative extreme, and $+1$, which denotes the positive extreme. The next step was to establish the threshold values for classifying tweets as negative, neutral and positive. More specifically, negative sentiment was defined as having compound scores ≤ -0.05, neutral sentiment as having compound scores between -0.05 and 0.05, and positive sentiment as having compound scores ≥ 0.05. These numbers correspond the typical threshold values used by many other researchers [31, 33, 41].

---

[4] https://pypi.org/project/textblob/0.9.0/.

[5] https://pypi.org/project/vaderSentiment/.

3.4.3.2 Machine Learning-Based Sentiment Analysis

One of the initial steps towards building a classifier is text representation, during which we need to identify a suitable method to transform text data into a numerical feature vector. We implemented the vector space representation model along with the term frequency—inverse document frequency approach (TF-IDF). TF-IDF represents the significance of a word in a document, by assigning its TF and IDF score, where TF determines how frequently the word occurs in a document and IDF indicates how rare the word is across all documents. Python library sklearn offers the TfidfVectorizer[6] to accomplish the feature extraction step.

Prior to applying each algorithm, we used exhaustive grid search to tune its hyperparameters and determine the set that optimizes performance. During the grid search process, a user-specified set of an estimator's parameter values was exhaustively searched.[7] When the best parameter set was identified, and the training data were divided into 70% training and 30% testing data, the estimator could be applied. The next paragraphs provide more detail on each estimator employed for the classification problem, including information about Logistic Regression, Naïve Bayes and SVM.

Logistic Regression

Logistic Regression (LR) accounts for one of the most prominent supervised ML techniques for binary classification, with modifications to support multi-class modeling [44]. It is a simple to implement model that employs a logistic function to predict a binary output variable and delivers excellent performance when the classes are linearly separable [45, 46]. Since supervised sentiment classification involves discrete classes, the aim of LR is to identify the decision boundaries between them [47]. The LR model works as follows, it first assigns weights to each input vector and secondarily predicts which sentiment class each tweet belongs to [48].

Naïve Bayes

Naïve Bayes (NB) falls into the probabilistic classifiers category and is built on top of the Bayes theorem. It assumes that all independent variable features are conditionally independent, which is a concept that ensures the way one variable influences an output has no effect to the way another feature influences the same output [49]. Despite its simple nature and "naïve" assumption, NB classifier has been shown to operate efficiently across a wide range of applications. There exist three basic variations of this algorithm, depending on the attributes' nature, and these are Bernoulli (BNB),

---

[6] https://scikit-learn.org/stable/modules/generated/sklearn.feature_extraction.text.TfidfVectorizer.html.

[7] https://scikit-learn.org/stable/modules/generated/sklearn.model_selection.GridSearchCV.html.

Gaussian (GNB) and Multinomial Naïve Bayes (MNB) [50]. In our framework we implement the last variation (MNB), which is suitable for multinomial models.

Support Vector Machine

Support Vector Machine (SVM) estimator has been widely used in past studies for both regression and classification tasks. The goal of the algorithm is to find a hyperplane that best separates observations belonging to different classes. In order to do so, SVM makes use only of the observations that are on the margin's edges, known as support vectors [51]. One of the advantages of the SVM algorithm is that it allows for the consideration of the linearity issue, introducing kernel functions. Well-known kernels include linear, polynomial and radial basis function [52, 53].

Dealing with Class Imbalance Problem

While exploring the retrieved dataset, we observed a class imbalance problem which may have an impact on the performances of the ML algorithms. This occurs when the observations of one class outnumber those of the rest classes. Figure 3.2 depicts the distribution of the observations in the studied dataset. Working with imbalanced datasets presents a challenge in that most learning algorithms tend to ignore the minority class because they are overwhelmed by the majority class.

Oversampling the minority class is one of the existent methods to deal with imbalanced datasets. The simplest solution involves duplicating examples from the minority class, even though these examples add no new information to the model. Instead, new examples can be synthesized from the existing ones. The Synthetic Minority Over-Sampling TEchnique (SMOTE) is used in our case, to generate these extra samples. For comparison we conducted the same analysis as described above, after applying SMOTE to our training data. In that way we can see how the learning algorithm's performance changed after over-sampling.

3.5 Experimental Results

The results of each sentiment analysis tool and classifier after applying the grid search technique are shown in Tables 3.1 and 3.2.

The accuracy, precision, recall and f-score values of each tool and classifier when applied to the imbalanced dataset are mentioned in Table 3.1. Table 3.2, on the other hand, shows the results of the metrics, for each classifier applied to the balanced dataset provided by SMOTE.

Let us first examine the imbalanced dataset's sentiment analysis results. We implemented both TextBlob and VADER to gain a better understanding of which lexicon-based sentiment analysis tools works best for our Twitter dataset. Comparing the

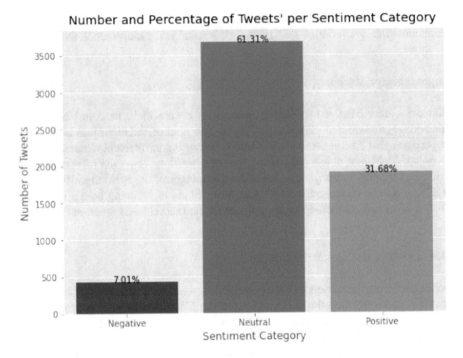

Fig. 3.2 Dataset distribution

Table 3.1 Classification performance analysis table (imbalanced dataset)

	Accuracy	Precision	Recall	F-score
TextBlob	0.479900	0.562000	0.479900	0.495800
VADER	0.476500	0.589100	0.476500	0.493800
Logistic regression	0.710234	0.694204	0.710234	0.673167
Naïve Bayes	0.698554	0.658705	0.698554	0.645336
SVM	0.711902	0.706722	0.711902	0.682989

Table 3.2 Classification performance analysis table (balanced dataset)

	Accuracy	Precision	Recall	F-score
Logistic regression	0.689099	0.695590	0.689099	0.692046
Naïve Bayes	0.615684	0.699108	0.615684	0.640510
SVM	0.690211	0.682389	0.690211	0.685498

results reported in the first two rows of Table 3.1, we find a similar performance between the tools which have nearly identical values for their performance metrics.

TextBlob, however, with an accuracy of 0.4799, outperformed VADER, which had an accuracy of 0.4765.

Moving on to the results of the machine learning-based component of our sentiment analysis framework, we find that LR had an accuracy score of 0.710234, Naïve Bayes had a score of 0.698554, and SVM had a score of 0.711902. As we can see the accuracy values, as well as the precision, recall and f-score values are very close to one another. SVM is the best performing classifier, closely followed by Logistic Regression, whereas Naïve Bayes is the worst performing classifier.

According to the results presented above, machine learning-based sentiment analysis achieved a greater performance than that of lexicon-based sentiment analysis. The SVM model, in particular, outperformed all other tools and classifiers tested, which is consistent with the literature findings discussed in Sect. 3.2. The superior performance of SVM model is also evident in Fig. 3.3, which shows the performance metric values for each sentiment analysis method examined.

After we employed SMOTE to deal with the imbalanced dataset, the results of the three ML algorithms slightly deteriorated. The accuracy of the LR algorithm has dropped to 0.689099, the accuracy of the Naïve Bayes algorithm has dropped to 0.615684, and the accuracy of the SVM has dropped to 0.690211. We observe that the accuracy score of the Naïve Bayes classifier decreased the most, remaining the worst performing classifier, whereas the SVM classifier continues to outperform the others even after its score decreased. Figure 3.4 illustrates the change in metrics values of each classifier, after being applied to the balanced dataset provided by SMOTE.

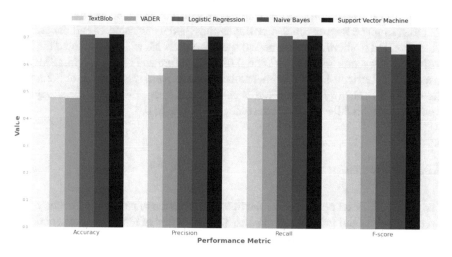

Fig. 3.3 Performance metrics comparison of different sentiment analysis methods

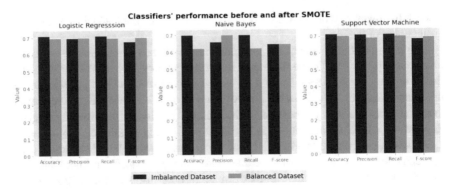

Fig. 3.4 Comparison of the performance metrics values of each classifier before and after applying SMOTE to the dataset

3.6 Conclusion

This chapter offers a detailed description of the two main sentiment detection techniques, known as lexicon-based and machine learning-based analyses. Following an extensive examination of both, a literature survey was conducted with a purpose to showcase some of the most recent studies where sentiment analysis has been used to detect public sentiments related to vaccines.

A Twitter vaccine-related dataset was retrieved and used by sentiment analysis methods to validate if the proposed framework can yield valuable insights. TextBlob, VADER, Logistic Regression, Naïve Bayes and SVM were tested. Significant results were obtained from ML algorithms and specifically SVM, which performed the best, with accuracy scores of 0.711902 and 0.690211 before and after applying SMOTE, respectively. Lexicon-based sentiment analysis tools were less accurate at predicting the sentiment category of the given tweets. Specifically, TextBlob's accuracy was equal to 0.4799, while VADER's accuracy was equal to 0.4765.

3.6.1 Discussion

The most significant challenge is related to the selection of a dataset with subjective tweets' labeling and imbalanced classes. The procedure of identifying the sentiment label of each tweet is subjective because subtly expressed opinions may be interpreted in different ways. Consequently, a model may fail to correctly classify tweets with sarcasm, irony and negation. Moreover, imbalanced datasets need to be cautiously addressed, since they can easily result in inaccurate findings.

The main objective of this study was to investigate different sentiment detection approaches experimentally and find the one that provides a sentiment analysis model capable of classifying Twitter messages about COVID-19 vaccines as accurately as possible. ML and lexicon-based techniques were evaluated, with accuracy scores ranging from 47.65% to 71.19%. The proposed framework involves a three-class classification scheme, that labels tweets as positive, negative or neutral, as well as four performance metrics for evaluating classification performance.

During the implementation of our strategy, we encountered a class imbalance problem in which the neutral class accounted for 61% of the total tweets in the dataset, the positive class for 32%, and the negative for only 7%. We used SMOTE to perform over-sampling and generate additional samples, because an imbalanced dataset, if not handled properly, could result in classifiers that ignore and perform poorly on the minority class, in our case the negative sentiment class.

Previous research on social media prediction analysis found that after a disease outbreak, the number of vaccine-related terms in social media posts increased [54]. Nowadays, the Twitter platform used in this study, as well as social media platforms in general, have become a common source of vaccine-related information and disinformation. Our effort aims to emphasize the importance of mining such readily available public attitudes, in order to forecast opinions and reactions related to vaccine uptake in near real-time. Such insights could be critical in dealing with health emergency situations like the ongoing coronavirus pandemic.

3.6.2 Overview of Contribution

In this chapter, we investigated the issue of inferring insights into COVID-19 vaccines public perceptions using sentiment analysis techniques. We first discussed sentiment analysis background, and processes and then we reviewed sentiment detection approaches including ML and lexicon-based analyses. Furthermore, we identified and examined the most widely employed ML algorithms and sentiment analysis tools, such as Logistic Regression, Naïve Bayes, SVM, TextBlob, and VADER. The significance of sentiment analysis in vaccine research, for vaccines such as Mumps-Measles-Rubella (MMR), HPV, and COVID-19, was also emphasized. We can therefore safely conclude that sentiment analysis has been widely used in the field of healthcare, demonstrating the power of such automatic techniques in extracting meaningful sentiments values from data and preventing negative reactions to vaccination campaigns, as well as refusal to vaccination.

Moreover, we applied various sentiment analysis methods on a real dataset in order to examine which were more efficient. Supervised and lexicon-based sentiment detection analyses were performed on the COVID-19 vaccination Twitter dataset with the help of Python Programming language.

3.6.3 Future Directions

Several aspects of our analysis require further exploration. To begin, a larger and more balanced dataset of annotated COVID-19 vaccine-related tweets can be studied in order to improve results. Furthermore, more COVID-19 vaccine-related datasets from different social media platforms can be integrated to gain a more complete overview of public attitudes toward vaccines.

Future research directions could include the development of better performing sentiment classification models through the examination and comparison of more models. In addition, it would be more interesting to apply the proposed sentiment analysis models to new tweets and monitor how public sentiment about vaccines changes over time. This could be accomplished by extracting a Twitter dataset based on specific vaccine-related keywords. It would also be informative if we could relate social events to each sharp increase or decrease in sentiment. As a result, scientists and health professionals will be able to better detect concerning trends in public COVID-19 vaccination awareness during the pandemic.

Acknowledgements We would like to thank the anonymous reviewers for their feedback which helped in improving this chapter.

References

1. Who.int.: Timeline: WHO's COVID-19 response. Available https://www.who.int/emergencies/diseases/novel-coronavirus-2019/interactive-timeline#event-72. Accessed: 07 Feb 2022
2. Covid19.who.int: WHO coronavirus (COVID-19) dashboard. Available https://covid19.who.int/. Accessed 07 Feb 2022
3. Worldometers.info: COVID live—Coronavirus statistics—Worldometer. Available https://www.worldometers.info/coronavirus/#countries. Accessed 07 Feb 2022
4. Roozenbeek, J., et al.: Susceptibility to misinformation about COVID-19 around the world. Roy. Soc. Open Sci. 7(10) (2020). https://doi.org/10.1098/rsos.201199
5. Petersen, E., et al.: Emergence of new SARS-CoV-2 variant of concern omicron (B.1.1.529)—Highlights Africa's research capabilities, but exposes major knowledge gaps, inequities of vaccine distribution, inadequacies in global COVID-19 response and control efforts. Int. J. Infect. Diseases **114**, 268–272 (2022). https://doi.org/10.1016/j.ijid.2021.11.040
6. Koukaras, P., Tjortjis, C.: Social media analytics, types and methodology. pp. 401–427 (2019). https://doi.org/10.1007/978-3-030-15628-2_12
7. Ni, M.Y., et al.: Mental health, risk factors, and social media use during the COVID-19 epidemic and cordon sanitaire among the community and health professionals in Wuhan, China: cross-sectional survey. JMIR Mental Health 7(5), (2020). https://doi.org/10.2196/19009
8. Merchant, R.M., Lurie, N.: Social media and emergency preparedness in response to novel coronavirus. JAMA **323**(20) (2020). https://doi.org/10.1001/jama.2020.4469
9. Mystakidis, A. et al.: Predicting covid-19 ICU needs using deep learning, XGBoost and random forest regression with the sliding window technique. Available https://smartcities.ieee.org/newsletter/july-2021/predicting-covid-19-icu-needs-using-deep-learning-xgboost-and-random-forest-regression-with-the-sliding-window-technique. Accessed 16 Feb 2022

10. Shofiya, C., Abidi, S.: Sentiment analysis on COVID-19-related social distancing in Canada using twitter data. Int. J. Environ. Res. Public Health **18**(11) (2021). https://doi.org/10.3390/ijerph18115993

11. Sanders, A.C., et al.: Unmasking the conversation on masks: natural language processing for topical sentiment analysis of COVID-19 Twitter discourse. medRxiv (2021). https://doi.org/10.1101/2020.08.28.20183863

12. Melton, C.A., et al.: Public sentiment analysis and topic modeling regarding COVID-19 vaccines on the Reddit social media platform: a call to action for strengthening vaccine confidence. J. Infect. Public Health **14**(10), 1505–1512 (2021). https://doi.org/10.1016/J.JIPH.2021.08.010

13. Alamoodi, A.H., et al.: Sentiment analysis and its applications in fighting COVID-19 and infectious diseases: a systematic review. Expert Syst. Appl. **167** (2021). https://doi.org/10.1016/j.eswa.2020.114155

14. Koukaras, P., et al.: Introducing a novel bi-functional method for exploiting sentiment in complex information networks. Int. J. Metadata Semant. Ontol. Indersci. (2022) (in press)

15. Cambria, E., et al.: New avenues in opinion mining and sentiment analysis. IEEE Intell. Syst. **28**(2), 15–21 (2013). https://doi.org/10.1109/MIS.2013.30

16. Medhat, W., et al.: Sentiment analysis algorithms and applications: a survey. Ain Shams Eng. J. **5**(4), 1093–1113 (2014). https://doi.org/10.1016/j.asej.2014.04.011

17. Liu, B.: Sentiment Analysis and Opinion Mining, vol. 5 (2012). https://doi.org/10.2200/S00416ED1V01Y201204HLT016

18. Chatzakou, D., Vakali, A.: Harvesting opinions and emotions from social media textual resources. IEEE Internet Comput. **19**(4), 46–50 (2015). https://doi.org/10.1109/MIC.2015.28

19. Feldman, R.: Techniques and applications for sentiment analysis. Commun. ACM **56**(4), 82–89 (2013). https://doi.org/10.1145/2436256.2436274

20. Wang, X., et al.: Public opinions towards COVID-19 in California and New York on twitter. medRxiv 2020.07.12.20151936 (2020). https://doi.org/10.1101/2020.07.12.20151936

21. Nousi, C., et al.: Mining data to deal with epidemics: case studies to demonstrate real world AI applications. Intell. Syst. Refer. Library **211**, 287–312 (2022). https://doi.org/10.1007/978-3-030-79161-2_12

22. Du, J., et al.: Optimization on machine learning based approaches for sentiment analysis on HPV vaccines related tweets. J. Biomed. Semant. **8**(1) (2017). https://doi.org/10.1186/s13326-017-0120-6

23. Du, J., et al.: Leveraging machine learning-based approaches to assess human papillomavirus vaccination sentiment trends with Twitter data. BMC Med. Inform. Decis. Mak. **17** (2017). https://doi.org/10.1186/s12911-017-0469-6

24. Yuan, X., Crooks, A.T.: Examining online vaccination discussion and communities in Twitter. In: ACM International Conference Proceeding Series, July 2018, pp. 197–206. https://doi.org/10.1145/3217804.3217912

25. Kunneman, F., et al.: Monitoring stance towards vaccination in twitter messages. BMC Med. Inform. Decis. Mak. **20**(1) (2020). https://doi.org/10.1186/s12911-020-1046-y

26. D'Andrea, E., et al.: Monitoring the public opinion about the vaccination topic from tweets analysis. Expert Syst. Appl. **116**, 209–226 (2019). https://doi.org/10.1016/j.eswa.2018.09.009

27. Cotfas, L.A., et al.: The longest month: analyzing COVID-19 vaccination opinions dynamics from tweets in the month following the first vaccine announcement. IEEE Access **9**, 33203–33223 (2021). https://doi.org/10.1109/ACCESS.2021.3059821

28. Villavicencio, C., et al.: Twitter sentiment analysis towards COVID-19 vaccines in the Philippines using Naïve Bayes (2021). https://doi.org/10.3390/info12050204

29. Kwok, S.W.H., et al.: Tweet topics and sentiments relating to COVID-19 vaccination among Australian twitter users: machine learning analysis. J. Med. Internet Res. **23**(5) (2021). https://doi.org/10.2196/26953

30. Raghupathi, V., et al.: Studying public perception about vaccination: a sentiment analysis of tweets. Int J. Environ. Res. Public Health **17**(10) (2020). https://doi.org/10.3390/ijerph17103464

31. Hung, M., et al.: Social network analysis of COVID-19 sentiments: application of artificial intelligence. J. Med. Internet Res. **22**(8), e22590 (2020). https://doi.org/10.2196/22590
32. Bhagat, K.K., et al.: Public opinions about online learning during COVID-19: a sentiment analysis approach. Sustainability **13**(6) (2021). https://doi.org/10.3390/su13063346
33. Sattar, N.S., Arifuzzaman, S.: Covid-19 vaccination awareness and aftermath: public sentiment analysis on twitter data and vaccinated population prediction in the USA. Appl. Sci. (Switzerland) **11**(13) (2021). https://doi.org/10.3390/app11136128
34. Hu, T., et al.: Revealing public opinion towards COVID-19 vaccines with Twitter data in the United States: spatiotemporal perspective. J. Med. Internet Res. **23**(9) (2021). https://doi.org/10.2196/30854
35. Yousefinaghani, S., et al.: An analysis of COVID-19 vaccine sentiments and opinions on Twitter. Int. J. Infect. Diseases **108**, 256–262 (2021). https://doi.org/10.1016/j.ijid.2021.05.059
36. Marcec, R., Likic, R.: Using Twitter for sentiment analysis towards AstraZeneca/Oxford, Pfizer/BioNTech and Moderna COVID-19 vaccines. Postgrad. Med. J. (2021). https://doi.org/10.1136/postgradmedj-2021-140685
37. Piedrahita-Valdés, H., et al.: Vaccine hesitancy on social media: sentiment analysis from June 2011 to April 2019. Vaccines **9**(1), 1–12 (2021). https://doi.org/10.3390/vaccines9010028
38. Khakharia, A., et al.: Sentiment analysis of COVID-19 vaccine tweets using machine learning. SSRN Electron. J. (2021). https://doi.org/10.2139/ssrn.3869531
39. Carter, S., et al.: Microblog language identification: overcoming the limitations of short, unedited and idiomatic text. Lang. Resour. Eval. **47**(1), 195–215 (2013). https://doi.org/10.1007/s10579-012-9195-y
40. Bird, S., et al.: Natural Language Processing with Python. O'Reilly, Beijing (2009)
41. Bonta, V., et al.: A comprehensive study on lexicon based approaches for sentiment analysis. Asian J. Comput. Sci. Technol. **8**(S2), 1–6 (2019). https://doi.org/10.51983/ajcst-2019.8.s2.2037
42. Hutto, C.J., Gilbert, E.: VADER: a parsimonious rule-based model for sentiment analysis of social media text. Available http://sentic.net/ (2014)
43. Elbagir, S., Yang, J.: Twitter sentiment analysis using natural language toolkit and VADER sentiment. In: Lecture Notes in Engineering and Computer Science: Proceedings of the International Multi Conference of Engineers and Computer Scientists, vol. 122, pp. 12–16, Mar. 2019
44. Bartosik, A., Whittingham, H.: Evaluating safety and toxicity. In: The Era of Artificial Intelligence, Machine Learning, and Data Science in the Pharmaceutical Industry, pp. 119–137, Jan. 2021, doi: https://doi.org/10.1016/B978-0-12-820045-2.00008-8.
45. Subasi, A.: Machine learning techniques. In: Practical Machine Learning for Data Analysis Using Python, Elsevier, pp. 91–202 (2020). https://doi.org/10.1016/B978-0-12-821379-7.00003-5
46. Belyadi, H., Haghighat, A.: Supervised learning. In: Machine Learning Guide for Oil and Gas Using Python. pp. 169–295. Elsevier (2021). https://doi.org/10.1016/B978-0-12-821929-4.00004-4
47. Gudivada, V.N., et al.: Cognitive analytics: going beyond big data analytics and machine learning. In: Handbook of Statistics, vol. 35, pp. 169–205 (2016). https://doi.org/10.1016/BS.HOST.2016.07.010
48. Prabhat, A., Khullar, V.: Sentiment classification on big data using Naïve bayes and logistic regression. In: 2017 International Conference on Computer Communication and Informatics, ICCCI 2017, Nov. 2017. https://doi.org/10.1109/ICCCI.2017.8117734
49. Rice, D.M.: Causal reasoning. Calculus of Thought, pp. 95–123 (2014). https://doi.org/10.1016/B978-0-12-410407-5.00004-0
50. Yeturu, K.: Machine learning algorithms, applications, and practices in data science. In: Handbook of Statistics, vol. 43, pp. 81–206 (2020). https://doi.org/10.1016/BS.HOST.2020.01.002
51. Xia, Y.: Correlation and association analyses in microbiome study integrating multiomics in health and disease. Prog. Mol. Biol. Transl. Sci. **171**, 309–491 (2020). https://doi.org/10.1016/BS.PMBTS.2020.04.003

52. Al-Amrani, Y., et al., Sentiment analysis using supervised classification algorithms. In: Proceedings of the 2nd International Conference on Big Data, Cloud and Applications, vol. 17, pp. 1–8, Mar. 2017. https://doi.org/10.1145/3090354.3090417
53. Malek, S., et al.: Ecosystem monitoring through predictive modeling. In: Encyclopedia of Bioinformatics and Computational Biology: ABC of Bioinformatics, vols. 1–3, pp. 1–8 (2019). https://doi.org/10.1016/B978-0-12-809633-8.20060-5
54. Rousidis, D., et al.: Social media prediction: a literature review. Multimedia Tools Appl. **79**(9–10), 6279–6311 (2020). https://doi.org/10.1007/S11042-019-08291-9

Chapter 4
Healthcare Support Using Data Mining: A Case Study on Stroke Prediction

Georgios Michailidis, Michail Vlachos-Giovanopoulos, Paraskevas Koukaras⬤, and Christos Tjortjis⬤

Abstract Data and information have become a valuable asset for small and big organizations in the past few decades. Data is the main ingredient for strategic decision-making, which could give businesses a significant advantage over their competitors, by providing customized services or overall experience to their customers and attracting new ones. For this purpose, data mining techniques are being utilized so that valuable information can be discovered and exploited. There is a vast amount of data generated in the field of healthcare that is not getting fully exploited by traditional methods, for reasons, such as their complexity, velocity, and volume. Therefore, there is a demand for the development of powerful automated data mining tools for the complete utilization of these data, and the uncovering of patterns and precious knowledge about patients, medical claims, treatment costs, hospitals, etc. This work focuses on exploiting the best-known data mining techniques: classification, clustering, and association rule mining, which are utilized extensively in the healthcare industry for incident prediction and general medical knowledge acquisition. The data mining process comprises several steps, such as data selection, pre-processing, transformation, interpretation, and evaluation. The section of the experimentation includes a stroke incidents dataset fetched from the Kaggle dataset provider. This chapter also provides a literature survey on data mining applications in the healthcare sector, while discussing the abovementioned machine learning concepts.

G. Michailidis · M. Vlachos-Giovanopoulos · P. Koukaras · C. Tjortjis (✉)
The Data Mining and Analytics Research Group, School of Science and Technology, International Hellenic University, 570 01 Thermi, Greece
e-mail: c.tjortjis@ihu.edu.gr

G. Michailidis
e-mail: gmichailidis@ihu.edu.gr

M. Vlachos-Giovanopoulos
e-mail: mvlachos@ihu.edu.gr

P. Koukaras
e-mail: p.koukaras@ihu.edu.gr

© The Author(s), under exclusive license to Springer Nature Switzerland AG 2023
C. P. Lim et al. (eds.), *Artificial Intelligence and Machine Learning for Healthcare*,
Intelligent Systems Reference Library 229,
https://doi.org/10.1007/978-3-031-11170-9_4

Keywords Data mining · Healthcare support · Machine learning · Stroke prediction

Term Definition Table

Term	Definition
Bmi	Body Mass Index
CRISP-DM	Cross-Industry Standard Process for Data Mining
CRM	Customer Relationship Management
Data mining algorithm	A set of heuristics and calculations that creates a model from data
DBSCAN	Density-Based Spatial Clustering of Applications with Noise
Feature	An independent variable that can be used as input of a machine learning model
FP-Growth	Frequent Pattern Growth
GDPR	General Data Protection Regulation
LEADERS	Lightweight Epidemiological Advanced Detection Emergency Response System
Machine learning model	An expression of an algorithm that processes data to explore patterns or make predictions
OLAP	Online Analytical Processing
Operator	In RapidMiner, a group of functions that perform actions on input data through parameters and outputs the results of said actions
Parameter	A special kind of variable used in an algorithm to refer to one of the pieces of data provided as input to it
Process	In RapidMiner, it is a set of sequentially connected operators represented by a flow design, where each operator provides its output as input to the next one
ROC	Receiver Operating Characteristic
SEMMA	Sample, explore, modify, model, assess
SVM	Support Vector Machine

4.1   Introduction

Over the last few decades, data analysis has become a vital tool for both small and large enterprises. Any business with a presence on the various types of social media platforms [1] and the web is collecting a vast amount of data about customers, user behavior, web traffic, demographics and more. The trajectory, as well as the success of any organization in the market, depends highly on the appropriate exploitation of these data. In other words, data is the main component for the strategic decision-making process, which could give the business a significant lead against their competitors by providing customized services or overall experience to their customers and attracting new ones [2].

The process of exploring and analyzing, by automatic or semi-automatic means, large quantities of data to summarize them into valuable information and discover meaningful patterns and extract useful knowledge, is called "data mining" (a.k.a. knowledge discovery) [2]. Consequently, data mining comprises functional elements that transform data stored into a data warehouse, manage them in a multidimensional database, make data access easier to experts, analyze data using tools and techniques, and present them in a way that valuable information can be discovered [2, 3].

4.1.1   Data Mining

The entire concept of data mining has been developed in the 90's and emerged as a powerful tool that is capable of discovering previously unknown patterns and valuable information from massive datasets comprised of thousands of records [3–6]. Previous studies mentioned that data mining approaches enable data owners to analyze and find unexpected connections in their data, which turn out to be supportive for decision making [7]. The data mining process is split into two parts, Data Preprocessing and Data Mining. During the data preprocessing phase, different algorithms and processes perform data cleaning, integration, reduction, and transformation. On the other hand, data mining phase involves pattern mining, evaluation, and knowledge representation, as shown in Fig. 4.1.

Skills and knowledge are necessary ingredients for implementing data mining since the performance depends on the person who is performing the procedure due to non-appearance of a basic structure. The Cross-Industry Standard Process for Data Mining (CRISP-DM) suggests a principle for data mining tasks, and splits them into six stages: business understanding, data understanding and preparation, modeling, evaluation, and deployment [8]. The first stage is rather crucial because it recognizes the business objectives and, therefore, the success standards of mining tasks. Data is unquestionably an essential component since it is the raw material. Without data we cannot mine information. Thus, according to CRISP-DM, data understanding and preparation are considered as prerequisites for modeling. Subsequently, modeling is the definite data analysis.

Most data mining operating systems contain Online Analytical Processing (OLAP). That is, non-traditional statistical analysis, like neural networks, decision trees, link and association analysis, and traditional statistical methods, like clustering, discriminant and regression analysis. This wide range of techniques is expected, given that data mining has been considered a descendant of three different disciplines, specifically computer science (also counting machine learning and artificial intelligence), statistics and database management. The evaluation phase allows models

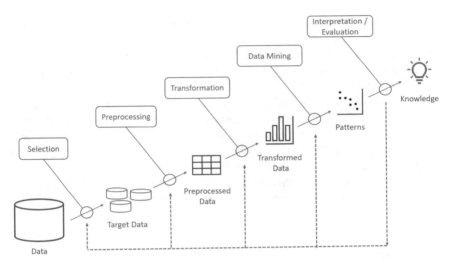

Fig. 4.1 Stages of data mining

and results to be compared based on a common criterion, such as lift charts, profit charts, or diagnostic classification charts. Finally, deployment is where data mining pays off. It has to do with the implementation and utilization of the models [4].

Data mining can be considered as a process, rather than a set of tools, and there is a methodology that illustrates this process. The SEMMA (Sample, Explore, Modify, Model, Assess) method splits data mining into five phases: (i) sample, to design a statistically representative sample of the data, (ii) explore, to apply exploratory, statistical and visualization techniques, (iii) modify, to select, create and transform the most important predictive variables, (iv) model, to model the variables to perform predictions, and (v) assess, to validate the model's accuracy. SEMMA is an iterative method. The internal stages can be performed repetitively based on the needs. Figure 4.2 illustrates the five stages of the SEMMA methodology [9].

4.1.2 Data Mining in Healthcare

Data mining applications are becoming more and more essential in healthcare [10, 11]. Various reasons have stimulated the use of data mining applications in healthcare. The enormous amounts of data generated by the healthcare industry are being under-utilized by using traditional methods due to the complexity, velocity, and volume of them. So, there is a need for developing powerful automated data mining tools for appropriate exploitation of these data, since they hide valuable information about patients, medical claims, treatment costs, hospitals, etc. [8].

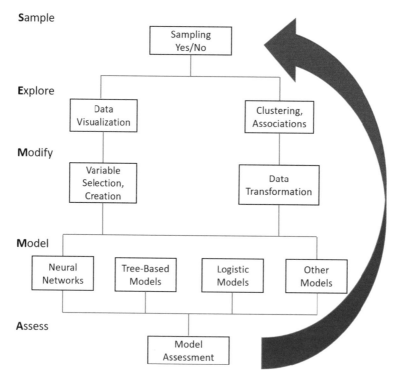

Fig. 4.2 SEMMA methodology

4.1.3 Applications of Data Mining in Healthcare

Various reasons have led to using knowledge discovery techniques in the healthcare sector. Data mining can upgrade decision-making by uncovering patterns and trends in huge amounts of complicated data. Financial burden has intensified the need for healthcare organizations to guide their management according to the analysis of clinical and financial data. Wisdom gain from knowledge discovery processes can motivate more sufficient and cost-effective operation and high-quality services.

Healthcare organizations adopting data mining techniques benefit and are better qualified for meeting future requirements. Another reason stimulating the utilization of data mining approaches in healthcare is the appreciation that they can produce knowledge that is supportive to every part of the healthcare system. For instance, data mining techniques can assist healthcare insurers to identify fraud and abuse. Medical centers, physicians and patients can benefit by finding better practices and treatments [4].

Such applications can be grouped as evaluation of treatment effectiveness, health-care management, fraud, and abuse detection in health insurance, causes of diseases detection, and more [4]. The analysis of health data upgrades the healthcare system by boosting the effectiveness of tasks that have to do with the management of the patients. Data mining techniques aim to support healthcare organizations on grouping patients with common health issues, so that they receive the appropriate treatment. They can also be used for predictions, such as predicting the length of hospitalization, predicting diagnosis, etc. Data mining technologies also provide benefits by analyzing various characteristics that cause a disease, like lifestyle, food, education, working environment etc. [8].

4.1.4   Chapter Overview

The following section, reviewing the literature, showcases various applications of data mining techniques in healthcare sector, as well as utilizes some of the most notable data mining methodologies. Such applications could be healthcare management, fraud and abuse detection, and treatment effectiveness, which are going to upgrade the overall healthcare quality. Moreover, machine learning concepts that are related with healthcare support are also discussed. With concepts like classification, regression, clustering and association rule mining, valuable predictions can be performed, such as to predict if a patient is likely to suffer from a particular disease.

Typically, various preparatory actions must be completed before reaching the stage where algorithms may be applied. First, data selection needs to be applied, in order to keep only the most relevant content. The steps that follow are data cleaning, integration, reduction, and transformation, which remove duplicate observations, outliers, noise, and deal with missing values, and data sampling to avoid overfitting. The next step is data mining, where the preprocessed data are fed into classification, regression, clustering, and association rule mining algorithms. It is a trial-and-error process, as there is no rule to choose the best algorithm for each data mining case. Finally, after running the data mining algorithms, some results are produced. From these results, the interpretation and evaluation step arise, when new useful knowledge is attained.

4.2   Literature Review

This section contains a description of several data mining applications in the healthcare sector, as well as machine learning concepts related with healthcare support. As already mentioned, information gained by utilizing data mining methodologies upgrade the overall healthcare quality, from both patient's and healthcare management's perspectives. In this chapter, the most noteworthy applications and machine learning concepts are reviewed.

4.2.1 Data Mining Applications in Healthcare

4.2.1.1 Healthcare Management

Data mining approaches can be used to detect and track the chronic disease states and high-risk patients, and make good use of hospital resources, which is an important task in healthcare [4, 8]. The main goal is to identify patients who need additional care, enhanced health quality, and cost-effective services. Other factors, such as physical condition and demographic details of patients, play a significant role in the appropriate utilization of the available hospital resources. These resources, both physical and human ones, are managed through an automated data mining procedure.

For instance, Group Health Cooperative, through data mining approaches, offer several cost-effective healthcare services. A non-profit organization enables patients to access their medical information through an online platform, where they can also fill the prescription form and securely communicate with the healthcare providers. Seton Medical Centre used knowledge discovery techniques to make information on the patient's health available, decrease admitted duration of patients in the medical centers, and thus improve healthcare quality. Blue Cross, through data mining, constructed a model which contributes to high-performance and cost-conscious management of diseases. With the help of data mining, Sierra Health Centre instructs appropriate management of the treatment and its cost and recognizes the prospects of upgrading health quality [8].

Data mining approaches can also be used to process big amounts of data and detect patterns related to bioterrorist attacks. For instance, the Lightweight Epidemiological Advanced Detection Emergency Response System (LEADERS) used knowledge discovery methods to reveal various epidemics [4].

4.2.1.2 Customer Relationship Management (CRM)

CRM is a central approach in managing interactions between commercial organizations and their customers, also in healthcare. When talking about customer interactions, we refer to interactions through call centers, billing departments, physicians' offices, inpatient settings, and ambulatory care settings [4]. Data mining can be used to identify preferences, usage patterns and current needs of individuals, to improve the relation with them [4, 8]. These approaches can also be used to predict future needs of individuals, and other products that a patient may purchase, whether a patient is likely to comply with prescribed treatment or whether preventive care is likely to decrease future use.

Customer Potential Management Corp. has established a Consumer Healthcare Utilization Index signifying how likely it is for a person to make use of healthcare services, defined by 25 major diagnostic categories, selected diagnostic related groups or medical service areas. With the help of healthcare transactions of millions of patients, this index can recognize the ones who can derive advantage from health-care services, support the ones who most need access to specific care, and constantly improve the means used to reach groups of people for enhanced health and long-term patient relationships. OSF Saint Joseph Medical Centre has used the index to deliver the appropriate messages and services to the appropriate patients at the right time. The outcome of this action were more efficient communications and higher earnings [4].

It was also suggested that knowledge discovery of patient survey data can define logical expectations about waiting times and uncover information about the kind of services patients anticipate from the providers, and how to improve these services [4].

On the other hand, pharmaceutical companies can derive advantage from health-care CRM and data mining, since by keeping track of physicians prescribing drugs along with the reason, they are able to recommend the most efficient and effective treatment plans, match physicians to specific groups of patients, and track the trajectory of an epidemic to better handle the situation. Moreover, such companies can also benefit from analyzing big amounts of genomic data to detect a link between a patient's genetic makeup and their response to a drug therapy [4].

4.2.1.3 Fraud and Abuse Detection

Healthcare insurers can use data mining to identify illegitimate prescriptions or referrals, fraudulent insurance and abnormal or fake patterns in medical claims by laboratories, clinics, physicians, or patients [8]. Many incidents were recorded when health insurance companies used these techniques and reported millions of dollars of annual savings. For instance, Texas Medicaid Fraud and Abuse Detection System which detected 1400 cases and saved $2.2 million in 1998, Australian Health Insurance Commission saved millions of dollars in 1997, and ReliaStar Financial Corp. has reported a 20% increase in annual savings [4].

4.2.1.4 Treatment Effectiveness

Data mining techniques may be used to compare causes, symptoms, and treatment plans to assess the efficacy of medical therapies [4, 12]. Physicians and patients are given the ability to analyze different treatments and their effectiveness to decide which technique is a better and cheaper choice [8]. For instance, the results of different groups of patients who received different medicines for the same health issue can be compared to decide which medicines perform better and are of lower cost. United HealthCare has analyzed its treatment data to find out how to offer more efficient medicine. It also created clinical profiles through which physicians can gain knowledge and compare their practice patterns with those of other physicians. Consequently, knowledge discovery techniques can uncover information about the appropriate therapy for particular diseases [4].

4.2.1.5   Improved Patient Care

Huge amounts of data are collected in the form of electronic health records. Digitized data regarding patients contribute to the enhancement of the healthcare system's quality. Using data mining, a predictive model was created in order to process and analyze these data and discover valuable information that lead to making appropriate decisions regarding the upgrade of the healthcare quality. Healthcare providers are able, through knowledge discovery processes, to recognize not only present, but also future needs and preferences of patients and offer more qualitative services. Data mining techniques can also equip patients with knowledge they need to have about diseases and their prevention, and they can also group patients with common features [8].

4.2.1.6   Hospital Infection Control

Data mining can be used to analyze and detect previously unknown or abnormal patterns in infection control data. Then, through association rules, unforeseen and useful information can be mined from the public surveillance and hospital control data. Finally, experts analyze this information and propose actions to control the infection in the hospitals [8].

4.2.1.7   Hospital Ranking

Through various data mining tools, several hospital details are examined and analyzed, in order to define their ranks. The ranking system considers the ability of taking care of high-risk patients. Higher ranked medical centers deal with high-risk patients on top priority. On the contrary, lower ranked hospitals are not able to handle such situations [8]. In addition, risk factors need to be considered from the healthcare providers' side when reporting information. This means that a hospital's rank will be lower because they reported a greater difference between predicted and actual death rate, no matter if their success rates are equal to those of other healthcare providers. So, it is important that the reports contain consistent and reliable information [9].

4.2.2 Machine Learning Concepts Related with Healthcare Support

4.2.2.1 Classification

Classification is one of the most popular techniques of data mining in healthcare. It splits data samples into training and test sets and predicts the target class of each observation. One good example of classification in the healthcare sector is the association of a risk factor to patients after analyzing their disease patterns. Classification belongs to the supervised learning methods (there are also semi-supervised approaches such as [13]), which means that the class categories are known.

According to the number of classes, it is characterized as binary classification, for two possible classes, such as "high" or "low" risk patient, and multiclass classification, for more than two possible classes, such as "high", "medium" and "low" risk patient. The initial dataset gets split into training and test dataset. The algorithm uses the training set and tries to explore the relationship between the attributes in the training set to predict the result. Then, the algorithm utilizes the test set, where the class attribute is not known yet, contrary to the training set. By analyzing the input, the algorithm performs the prediction. Finally, as for the evaluation of the performance, with the help of the accuracy is it defined how "good" predictions the algorithm achieved [14].

Some of the most popular classification algorithms are K-Nearest Neighbors, Decision Tree, Support Vector Machine (SVM), Neural Network, and Bayesian Methods [14, 15].

Das et al. tried to diagnose heart diseases with the help of data mining. For this purpose, they mainly used a neural networks ensemble model, which achieved almost 90% accuracy by utilizing data from Cleveland heart disease database. So, they managed to create an intelligent medical decision support system to help healthcare assistants [16].

Curiac et al. conducted an experiment analyzing psychiatric patient data to examine the most important factors and their correlations with some diseases. They used the Bayesian Networks technique and they found that it is a very useful tool which can be used to support physicians in the process of prediction and diagnosis of psychiatric diseases [17].

4.2.2.2 Regression

Regression is another popular method of knowledge discovery, which is used to discover the significant variables in terms of correlation [8, 14]. It is a mathematical model which, similarly to classification, uses the training set to be constructed. There are two types of variables that are used in statistical modeling, that are called dependent (usually represented using "Y") and independent (usually represented using "X") variables respectively. Every model can have one or more independent variables, while the dependent variable is only one.

According to the number of independent variables, regression can be characterized as Linear or Non-linear. Linear regression refers to explaining the relation between a dependent variable and one or more independent ones and works only with numerical data. When the data are of categorical type, logistic regression can be used, which is a type of non-linear regression, and is divided into Binomial and Multinomial types. Binomial regression's role is to predict the outcome for a dependent variable when there are two possible outcomes, while multinomial deals with three or more possible outcomes [14]. Other common regression methods are Support Vector Regression, Decision Tree Regression, and Multilayer Perceptron [14].

Tomar and Agarwal analyzed real time body information through sensors and predicted the activity to provide continuous monitoring and better healthcare services. Based on their experiment, they proved that Least Square Support Vector Regression achieved more accurate results than other Support Vector Regression techniques examined [18].

Alapont et al. presented a research project related to hospital management, where they examined various machine learning techniques, such as Linear Regression, Least Med Squared Linear Regression, SVM for Regression, Multilayer Perceptron, K Star, Locally Weighted Learning, Tree Decision Stump, Tree M5P, and IBK. After executing the algorithms, they found that Linear Regression and Tree M5P produced the best results in terms of hospital management, such as human and physical resources, ward management, emergencies, etc. [19].

4.2.2.3 Clustering

Another popular data mining method is Clustering, which is an unsupervised learning, meaning that there are not predefined classes [8, 20]. It is used mainly in cases where there is not adequate knowledge about the objects of large datasets, trying to group them based on similar characteristics [5]. The groups that will be formed are called clusters, and data points within the same cluster are characterized by higher similarity, while those assigned to different clusters have lower similarity [8]. The most common clustering techniques used in healthcare are Partitional, Hierarchical, and Density-Based Clustering [14].

Bertsimas, et al. attempted to predict healthcare costs by utilizing medical and cost data over three years for 800,000 insured people. For their experiment they first set a baseline method by using the healthcare cost of the last 12 months of the period of examination as the forecast of the overall healthcare cost in the result period. Then, they used classification trees and clustering. The clusters that were formed contained groups of people with similar cost characteristics and often similar medical characteristics. They concluded that knowledge discovery methods significantly improved performance compared to the baseline method, with the classification tree algorithm performing better on the lowest-cost buckets, while clustering doing better on the higher-cost buckets. Moreover, clustering achieved better results when utilizing both cost and medical data [21].

Peng et al. applied clustering to understand the data and detect suspicious healthcare frauds from large amounts of real-life health insurance data. To reach their goal, they used two clustering techniques, SAS EM and CLUTO. After conducting their experiment, they concluded that the second method needs less time, while the clusters formed by the first method are more valuable for their purpose [22].

4.2.2.4 Association Rules

Association rules is one of the most important knowledge discovery techniques used to detect valuable links and recognize frequent patterns among data objects [23]. It plays a significant role in the healthcare sector as it helps in detecting relationships among diseases, health state and symptoms. Health insurance companies also use association approach to analyze data and detect fraud and abuse. The most common association algorithm is Apriori [14].

Patil et al. introduced a new approach to classify whether a patient is likely to suffer from diabetes or not [24]. For this purpose, they first used equal interval binning based on medical expert opinion, and then they used association to produce rules and understand the relationship among their data.

Kai et al. used association rule mining to develop a support system for clinical decisions. The goal of their project was to support healthcare assistants identify and offer appropriate lifestyle guidance [25].

4.3 Methodology and Results

In the previous literature review section, we specified some interesting case studies of data mining applications in the field of healthcare support. In this experimentation section, we present various data mining tools and algorithms, either predictive ones, like classification, or descriptive ones, such as clustering and association rule mining. That was intended to extract valuable knowledge, information and patterns with the aim to predict stroke incidents from medical records.

4.3.1 Methodology Outline

We used a dataset from Kaggle that contains stroke incident records to perform several experiments. Our main objective was to use data mining tools to extract useful knowledge from the dataset and develop a predictive tool that will predict whether a person will suffer from stroke.

For the experimentation, we used classification, clustering, and association rule mining. Decision Tree, Random Forest and Naïve Bayes were used for classification, k-means, k-medoids and DBSCAN for clustering and FP-Growth for association rule mining. During these experiments, it was necessary to perform some pre-processing to filter out invalid records or fix wrong values.

4.3.2   Experiments

4.3.2.1   Dataset

We utilized a dataset named "Stroke Prediction Dataset" which contains medical records about stroke incidents, retrieved from the open-source dataset provider Kaggle. In total, the dataset consists of 5110 records and 12 attributes of all attribute types, such as categorical, real, integer or binary. As mentioned earlier, the general purpose was to use data mining to develop a predictive tool to predict whether a person will suffer from stroke. Therefore, the class attribute, which is also provided by the dataset, must be of binary type and take two values, "suffered from stroke" and "not suffered from stroke". As for the other attributes, integer ones are "id" and "age", real ones are "average glucose level" and "body mass index (bmi)", categorical ones are "gender", "work type", "residence type" and "smoking status" and binary ones are "hypertension", "heart disease" and "ever married". All experimentations with the different data mining techniques were performed with RapidMiner.

4.3.2.2   Classification

With regards to classification, our goal was to learn a classifier that correctly predicts cases of people who might suffer from stroke. Before proceeding to performing experiments, it was necessary to pre-process the data. First, the class attribute as well as the attributes "heart_disease" and "hypertension" were converted from integer to binominal, because according to the dataset description, they take values 0 or 1, meaning false or true.

Then, we set the label role to the class attribute and id role to the "id" attribute and handled the missing values either by changing any "N/A" and "Unknown" text to blank value to turn them into actual missing values and then with the "Replace Missing Values" operator, the missing values were replaced with the average of the attribute or filtered out in case the average could not be calculated. With regards to "bmi" attribute, it was of polynomial type, so in order to be converted to real, we applied the "Parse Numbers" operator. Finally, to balance the dataset, the Sample operator was used to filter the dataset up to 280 records per class, almost as much as the smallest set, to avoid learning a biased classifier. The pre-processing task can be seen in RapidMiner application in Fig. 4.3.

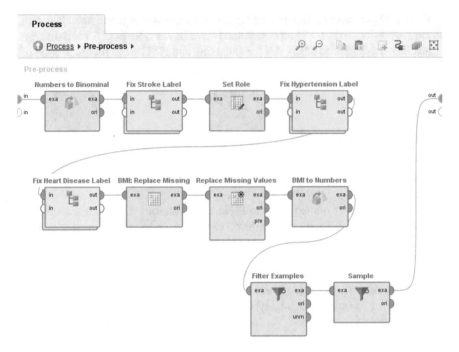

Fig. 4.3 Pre-processing process

Table 4.1 Decision Tree
accuracy per criterion

Criterion	Accuracy (%)
Gain ratio	69.69
Information gain	70.75
Gini index	66.19

Then, the dataset was ready to be used for classification to train different classifiers and measure their prediction accuracy. The classification algorithms that were used were Decision Tree, Random Forest, and Naïve Bayes. For each one, it was important to perform a tenfold cross validation, with the use of "Cross Validation" operator, using accuracy as the main criterion of performance evaluation.

Decision Tree

Inside the "Cross Validation" operator, the "Decision Tree" was used with the default parameters except the criterion. We performed the classification for gain ratio, information gain and gini index criterion values. Table 4.1 presents the accuracy results for each criterion. As it seems, with the information gain criterion the learned classifier has the highest accuracy.

Table 4.2 Random Forest accuracy per criterion

Criterion	Accuracy (%)
Gain ratio	74.48
Information gain	74.26
Gini Index	75.10

Table 4.3 Classifier accuracy comparison

Classifier	Accuracy (with best criterion)
Decision Tree	70.75% (with information gain)
Random Forest	75.10% (with gini index)
Naïve Bayes	77.59%

Random Forest

Similarly, with the previous experiment, by swapping the "Decision Tree" operator with the "Random Forest" one, inside "Cross Validation", we performed classification with random forest and used the same criterion values, to test and find which one produces the best results. This time the gini index criterion produces the classifier with the highest prediction accuracy, from what can be seen in Table 4.2.

Naïve Bayes

Finally, we swapped "Random Forest" with "Naïve Bayes" operator. This methodology does not have any parameters, like the criterion from the previous ones, to modify, test and get the best results. So, it always produces a classifier with accuracy of 77.59%.

Classifiers Comparison

The results of our experimentations showed that the Naïve Bayes produces the best classifier with overall accuracy of 77.59%, as shown in Table 4.3.

However, the accuracy by itself may not be enough to prove that a classifier is the best. For the classifier comparison to be more prestigious and since we are dealing with matters in the medical domain, we used the Receiver Operating Characteristic (ROC) curve, to find the most accurate classifier [26]. The ROC curves of the three classifiers shown in Fig. 4.4, validate that the Naïve Bayes classifier is indeed the most accurate.

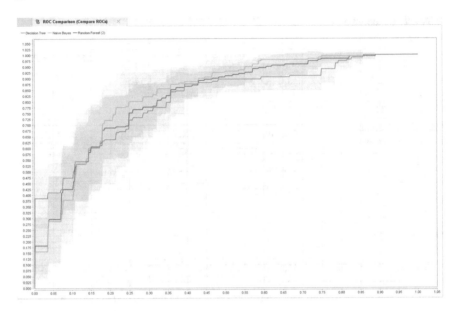

Fig. 4.4 ROC curve comparison

4.3.2.3 Clustering

Clustering is a data mining methodology which partitions data in different groups
or clusters based on similarity criteria. That is, data in the same cluster bear some
conceptual resemblance and those from different clusters are dissimilar [27]. For
the clustering experiments, we used the same stroke incident dataset and the k-
means, k-medoids and Density-Based Spatial Clustering of Applications with Noise
(DBSCAN) algorithms. Similarly with the classification experimentation, some
pre-processing was also applied to the dataset before running the clustering algorithm, to select the appropriate attributes, clear missing values or outliers and transform the data. The attributes that were selected for all experiments, were "bmi",
"average glucose level" and age, since those are the only numerical ones, hence
being interesting for clustering purposes.

k-Means

After pre-processing the data, the k-means algorithm was used for the initial experiment. Given that the dataset has two classes, "had stroke" and "not had stroke", we
set the parameter k = 2 for the cluster number, meaning that 2 clusters would be
produced. After clustering, the first cluster had 4355 records, while the second one
had 755, as shown in Table 4.4.

Table 4.4 K-means clustering

Clusters	Records
Cluster 0	4355
Cluster 1	755

Table 4.5 k-medoids clustering

Clusters	Euclidean distance	Manhattan distance
	Records	
Cluster 0	973	983
Cluster 1	4137	4127

Table 4.6 DBSCAN clustering

Epsilon parameters	Number of clusters	Number of noise records
1	0	5110 (all records)
2	2	5108
2.5	22	5017
3	38	4607
3.5	17	3533
4	9	2702
4.5	8	2104
5	5	1705
5.5	8	1368
6	4	1117

k-Medoids

The following experiment utilized k-medoids, which is similar to the k-means. For this experiment, we used the same cluster size as before, meaning that we set the parameter k = 2, but this time for the "Measure Types" parameter, we used two different types, Euclidean and Manhattan distance. The results of clustering can be seen in Table 4.5.

DBSCAN

For the third and final clustering experiment, we used the DBSCAN. In contrast with k-means and k-medoids, for this algorithm the initial cluster size parameter k cannot be set, and it accepts only one parameter, the epsilon parameter. We tried different values for the epsilon parameter, and it produced interesting results, where a lot of this values produced clusters with only a few records while considering most of the records as noise. The results of this experiment can be viewed in Table 4.6.

4.3.2.4 Association Rule Mining

As a final step, we used association rule mining [28]. With this technique, one can extract useful patterns, relations, and associations between records of large datasets [29]. For this purpose, we used Frequent Pattern (FP)-Growth and the "Create Association Rules" operator in RapidMiner, with various values for support and confidence, after applying once more some pre-processing to the dataset. Figure 4.5 shows the RapidMiner process that was developed for this experiment.

The results of an experimentation example can be seen here, with support level being at 60% and confidence at 70%. A total of 50 different rules were produced and the more interesting one are presented in Table 4.7.

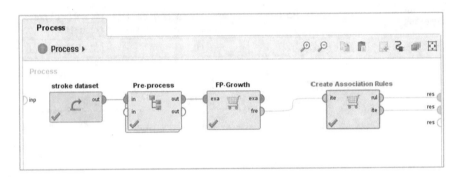

Fig. 4.5 Association rule mining process

Table 4.7 Association rules

Premises	Conclusion	Support (%)	Confidence (%)
No hypertension	No heart disease	83	95
Married	No heart disease	70	93
No heart disease	No hypertension	83	88
Married	No hypertension	65	85
No heart disease	Married	70	75
No hypertension	Married	74	88
No heart disease, No hypertension	Married	73	88

4.4 Conclusion

4.4.1 Discussion

Several experiments were carried out using a dataset that included stroke incidence records. The main goal was to employ data mining methods to acquire meaningful knowledge and predict if a patient would have a stroke. To that end, classification, clustering, and association rule mining were utilized. It was also necessitated to undertake some data pre-processing steps to filter out invalid or rectify incorrect values. Therefore, for classification, Decision Tree, Random Forest, and Nave Bayes were employed achieving a stroke prediction accuracy of 70.75%, 75.10% and 77.59%, respectively. For clustering we incorporated k-means, k-medoids and DBSCAN showcasing controversial results with the best ones forming 2–4 clusters of patients with strokes or not. Finally, for mining association rules we used FP-Growth retrieving a few strong rules with the top three associating "No hypertension" with "No heart disease" (Support 83% and Confidence 95%), "Married" with "No heart disease" (Support 70% and Confidence 93%) and "No heart disease" with "No hypertension" (Support 83% and Confidence 88%).

Even though data mining is relatively new, it has become a useful asset for any organization because of its ability to extract new knowledge from enormous databases fast. This is very important in healthcare, since we are dealing with records from patients. But also, there is the potential to extract useful knowledge and information by carefully evaluating and mining such data.

Data mining could be applied to many different healthcare domains, such as measuring the treatment effectiveness provided from medical stuff, helping with decision making with regards to healthcare management, detecting fraudulent cases in the healthcare insurance domain, finding out about the preferences of patients to provide better services, discovering new patterns for better infection control, improving patient care and ranking hospitals based on their ability to handle high-risk patients.

4.4.2 Issues and Challenges of Data Mining in Stroke Prediction and Healthcare

Performing experiments on patient stroke records to produce a classifier that predicts stroke incidents was challenging. The need for knowledge in healthcare, especially in the stroke domain, slows down experimentation, as it is required to study material and perform a targeted data mining analysis. Data mining needs specific attributes to be selected, based on relations between them and how they co-relate with the stroke incident.

Another challenge with stroke prediction process was the data format. The dataset has a lot of missing values, and those missing values are not just blank entries, but they are represented by terms like "N/A" or "Unknown". This can cause some analysis barriers in the application environment of RapidMiner. RapidMiner's "Replace Missing Values" operator only works on actual blank values and when a record is filled with "N/A" or any kind of text, it is not considered blank. The solution is to first use the "Replace" operator and replace the "N/A", "Unknown" and every word that implies missing values with the actual empty value. Then the "Replace Missing Values" operator can be used correctly.

In conventional data mining applications, data scientists are interested in discovering useful patterns in datasets and describing those patterns in simple terms. On the other hand, in the healthcare domain, data scientists may aim to identify irregular cases present in a small number of records, which do not follow the usual patterns. In contrast with conventional data mining, in most healthcare applications it is of critical importance to detail every piece of new-found knowledge as thoroughly as possible. Even minor mistakes could have fatal results on peoples' lives [5].

The General Data Protection Regulation (GDPR) is another challenge. Health related data are sensitive and private and must not be accessed by anyone without sufficient authorization [30]. Additionally, for data mining to be able to produce accurate and useful results, a vast amount of different, real data from many different patients is required. Those two obstacles combined hinder data mining related applications and can be critical in any healthcare related data analysis [5].

One more obstacle after knowledge extraction is that healthcare specialists may not modify their working routines because of some computer-assisted acquired knowledge. Even if data mining results provide major improvements on healthcare professionals' routines, they may be reluctant to change their practices [4].

Moreover, the actual quality of data poses a great challenge. Since data mining requires many records, such data are gathered from many different sources, organizations, or data warehouses. All these sources do not use the same schemas. When collecting non-uniform data, difficulties may arise, as the same type of data are stored differently [14]. It is also possible for a data scientist to deal with missing values or noisy data that do not provide useful knowledge results [31]. The pre-processing required to deal with all these issues slows down the entire process [5].

In addition to the previous challenges, there is also the question of trustworthiness of data mining models. These models are predictive, meaning that they produce an estimated conclusion of some input data, and the conclusion is by no means to be taken for granted. They should be used by medical staff as an extra tool that provides a second opinion. Therefore, predictive models should be used wisely for critical decisions on patients' health, as the estimated decision produced by the model could potentially endanger lives [5].

4.4.3 Future Directions and Insights

As mentioned above, a critical challenge of data mining is the quality of the data in healthcare. That is the reason why it is of importance for healthcare to find a more efficient way to handle its data. With regards to (i) how those data are collected, (ii) stored in databases or data warehouses, (iii) pre-processed and finally (iv) what mining techniques can be used on them. These points may be considered as future work of this study.

To achieve that, a solution would be the standardization on how to handle healthcare data, as well as the implementation of a secure and efficient infrastructure that supports sharing of these private, personal data.

It is also important to mention that healthcare data could be either quantitative or qualitative. Quantitative are data that can be counted, measured, or expressed in a numerical format, while qualitative are more conceptual and descriptive. Normally, qualitative data can be considered notes, documents, any kind of text in general and even media files, like audio, video, and images. In the healthcare domain, qualitative data can be a doctor's notes from his/her patients, some clinical records or even diagnostic or x-ray images. Those data should also be included in a data mining process along with quantitative ones, in order to achieve even better results.

Finally, in data mining, it is important to perform some pre-processing and filter the available attributes. Outliers and noise should be filtered out, as they negatively impact on both accuracy and speed. Data mining provides statistical techniques that can detect such attributes and there are feature selection algorithms that can identify the most suitable attributes.

Acknowledgements We would like to express our gratitude to the anonymous reviewers who provided critical feedback during the preparation of this manuscript. Their remarks and recommendations significantly improved the quality of this work.

References

1. Koukaras, P., Tjortjis, C., Rousidis, D.: Social Media Types: introducing a data driven taxonomy. Computing **102**(1), 295–340 (2020). https.//doi.org/10.1007/s00607-019-00739-y
2. Baitharu, T.R., Pani, S.K.: Analysis of Data Mining Techniques for Healthcare Decision Support System Using Liver Disorder Dataset. Procedia Computer Science **85**, 862–870 (2016). https://doi.org/10.1016/j.procs.2016.05.276
3. Tjortjis, C., Saraee, M., Theodoulidis, B., Keane, J.A.: Using T3, an Improved Decision Tree Classifier, for Mining Stroke-related Medical Data. Methods Inf. Med. **46**(05), 523–529 (2007). https://doi.org/10.1160/ME0317
4. Koh HC, Tan G. "Data mining applications in healthcare", J Healthc Inf Manag, 2005 Spring;19(2):64–72. PMID: 15869215.
5. M. H. Tekieh and B. Raahemi, "Importance of data mining in healthcare: A survey," in Proceedings of the 2015 IEEE/ACM International Conference on Advances in Social Networks Analysis and Mining, ASONAM 2015, Aug. 2015, pp. 1057–1062. doi: https://doi.org/10.1145/2808797.2809367.
6. Zhang, S., Tjortjis, C., Zeng, X., Qiao, H., Buchan, I., Keane, J.: Comparing Data Mining Methods with Logistic Regression in Childhood Obesity Prediction. Inf. Syst. Front. **11**(4), 449–460 (2009). https://doi.org/10.1007/s10796-009-9157-0

7. Glover, S., Rivers, P.A., Asoh, D.A., Piper, C.N., Murph, K.: Data mining for health executive decision support: An imperative with a daunting future! Health Serv. Manage. Res. **23**(1), 42–46 (2010). https://doi.org/10.1258/hsmr.2009.009029
8. Tomar, D., Agarwal, S.: A survey on data mining approaches for healthcare. International Journal of Bio-Science and Bio-Technology **5**(5), 241–266 (2013). https://doi.org/10.14257/ijbsbt.2013.5.5.25
9. Obenshain, M.K.: Application of Data Mining Techniques to Healthcare Data. Infect. Control Hosp. Epidemiol. **25**(8), 690–695 (2004). https://doi.org/10.1086/502460
10. T. Chatzinikolaou, E. Vogiazti, A. Kousis, and C. Tjortjis, "Smart Healthcare Support Using Data Mining and Machine Learning," in EAI/Springer Innovations in Communication and Computing Book: "IoT and WSN based SmartCities: A Machine Learning Perspective," 2022.
11. P. Koukaras, D. Rousidis and C. Tjortjis, "Forecasting and Prevention Mechanisms Using Social Media in Health Care", in Maglogiannis I., Brahnam S., Jain L. (eds) Advanced Computational Intelligence in Healthcare-7. Studies in Computational Intelligence, vol 891, March 2020, Springer, Berlin, Heidelberg. https://doi.org/10.1007/978-3-662-61114-2_8.
12. S. El-Sappagh, S. El-Masri, M. Elmogy, S. H. El-Sappagh, and A. M. Riad, "Data Mining and Knowledge Discovery: Applications, Techniques, Challenges and Process Models in Health-care," International Journal of Engineering Research and Applications (IJERA), vol. 3, no. 3, pp. 900–906, May 2013, [Online]. Available: https://www.researchgate.net/publication/250612388.
13. P. Koukaras, C. Berberidis and C. Tjortjis, "A Semi-supervised Learning Approach for Complex Information Networks", in Hemanth J., Bestak R., Chen J.IZ. (eds) Intelligent Data Communication Technologies and Internet of Things. Lecture Notes on Data Engineering and Communications Technologies, vol 57, February 2021, Springer, Singapore. https://doi.org/10.1007/978-981-15-9509-7_1.
14. Ahmad, P., Qamar, S., Qasim, S., Rizvi, A.: Techniques of Data Mining In Healthcare: A Review. International Journal of Computer Applications **120**(15), 38–50 (2015). https://doi.org/10.5120/21307-4126
15. Tzirakis, P., Tjortjis, C.: T3C: improving a decision tree classification algorithm's interval splits on continuous attributes. Adv. Data Anal. Classif. **11**(2), 353–370 (2017). https://doi.org/10.1007/s11634-016-0246-x
16. Das, R., Turkoglu, I., Sengur, A.: Effective diagnosis of heart disease through neural networks ensembles. Expert Syst. Appl. **36**(4), 7675–7680 (2009). https://doi.org/10.1016/j.eswa.2008.09.013
17. D. I. Curiac, G. Vasile, O. Banias, C. Volosencu, and A. Albu, "Bayesian network model for diagnosis of psychiatric diseases," in Proceedings of the International Conference on Information Technology Interfaces, ITI, 2009, pp. 61–66. doi: https://doi.org/10.1109/ITI.2009.5196055.
18. Divya, D., Agarwal, S.: Weighted support vector regression approach for remote healthcare monitoring. International Conference on Recent Trends in Information Technology, ICRTIT **2011**, 969–974 (2011). https://doi.org/10.1109/ICRTIT.2011.5972437
19. J. Alapont, A. Bella-Sanjuán, C. Ferri, J. Hernández-Orallo, J. D. Llopis-Llopis, and M. J. Ramírez-Quintana, "Specialised Tools for Automating Data Mining for Hospital Management," in Proc. First East European Conference on Health Care Modelling and Computation, Aug. 2005, pp. 7–19.
20. Kanellopoulos, Y., Antonellis, P., Tjortjis, C., Makris, C., Tsirakis, N.: k-Attractors: A Partitional Clustering Algorithm for Numeric Data Analysis. Appl. Artif. Intell. **25**(2), 97–115 (2011). https://doi.org/10.1080/08839514.2011.534590
21. Bertsimas, D., et al.: Algorithmic prediction of health-care costs. Oper. Res. **56**(6), 1382–1392 (2008). https://doi.org/10.1287/opre.1080.0619
22. Y. Peng, G. Kou, A. Sabatka, Z. Chen, D. Khazanchi, and Y. Shi, "Application of Clustering Methods to Health Insurance Fraud Detection," in 2006 International Conference on Service Systems and Service Management, Oct. 2006, pp. 116–120. doi: https://doi.org/10.1109/ICSSM.2006.320598.

23. S. M. Ghafari and C. Tjortjis, "A survey on association rules mining using heuristics," WIREs Data Mining and Knowledge Discovery, vol. 9, no. 4, Jul. 2019, doi: https://doi.org/10.1002/widm.1307.

24. B. M. Patil, R. C. Joshi, and D. Toshniwal, "Association rule for classification of type -2 diabetic patients," in ICMLC 2010 - The 2nd International Conference on Machine Learning and Computing, 2010, pp. 330–334. doi: https://doi.org/10.1109/ICMLC.2010.67.

25. E. Kai et al., "Empowering the Healthcare Worker Using the Portable Health Clinic," 2014 IEEE 28th International Conference on Advanced Information Networking and Applications, 2014, pp. 759–764, doi: https://doi.org/10.1109/AINA.2014.108.

26. Maroco, J., Silva, D., Rodrigues, A., Guerreiro, M., Santana, I., de Mendonça, A.: Data mining methods in the prediction of Dementia: A real-data comparison of the accuracy, sensitivity and specificity of linear discriminant analysis, logistic regression, neural networks, support vector machines, classification trees and random forests. BMC Res Notes. **17**(4), 299 (2011). https://doi.org/10.1186/1756-0500-4-299.PMID:21849043;PMCID:PMC3180705

27. P. Berkhin, "A Survey of Clustering Data Mining Techniques," in Grouping Multidimensional Data, Berlin/Heidelberg: Springer-Verlag, pp. 25–71. doi: https://doi.org/10.1007/3-540-283 49-8_2.

28. Kotsiantis, S., Kanellopoulos, D.: Association Rules Mining: A Recent Overview. GESTS International Transactions on Computer Science and Engineering **32**(1), 71–82 (2006)

29. Y. Liu, Institute of Electrical and Electronics Engineers, and IEEE Circuits and Systems Society, ICNC-FSKD 2017: 13th International Conference on Natural Computation, Fuzzy Systems and Knowledge Discovery : Guilin, Guangxi, China, 29–31 July, 2017.

30. Abouelmehdi, K., Beni-Hessane, A., Khaloufi, H.: Big healthcare data: preserving security and privacy. Journal of Big Data **5**(1), 1 (2018). https://doi.org/10.1186/s40537-017-0110-7

31. B. Milovic, "Prediction and decision making in Health Care using Data Mining," International Journal of Public Health Science (IJPHS), vol. 1, no. 2, Dec. 2012, doi: https://doi.org/10.11591/ijphs.v1i2.1380.

Chapter 5
A Big Data Infrastructure in Support of Healthy and Independent Living: A Real Case Application

Valerio Bellandi

Abstract This chapter illustrates how the SMART BEAR project aims to integrate heterogeneous smart devices, including wearables and environmental sensors, to enable the continuous data collection from the everyday life of the elderly, which will be processed by an affordable, accountably secure, and privacy-preserving eHealth platform applying Machine Learning algorithms to deliver interventions such as personalized notifications and alerts to each patient, thus promoting their healthy and independent living.

Keywords Smart healthcare · Machine learning · Analytics · Cloud computation

5.1 Introduction

A rapid increase in the elderly European population is predicted for the coming decades, due to the ageing of those born after WWII. Within Europe's ageing population, Hearing Loss, Cardio Vascular Diseases, Cognitive Impairments, Mental Health Issues, and Balance Disorders, as well as Frailty, are prevalent conditions, with tremendous social and financial impact. Preventing, slowing the development of, or dealing effectively with the effects of the above impairments can have a significant impact on a person's quality of life and lead to significant savings in the cost of healthcare services at the same time.

This chapter describes the approach adopted by the SMART BEAR (**Smart Big Data Platform to Offer Evidence-based Personalised Support for Healthy and**

Contributing authors are listed in the Acknowledgements Section.

V. Bellandi (✉)
Computer Science Department, Universitá degli Studi di Milano, Via Celoria 18, Milano 20133, Italy
e-mail: valerio.bellandi@unimi.it

© The Author(s), under exclusive license to Springer Nature Switzerland AG 2023
C. P. Lim et al. (eds.), *Artificial Intelligence and Machine Learning for Healthcare*,
Intelligent Systems Reference Library 229,
https://doi.org/10.1007/978-3-031-11170-9_5

Independent Living at Home) project [1,2] to design the data-driven decision-making process supporting the creation of personalized interventions, in order to sustain the healthy ageing of people.

SMART BEAR (SB) targets participants who are between 67 and 80 years old and have a clinical history including at least two of the following conditions: Hearing Loss, Cardio Vascular Diseases, Cognitive Impairments, Mental Health Issues, and Balance Disorders, as well as Frailty. In addition to the conditions mentioned above, during the initial testing phase, which is hereby called "**Pilot of the Pilots**" and has been set up **in Madeira** as the trial scenario for technical requirements, *low back pain* is also targeted.

The aim of the SMART BEAR platform is to integrate heterogeneous sensors, assistive medical and mobile devices to enable the continuous data collection from the everyday life of the participants, which will be analysed to obtain the evidence needed in order to offer personalised interventions promoting their healthy and independent living [1].

eHealth platforms hold promise for many health benefits that can enhance the overall well-being of the elderly,through promotion of a healthier lifestyle and facilitation of the self-monitoring and self-management of their comorbidities. SMART BEAR is built on the eHealth platform developed by the H2020 project EVOTION[3] to support evidence-based public health policies formation and monitoring, which supports: (a) the continuous collection of medical, physiological and lifestyle data from heterogeneous resources (hospitals, biosensors,advanced hearing aids and mobile phones), and (b) the analysis of these data, driven by high level big data analytics and decision models to generate evidence useful for making public health policy level interventions [2].

The data processing schema encompasses a collection phase, where data are transmitted from the smart devices to the repositories in the SMART BEAR platform, and a data analysis phase, where the data are ingested by the Big Data Analytics (BDA) engine. The engine is designed to manage Data Analysis Workflows (DAWs), whose results are eventually relayed to the Dashboard, where overview charts are visualized for the clinicians. Finally, the Decision Support System (DSS) component provides suggestions for the personalized interventions to be delivered to the patients in form of app or dashboard alerts.

The raw data collected from the environment, the wearable devices, and the SB@App are continuously ingested in the FHIR and non-FHIR Data Repositories. In particular, the former is built based on the FHIR (Fast Healthcare Interoperability Resources) framework[4] and provides also the developers with a standard code based

---

[1] https://www.smart-bear.eu.

[2] https://cordis.europa.eu/project/id/857172.

[3] https://h2020evotion.eu.

[4] https://www.hl7.org/fhir/.

on HL7[5], which can be complemented with medical terminologies defined in the standards SNOMED-CT,[6] LOINC,[7] and MeSH.[8]

Then, the **BDA Engine**, based on the Hadoop stack,[9] exposes a set of APIs to get raw data from the Data repositories and to perform pre-processing procedures such as aggregations or filtering, the outcome of which supports the execution of Machine Learning (ML) analytics in scheduled jobs to run periodically at fixed times, dates, or intervals. This allows the execution of multiple data-driven procedures that, after an evaluation step, can be eventually selected to support decision making.

The **DSS component** is designed to assist the clinicians in the initial assessment of every patient in terms of the optimal clinical tools (i.e., questionnaires, exams) that must be used to assess a patient and then provide them with the optimal combination of the devices to monitor their health during the monitoring phase. The DSS will continuously be trained by the data that will be digested into the platform.

The **Dashboard** is the component aimed at providing a user-friendly graphical interface for the clinicians involved in the project. The Dashboard supports the clinicians to register, create, and manage a patient, taking into account his/her devices and medication, conduct the first visit and the checkup, verify patient's questionnaire score and medical history, in addition to the delivered interventions, perform analytics on medical data, and create interventions to be delivered.

Finally, all the components need to be integrated into the SMART BEAR cloud platform. The complexity of the project and the necessity of delivering new releases of the components at high velocity require a DevOps-like integration culture.[10] That is specially important when the pilots are running and the initial requirements are evolving and functionalities need to be improved, testing and released in a very short period of time.

5.2 Architecture

The SMART BEAR platform leverages big data analytics and learning capabilities, allowing for large scale analysis of the data collected, to generate the evidence required for making decisions about personalised interventions.

The SMART BEAR platform architecture consists of the following main components: the *HomeHub*, the *SB@App*, and the *SB@Cloud* (Fig. 5.1). The SB@Cloud is the core system of the architecture and covers the main functionalities of SMART BEAR such as: secure storage, collection, and analysis of medical data.

---

[5] https://hl7.org/fhir/.

[6] https://www.snomed.org.

[7] https://loinc.org/.

[8] https://www.nlm.nih.gov/mesh/meshhome.html.

[9] https://hadoop.apache.org/.

[10] https://about.gitlab.com/topics/devops/.

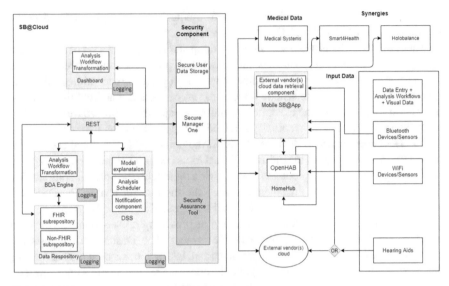

Fig. 5.1 The architecture of the SMART BEAR platform

In turn, it consists of the following modules: *Dashboard, BDA engine, Data Repository, Decision Support System (DSS)*, and *Security Component (SC)*.

The Dashboard is the entry point of user interaction with the SMART BEAR system for configuration and data visualization. The user interface allows to input data, set up Analysis Workflow data models and interventions, register or disconnect external data sources, execute data analytics workflows, and retrieve executions results.

The BDA Engine is responsible for the actual data analysis and retrieves the data from the Data repository for further processing, the results are written back to be accessed by users via the Dashboard. The Data repository includes FHIR and non-FHIR compliant sub-repositories. The FHIR component provides the storage for the medical data. The rest of the information is stored in the non-FHIR component. Some clinical repository interfaces allow data collection from external Electronic Health Records (EHRs) and synergistic projects (such as Smart4Health,[11] Holobalance.[12]).

The DSS provides the functionalities for interventions, reasoning behind the decisions proposed, and analysis scheduling and notifications, while the SB@App is responsible for the data collection from all portable devices connected to the patient's smartphone, such as pulse/steps measurements and portable medical sensors.

Finally, the HomeHub accumulates data from home-based devices, like smart weight scales and movement sensors. It collects data directly as well as from the device's vendor private clouds. On the backend level, all components are communicating via REST interfaces. The information exchange between components,

---

[11] https://smart4health.eu/en/.

[12] https://holobalance.eu/.

as well as authentication at the Dashboard, is secured according to GDPR through the Security Component. In particular, the Security Assurance Tool module put in place all mechanisms to enforce security policies.

eHealth platforms can actually support the overall well-being of the elderly, yet, their use is often perceived to have technological and privacy risks. Being SMART BEAR an eHealth platform, but like the majority of platforms integrating external solutions that interconnects software and hardware components, it presents challenges in relation to how to cope with security and privacy issues that could emerge due to different underneath technologies and different levels of compliance. In particular, external devices serve different purposes and, consequently, the aggregated system of devices is not implemented as a whole. In fact, each specific implementation considered a variety of protocols and best practices, not necessarily targeting security and privacy.

In this context, and in addition to the well-known security/privacy provisions [3] any modern eHealth system should support (e.g., Role-based access control, Data validation and encryption, end-users authentication, authorisation of users and M2M services, security monitoring and audit, logging mechanisms), developers must take into consideration the legislation that imposes tough obligations in the framework of the European General Data Protection Regulation (GDPR) [4], technical guidelines for minimum security measures suggested by organisations (e.g., Security and Resilience in eHealth Infrastructures and Services guidelines of ENISA [5], encryption guidelines of NIST [6]), and best practices for privacy like the one described in [7]), along with encryption, protocol e.g., the Bluetooth 4.0 Security Modes [8]) and vendor-specific data integrity advancements in Io(M)T.

5.2.1   HomeHub

The SB HomeHub defines both the hardware and the software that is installed inside the patient's home. In the case of SB, the HomeHub integrates the following sensors: a motion sensor, one or more smart bulbs, and a temperature sensor. These sensors are grouped in the SB@Home kit. In order to control sensors and devices from a central access unit, a *hub* is required. SMART BEAR must use and integrate multidisciplinary devices and sensors in the simplest and more robust way. For this purpose, the OpenHAB3[13] architecture is implemented in a Raspberry PI4[14] aiming to serve the technology-agnostic integration and functionality through a unified way by a single management and access interface, common to all actors of the process.

The architecture of the SB HomeHub can be abstracted in the following layers:

(a) *Sensors' installation Layer*: The physical sensors that are installed by a technician (or the person itself) in the patient's house.

---

[13] https://www.openhab.org/blog/2020-12-21-openhab-3-0-release.html.

[14] https://www.raspberrypi.com/products/raspberry-pi-4-model-b/.

(b) *Sensors' communication Layer*: This is a layer hidden from the user that explicitly defines the communication protocol that a sensor is using to communicate with the hub. The communication in most cases is based on ZigBee5 or WiFi6 protocols.
(c) *Sensors' configuration Layer*: This layer includes all the devices. The sensors cannot operate without the appropriate hardware that fits their communication protocol.
(d) *Home Local Area Network (LAN) Layer*: This layer explicitly defines the communication of the Raspberry PI board with the gateways and bridges. In this way, Raspberry interconnects and unifies all different devices and sensors. In SMART BEAR this means that the network communication with at least a LAN switch and a ZigBee USB stick, plugged in the Raspberry PI, is considered a requirement.
(e) *Home Control Layer*: This is the high-level layer and the actual HomeHub. The main building block is a Raspberry PI equipped with the openHAB software, actually hosting the HomeHub. In particular, the heart of the HomeHub is the openHAB technology-agnostic platform that unifies all home installations and allows access through the REST API by the SB@App (that in turn integrates the HomeHub with the SB@Cloud).

5.2.2 SB@App

The SMART BEAR mobile application (SB@App) is a component aimed at providing a user-friendly graphical user interface for the participant. The application handles the communication between the wearable devices and the SMART BEAR platform while accessing the Platform utilities and functionalities. Through the SB@App, a patient has access to all the data being collected by the wearable devices and the SB@Home kit An example of a usage scenario is depicted in Fig. 5.2a, b, where a patient with Cardiovascular Diseases **CVDs** can select a device and take a measurement, in this case, a Blood Pressure monitor to measure Systolic and Diastolic Blood Pressure.

The SB@App has also been designed to deliver to the patient alerts and notifications as part of an Intervention. In Fig. 5.2c, alerts and notifications concerning Blood Pressure are shown. The alerts and notifications feature a color coding based on the severity gradation that is described in Sect. 5.2.3.3.

5.2.2.1 Wearable Devices and IoT

All the patients receive a set of the following devices based on their clinical history considering the medical conditions that are targeted in SMART BEAR and are indicated in Sect. 5.1:

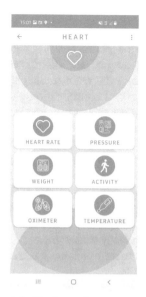

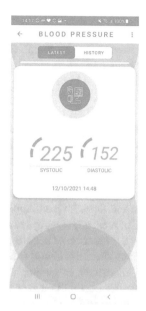

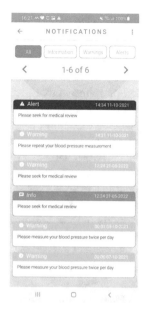

(a) Device selection in the case of Cardiovascular Diseases.

(b) Blood Pressure measuring.

(c) Cardiovascular Diseases notifications and alerts.

Fig. 5.2 SB@App interface

- *Smartphone* (all conditions), which is equipped with the SB@App and used by the patients to execute exercises and receive notifications.
- *Smartwatch* (all conditions), which is used to measure the steps walked by the patient and his/her location.
- *Smart thermometer* (all conditions), whose functionalities are exploited once a day to monitor the user's body temperature and check COVID-19 symptoms.
- *Smart pulse oximeter* (all conditions), which is used to measure the Blood Oxygen saturation and check COVID-19 symptoms.
- *Smart Blood pressure monitor* (CVDs), which retrieves the patient's vital signs about systolic and diastolic pressure and heart rate data.
- *Smart weight scale* (CVDs), which is used to retrieve a patient's data about body weight and composition.
- *SB@Home kit* (Cognitive Disorders), which is used to monitor the environment where the patient lives, more in detail air pressure, temperature, and light level are detected.
- *Hearing Aids* (Hearing Loss), which are used to retrieve patient's data about the usage time and to perform auditory training. The training procedure is described in Sect. 5.3.

5.2.3   Security Component

Concerning security and privacy at the backend, since the platform deals with the distribution of sensitive data and its processing, it adopts new distributed and/or collaborative paradigms of cloud computing. Among the main techniques to prevent sensitive cloud information leakage, we can cite the obfuscation and pseudonymization of uploaded data. Such cryptographic mechanisms are used not only for protecting data in the cloud but also as end-to-end mechanisms for protecting data in transit. However, cryptography alone cannot sufficiently preserve user privacy therefore additional forms of privacy enforcement are employed such as proper identity and authorization management, by specifying and enforcing security, access control, and privacy policies [9]. The SMART BEAR Security Component (SC) supports authentication of the entities (devices, applications, end-users, etc.) and protection of their data and resources, addressing security and privacy concerns.

Supported workflows allow the creation of secure and privacy-preserving communications within and from the SB@Cloud infrastructure to uniquely paired smartphones in an end-to-end manner. In this context:

Pseudonymisation a process that ensures that a record *after-the-fact* can no longer be attributed to a specific data subject without having previously been associated with additional information, is utilised to separate any key information (i.e., personal data, Personal Identifiable Information—PIIs) that may lead to subject's identification. This small critical dataset is stored encrypted in a separate repository, whose use is monitored continuously (i.e., usage logs can provide evidence in case of a GDPR audit), and it is the one that allows data controllers to meet specific GDPR obligations. Subsequently, its existence (during SMART BEAR project's lifecycle) allows the exercise of all GDPR individual rights (such as subject's request to know who viewed his/her pseudonymised data, also known as "Right to be informed") or the data controller's obligation to keep records, while its absence will convert all big data collected and produced to a fully anonymised dataset and as such it can be used under specific conditions ("appropriate safeguards") even beyond the duration of the project ("storage limitation"). A unique identifier (Pseudo-ID1) provided by the SC, is used to configure all the devices (e.g., smartwatch, (m)IoT, sensors, wearables) handed to a particular patient, while all associated data (PIIs have been removed or altered prior to this) reside in the main repository having a different identificator (Pseudo-ID2), allowing any analysis without revealing end-users identity. Since the SC is the only component that maintains encrypted this association, whenever it will be necessary to send or receive data, changes are made by the SC prior to transmission or digestion respectively, while the real ID of the patient will not be conveyed to SB@Cloud. The full process is depicted in Fig. 5.3.

Pseudonymised data personal health records, devices/sensors big data, questionnaires, interventions, usage data from synergies projects, stored in the Data Repository are subjected to different types of analysis, including statistical analysis techniques and data mining techniques, to obtain the evidence needed in order to offer personalised interventions promoting their healthy and independent living.

PIIs removal techniques used were introduced in [10] and properly enhanced to meet SMART BEAR needs. By design, data kept in the SC will no longer be needed to conduct the research (e.g., analytics, interventions), and consequently will be erased and not further used for any data processing.

Device security two main components are exploited for authenticating a device (SMART BEAR smartphone, or devices of any collaborating project): (*i*) a unique identity key or security token for each device; (*ii*)) an on-device X.509 certificate and private key. In a typical operation, the token is used for authentication for each message transmitted. The certificate file and private key are used to secure the communication among devices by validating the transmitted messages and encrypting data at rest.

Connectivity security seamless communication is supported by relevant protocols, such as the Advanced Message Queuing Protocol (AMQP),[15] Message Queuing Telemetry Transport (MQTT),[16] and HyperText Transfer Protocol (HTTP), and is safeguarded by their own security mechanisms, like for instance TLS for HTTP (HTTPS).

Within the SC, a security/privacy platform provides privacy-preserving and secure by design data handling capabilities, covering data at rest, in processing, and in transit, and all components and connections, offering a real-time healthcare monitoring framework, under which key functional, quality, usability, security and privacy conditions will be fulfilled to ensure the acceptability of SMART BEAR by its targeted users.

In conclusion, the SC provides a service to manage *privacy-related requests* issued by the end-users and forward them to the responsible System Administrators for processing. The end-users may issue a request via the mobile application (SB@App) by which they can also track status, follow-up, and provide feedback to those handling their requests. In this context, an Auditor may also track the progress of the request and see who is currently working on it.

5.2.3.1 Data Repository

The Data Repository component of the SB@Cloud exploits a combination of FHIR-compliant and non-FHIR databases. All the data that represent medical entities are stored in the FHIR database while data related to non-medical entities are stored in a relational database of the Cloud back-end. The latter contains elements that are not mapped to FHIR models (such as the SB Dashboard user settings), and intermediate results of the analytic models, which in turn can relay data back to the FHIR database after additional processing. The SMART BEAR FHIR database stores HL7 FHIR standardized medical data. HL7 FHIR is based on the concept of "resource", which are medical-related concepts; being the basic pieces of information that makes sense

---

[15] https://www.amqp.org/.

[16] https://mqtt.org/.

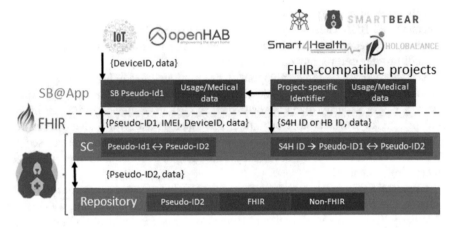

Fig. 5.3 SMART BEAR pseudonymisation supported mechanism

to exchange. The HL7 FHIR integrates medical terminologies such as SNOMED-CT and LOINC that complement the FHIR HL7-based coded values.

5.2.3.2 BDA Engine

The BDA Engine mainly addresses the functionalities required for processing Data Analysis Workflows (DAWs) and providing/storing their execution results. The BDA engine exposes a set of APIs to compute and get raw data in order to perform analyses from the FHIR and non-FHIR repositories. In terms of Machine Learning (ML), a preliminary extraction of data analytics, that will be carried out on pre-processed datasets, are going to indicate variables or combinations of variables for the feature selection approaches.

The preliminary extraction of data analytics is performed by the following sub-components, featured in the BDA Engine architecture: Delta Lake,[17] Spark,[18] Trino,[19] and Airflow.[20] The components are described below by following a bottom-up approach, the layer at the bottom being the closest to the data repositories. The architecture is shown in Fig. 5.4 and is an extended version of the one presented in [11].

Delta Lake is an ACID table storage layer over cloud object stores and is the component closest to the repositories. Delta Lake enables incremental data update, data versioning, and schema evolution.

---

[17] https://delta.io/.

[18] https://spark.apache.org/.

[19] https://trino.io/.

[20] https://airflow.apache.org/.

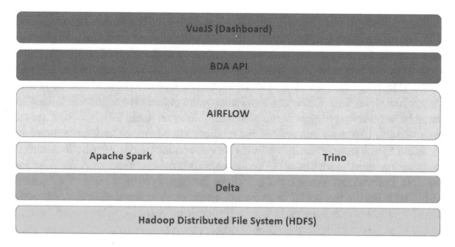

Fig. 5.4 The SMART BEAR BDA engine architecture

Spark and Trino are the components that provide the capability to access data and perform queries on the datasets. Concerning Spark, it is a multi-language engine for executing data processing and ML routines on single-node machines or clusters. Spark was chosen thanks to its capability of processing tasks that encompass custom analytics on large data volumes. In addition, it features many bindings with other commonly used Data Science and ML libraries. Spark is also capable to work both on batch and stream data.

Trino is the component providing the capability to access and perform parallel and distributed queries on data from multiple systems. Trino was chosen because it provides the BDA Engine with the capability of managing On-Line Analytical Processing (OLAP) queries and data warehousing tasks, and also because it can operate on many data sources in addition to data that is stored on HDFS.

Finally, Airflow is the component providing the capability to programmatically author, schedule, and monitor workflows written in Python language.

5.2.3.3 Decision Support System

The DSS provides functionalities for managing the Interventions, reasoning behind decisions proposed, analysis scheduling, and notifications for the clinicians and the patients.

Starting with the initial assessment, the DSS will assist the clinicians in terms of choosing the optimal set of clinical tools (i.e. exams, questionnaires, measurements) that will be used to assess each patient. Subsequently, by setting personalized thresholds for each patient individually, the clinicians configure the variables that will trigger the generation of Interventions for the patients.

For the first pilot of SMART BEAR, named Pilot of the Pilots (PoP), the DSS will rely on standard clinical practice, based on the clinical guidelines, to generate interventions for the patients, that will be delivered in the form of notifications and alerts to the smartphone of the participant. For each condition targeted in SMART BEAR (Hearing Loss, Cardio Vascular Diseases, Cognitive Impairments, Mental Health Issues, Balance Disorders, and Frailty), the clinicians are providing the rule-based conditions that trigger the corresponding Interventions, which act as a ground truth system, based on state-of-the-art medical knowledge. The interventions are regulated by the personalized thresholds for each patient and trigger notifications or alerts with severity gradation to both patients and clinicians as shown in Fig. 5.2c. For example, optimal and extreme cut-off values for Blood pressure are set for a patient with CVDs during the initial assessment, leading to a green notification when the Blood pressure measurement is within the optimal range, a yellow alert when a measurement is outside of the optimal range, and red alert when the measurement exceeds the extreme cut-off values. Utilizing the color coding for the generated notifications, the patients are getting feedback from the platform to stay healthy or seek medical advice in case the measured values are detected to be out of the limits set by the clinicians.

This initial version of the DSS is designed to evolve throughout the project, towards an ML-assisted DSS. Starting with the PoP, this evolution will be accomplished through the continuous training of the DSS by feeding the collected data to the models of the BDA engine. The outcome of the analytics following the measured parameters will provide suggestions on Interventions, targeting individuals or subgroups of patients, such as personalised thresholds modifications. For these suggestions to be integrated into the system, clinicians' approval will be required.

5.2.3.4 Dashboard

The SMART BEAR Dashboard is a component aimed at providing a user-friendly graphical user interface for the clinicians of the platform. The application is responsible for managing the interactions between the cloud platform and the users who must use it, to introduce patients into the system, enter clinical data, perform analytics on aggregated data and set the threshold value of parameters (e.g. Blood Pressure in the case of CVDs) that trigger the corresponding Interventions. For instance in Fig. 5.5 the Home page of the Dashboard is shown, and in Fig. 5.6 the form for creating Intervention is shown.

5.2.3.5 Continuous Integration and Continuous Deployment

The implementation of the above-described components and full platform integration process is performed by using well-known DevOps tools. This includes GitLab[21] for

---

[21] https://about.gitlab.com/.

Dashboard
EN
CCM
CARLOS AGOSTINHO
Home
Patients
Notebooks
Inbox
GDPR
Dashboard
UPDATE DATA
Resources recorded
Patient
Observation
Condition
Questionnaire
Family Member History
Research Subject
Medication
Diet Supplement
Profiling of patients
Back pain
Life habits data per patient
Body Mass Index
30.58
Cigarettes smoked
19.00
Physical activity
197.22
Falls
2.00
Blood Pressure Observations
Weight Observations
Moca Distribution Age group

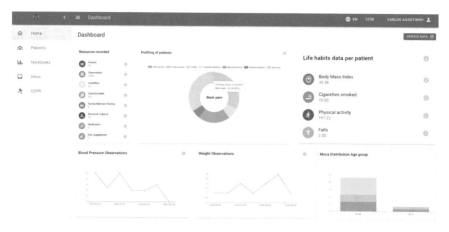

Fig. 5.5 The SMART BEAR dashboard

Create Intervention
Systolic Blood Pressure
Extreme Low Value
75
mmHg
Extreme High Value
140
mmHg
Optimal Low Value
125
mmHg
Optimal High Value
134
mmHg
Threshold Value
110
mmHg
Diastolic Blood Pressure
Extreme Low Value
50
mmHg
Extreme High Value
85
mmHg
Optimal Low Value
70
mmHg
Optimal High Value
79
mmHg
Threshold Value
110
mmHg
CANCEL
SAVE

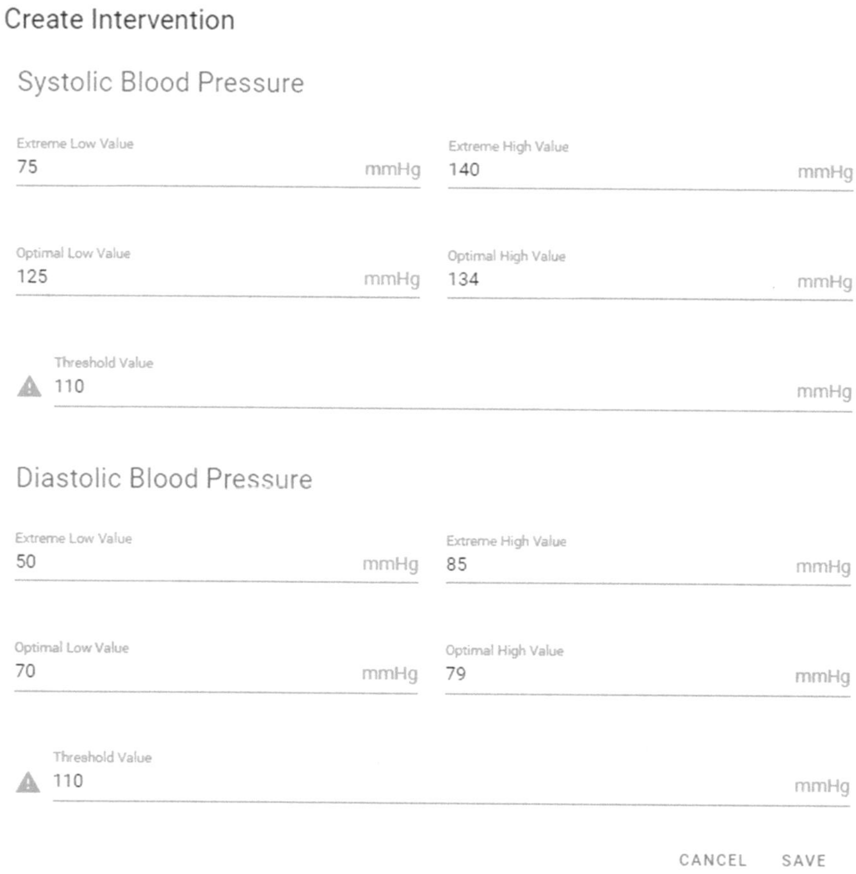

Fig. 5.6 The create intervention form on the SMART BEAR dashboard

source code repository and manage CI/CD practices, and the use of Kubernetes[22] clusters set up to provide test and production environments and managing the resulting containerized application. The SMART BEAR Gitlab repository[23] and CI/CD setup is administrated and maintained by Atos and the GitLab runner, that carries the process load needs, is installed in the Kubernetes cluster taking advantage of the same infrastructure.

CI/CD processes are based on the concept of pipelines, which describes the actions to be executed (build, test, deploy, etc.) and that are triggered automatically or manually when a component changes, automating those repetitive and worthless processes during development. Most of the configuration is concentrated in a component .gitlab-ci.yml description file.

Kubernetes is a portable, extensible, open-source platform for managing containerized workloads and services (containers orchestration), that facilitates both declarative configuration and automation. The clusters for test and production environments are each based on three nodes (independent Virtual Machines based on Ubuntu), one in the role of master (*smartbear-k8s-master*, control-plane node) and two others with the effective load of the application (*smartbear-k8s-node-0* and *smartbear-k8s-node-1*, worker nodes). In addition, the system itself provides security tools and permissions management via role-based access control, as well as resources grouping and isolation based on *namespaces*.

Having two worker nodes also allows the flexibility to reallocate resources, balance the load, perform any maintenance independently and, in the event of failure of one of them, keep the service available.

In practice, by preparing the appropriate manifest files and making them available to the CD mechanism, the rebuild and deployment of the platform are fully automatized to the cluster, which can be also monitored. In the case of needing to scale the infrastructure, along with providing the necessary resources, only minimal configuration adjustments would be necessary.

Another advantage of using this type of environment is the incorporation of the configuration and auxiliary infrastructure modules into the platform. For example, installing the GitLab runner or the NFS service that provides the persistence is performed via *Helm Charts*, which is a system that facilitates the installation of packages with the only need of informing the necessary variable parameters. In the case of the GitLab runner is enough to inform the *gitlabUrl* and a *runnerRegistrationToken*.

During the development of new functionalities for the platform as well as making corrections, the two differentiated environments allow the application to evolve with greater agility and less risk, facilitating the validation of changes and fixes before moving the changes and affecting the production environment.

---

[22] https://kubernetess.io/.

[23] https://scm.atosresearch.eu/ari/smartbear.

5.3 Clinical Interventions

As it has been mentioned in Sect. 5.1, SMART BEAR is a platform for elaborating and delivering personalized interventions, supporting Healthy Ageing through the monitoring of everyday activities. In the case of the Pilot of the Pilots, which serves as the scenario for testing the technical requirements, *Low back pain* is also targeted in addition to the six medical conditions mentioned in Sect. 5.1. The results from the Pilot of the Pilots are described in more detail in Sect. 5.4.

In general, from a clinical point of view the personalised interventions cannot substitute or replace the medical prescriptions and therapies doc in any way, instead, they will support both the patients in doing their daily activities and the clinicians or caregivers assisting them. Also, the SMART BEAR platform will deliver messages inviting the user to schedule an appointment with a doctor in the worst cases.

The description of Hearing Loss and its treatment is provided here in Sect. 5.3.1, demonstrating how the clinical knowledge is exploited in SMART BEAR to perform a specific training or collecting massive data from the devices in a fully transparent way for the patients. In the case of Balance Disorders, some patients will benefit from HOLOBalance https://holobalance.eu/., which is a virtual coaching platform for performing physiotherapy sessions and the description is provided here in 5.3.2.

5.3.1 Hearing Loss

Hearing Loss (HL) is affecting one out of three people over 65, while debilitating HL is observed in 6% of the global population (466 million people) [12]. It is currently estimated that, by 2050, HL will affect more than 900 million people, reaching 10% of the global population. Its management cost is estimated at 213 billion Euros for the European countries and 750 billion dollars, per annum, globally.

HL should not be considered an isolated health problem. Apart from the associated financial cost, HL is related to significant comorbidities as well. According to the Global Burden of Disease study, it is one of the 8 leading causes of living years with disability [13]. Multiple studies imply association of hearing impairment with psychological and physical diseases, such as cognitive disorders and dementia (reduction in cognitive performance associated with a 25 dB elevation of hearing threshold is equivalent to the reduction associated with an age difference of 7 years [14]), anxiety and depression [15] and higher mortality rate [16].

Although the only available and validated management solution that currently exists for HL is the fitting and use of hearing assistive devices, only 20% of the people needing one will seek, acquire, and continue using it [17, 18]. Key points to the efficacy of the use of such assistive devices, to the satisfaction and improvement of quality of life of their users and thus the minimization of drop-out risk is their proper fitting, the affordability, and accessibility of the follow-up services, and their proper combination with thorough and evidence-based personalized counseling and training.

   The principal goal in current hearing aid fitting practices is the improvement of patients' overall quality of life. This improvement is significantly related to patients' participation in daily activities and to their listening ability [19]. Modern counseling is trying to take into account both these parameters, which are not static but rather change over time, by means of extensive interviews and frequent follow-ups. Nevertheless, recall bias, assessment in office conditions and limited time make optimal HAs configuration according to patients' individual needs still very challenging [17, 20, 21]. Therefore, "real-life" monitoring of patients' hearing and cognitive capacity, medical, and behavioral assessment in a continuous way is an important element of HA fitting, fine-tuning, and counseling [22, 23]. Consequently, it is evident that achieving the goal of hearing aid fitting and thus hearing rehabilitation demands knowledge, active monitoring, and dynamic adaptation of many more factors than the pure tone audiogram of the patients. Furthermore, although hearing assisting devices remain the main current approach for hearing rehabilitation and improvement of communication and life quality in Hearing Loss, there is evidence that additional practices, such as Auditory or cognitive Training (AT), may be able to elicit optimal conditions for neural plasticity and associated improvements in cognitive function [24]. SMART BEAR is by default designed to address all the aforementioned requirements for optimal hearing loss management and rehabilitation.

   In SMART BEAR, we are addressing Hearing Loss through 12-month continuous monitoring of each HL participant (collection of heterogeneous data, such as demographics, audiometric data, information about the use of their HA or their performance on serious cognitive games or the auditory training, cognitive status, mental status, habits, biological and other information) through sensors and face-to-face and remote counseling and fitting/remote fine-tuning sessions with the audiologists of the project. A total of 1000 HL patients (200 patients per pilot) will be included in the study during a 2-year period. During their initial assessment, those HL participants will undergo otoscopy, tympanometry, pure tone audiometry (according to the British Society of Audiology standards). Moreover, their lifetime noise exposure will be estimated through a structured interview with the help of the clinician. According to the observations of this assessment, SMART BEAR audiologists will fit the SMART BEAR hearing aid unilaterally or bilaterally, according to each participant's needs. Fitting protocol and HA model will be common for all 1000 HL participants and will follow the common fitting practices. Moreover, HL participants will have access to the SMART BEAR Auditory Training mobile application and will be encouraged to complete a certain number of sessions (minimum 1 per week). During the project, according to predefined rules set by the SMART BEAR clinical researchers and based on previous literature and EVOTION experience, participants will be notified about how efficiently they are using their HA and about their performance on auditory training. According to the same rules, they will also receive notifications on how to improve their overall adherence to their hearing rehabilitation program (hearing aid +/− AT +/− serious cognitive games, etc). Predefined rules are currently based on established clinical guidelines. An example of such an evidence-based, predefined management scenario

Table 5.1   Interventions of the SMART BEAR platform for patients with HL

Scenarios*	Intervention	Frequency
Module A—HA compliance (Hours of usage)		
A1. Hours of usage within the target (>=10h per day)	A1. Green code: congratulating message through the SMART BEAR App	A1. Daily
A2. Hours of usage below the target (<10h per day)	A2. Yellow code: reminder of target hours of HA usage	A2. Daily
A3. Hours of usage below the target (<10h per day) on weekly average	A3. Yellow code: advice to consult SMART BEAR audiologist	A3. Weekly
A4. Hours of usage below the target (<10h per day) on weekly average for 2 consecutive weeks	A4. Red code: advice to consult SMART BEAR audiologist and repeat counselling or fine tuning	A4. Biweekly
PM1, PM4 and PM5 may affect this scenario: e.g., High levels of satisfaction in correlation with other than 10h of usage could modify this scenario; 10h is based on previous literature		
Module B—manual changes of HA program		
B1. Average number of manual changes of HA program per day over week, within accepted limits	B1. Green code: congratulating message	B1. Weekly
B2. High average number of manual changes of HA per day over a week	B2. Yellow code: Advice to consult SMART BEAR Audiologist and repeat counselling or fine tuning	B2. Weekly
* PM9 may affect this scenario: e.g., limits of number of manual changes of program may be altered during the project, according to their relationship to (GHABP) [24] satisfaction scores degrees of hearing loss, hours of usage, hours of usage in environments with various noise levels or other hearing-related factors and according to their relationship with other parameters, such as participant' comorbidities, age, sex, etc.		
Module C—auditory training (AT) compliance		
C1. Completion of target number of AT sessions per week	C1. Green code: congratulating message	C1. Weekly
C2. Omission of one AT session	C2. Green code: reminder that one AT session was missed. Reminder of benefits of AT	C2. Daily
C3. Omission of the AT sessions for a week	C3. Yellow code: advice to consult SMART BEAR audiologist	C3. Weekly
C4. Omission of the AT sessions for two consecutive weeks	C4. Red Code: advice to consult SMART BEAR audiologist	C4. Biweekly
* PM2, PM3 and PM6 may affect this scenario: e.g., the number of target AT sessions per week could be adjusted according to relations discover between AT adherence and satisfaction scores (GHABP), degrees of hearing loss, hours of usage, hours of usage in environments with various noise levels or other hearing-related factors and according to their relationship with other parameters, such as participant's comorbidities, age, sex, etc.		

for patients with Hearing Loss is provided in Table 5.1, along with the possible clinical implications ML-analysis outcomes could have. Variables that will be assessed throughout the project are reported in Tables 5.2, 5.3, 5.4, 5.5, and 5.6.

In particular, during the project, dynamic analysis of the collected data prediction models will be developed in order to enable a better understanding of those factors that play a significant role in the success of a hearing rehabilitation program:

PM1   Identification of those characteristics that make patients more prone to drop out and quit using their hearing aid (*Prediction model for HA dropouts*).

PM2   Identification of those characteristics that make patients more prone to drop out from their rehabilitation program (AT) (*Prediction model for hearing rehabilitation dropouts*).

PM3   Identification of those characteristics that can predict patients' adherence (number of sessions) to AT (*Prediction model for AT adherence*).

PM4   Identification of those characteristics that make patients more prone to use their hearing aid efficiently long during the day (*Prediction model for hearing aid hours of usage*).

PM5   Identification of those factors augmenting the satisfaction of patients from using their hearing aid (*Prediction model for HA usage satisfaction*).

PM6   Identification of those characteristics that make patients more prone to perform better in AT tasks (*Prediction model for AT performance*).

PM7   Identification of those factors decreasing the number of needed face-to-face sessions with their Audiologist for counseling and/or hearing aid fine-tuning (*Prediction model for a number of visits at the Audiologist's office*).

PM8   Identification of those factors decreasing the number of needed remote sessions with their Audiologist for counseling and/or hearing aid fine-tuning (*Prediction model for some remote fine-tuning sessions with the Audiologist*).

PM9   Identification of those factors decreasing the number of manual changes of hearing aid program (as an indication of poor sound quality and bad adaptation of hearing aid configuration to patients' real needs and daily challenges, *Prediction model for a number of changes of hearing aid program*).

As a results, our findings shall provide insights on the optimal way patients with hearing loss should be classified into patients of high or low risk of hearing rehabilitation dropout, patients with higher probability to benefit from the hearing aids or the AT, patients that will likely seek more frequently the remote or face-to-face help of their Audiologist. This newly gained insight will help the SMART BEAR clinical researchers in two directions:

1. Optimization of the SMART BEAR DSS will be considered. Following validation for their safety and relevance by SMART BEAR clinicians, models will be evaluated in the production environment. In other words, knowledge gained through the analysis will be evaluated by the SMART BEAR clinical researchers for its relevance and its safety and then it will be directly implemented in the SMART BEAR project.

2. New research hypotheses will be created and shall be tested in the context of future clinical trials.

Table 5.2 Outcome variables for hearing loss—related prediction models

Prediction models	Outcome variables	Acronym	Description	Value type
PM1 dropouts	Dropout number	DROPOUT	No. participants who stopped using the hearing aid (HA)	Integer
	Dropout	DROP	Dropout of HA usage, as no usage for more than 7 consecutive days	YES/NO
PM2 hearing rehabilitation dropouts	Drop out of auditory train. (AT)	DROPAT	No. session of AT for 3 consecutive days	YES/NO
PM3 AT adherence	AT sessions per week	AT	no. AT sessions per week	Integer
PM4 hearing aid active use	Time of HA usage	HAUSAGE	Average time of usage	Minutes/day
PM5 hearing aid satisfaction	Overall HA usage satisfaction satisfaction	GHABP	Score on GHABP	Integer
PM6 AT performance	AT score	ATSCORE	Average score of AT sessions till that particular point	Integer
PM7 no. visits at the Audiologist's office office	Visits to audiologist's office	VISIT	No. necessary audiologist's visits to the audiologist's office	Integer
PM8 Remote fine tuning sessions with the audiologist	Remote sessions with the audiologist	FINETUN	No. necessary remote meetings for counselling or remote fine tuning with the audiologist	Integer
PM9 changes of HA program	Need for manual change of HA program by the user	PROGR	No. changes of HA program per day till that point	Integer

5.3.2   Balance Disorders

Basic human behaviors such as maintaining posture at rest and in motion, keeping clear vision while moving and navigating through complex urban environments, are highly sophisticated functions. They rely on the harmonized integration of afferent sensory signals, mainly from visual, vestibular and musculoskeletal systems, within the Central Nervous System. Common everyday activities, such as walking and talking to the phone, demand additional attention, and thus specific cognitive functions, named as executive function, plays a crucial role for normal postural control.

Unavoidably entropy forces these functions to decline over the years, making age related progressive loss of sensory information one of the major factors responsible for the increase in fall risks in older adults [43]. Comorbidities like sarcopenia, cognitive impairment, neurogenerative diseases, ageing vision, polypharmacy, mood disorders, decreased intrinsic motivation, deprives elderly from proper sensory re-weighting. As a result, physical inactivity and increased sedentary time produce a continuous spiral of organs degeneration leading to additional functional impairments, fear of falling and eventually frailty [44]. These factors raise the risk of injury-related falling and interfere with the body's effort to restore homeostasis [45].

Table 5.3 Covariates—predictor variables for hearing loss

Covariates	Acronym	Description	Value type
Time	TIMEC	Time as continuous variable in order to link each data item to specific time points	Continuous
Age	AGE	Years of age	Years
Biological gender	SEX	Female or male	F/M
Hearing loss type	HLTYPE	Predefined text for specific types of hearing loss	–
Hearing loss chronicity	HLCHRNCTY	Years since diagnosis of hearing loss	Years
Side of hearing loss	SIDE	Right, left, bilateral	–
Ear side	EAR	Right/left (in	Order to correspond HL/fitting)
Fitting side	FIT	Right/left/bilateral	–
Degree of hearing loss	HLDGREE	Predefined text for clinician to choose according to part. pure tone audiogram	–
Baseline pure tone threshold per frequency for right ear	PTAR	Mean value of PTA threshold at 0.5–4 kHz (right ear)	dB HL
Baseline pure tone threshold per frequency for left ear	PTAL	Mean value of PTA threshold at 0.5–4 kHz (left ear)	dB HL
Baseline pure tone threshold per frequency for right ear	PTAR0.5-8kHz	Mean value of PTA threshold at 0.5–8kHz (right ear)	dB HL
Baseline pure tone threshold per frequency for left ear	PTAL0.5-8kHz	Mean value of PTA threshold at 0.5–8kHz (left ear)	dB HL
Drop out	DROP	Dropout of HA usage	YES/NO
Time of HA usage	HAUSE	Average time of usage per day till that particular point	Minutes
Number of visits to audiologist's office	VISITS	Number of necessary visits to the audiologist's office	Integer
Overall HA usage satisfaction	GHABP	Total score on GHABP and per situation	Integer
Percentage of usage per environment	ENVRNMT	Average percentage of time spent in the predefined environments per day	%
Noise exposure	NOISE	Average noise exposure per day	dB SPL × Time AND dB TWA
Manual adjustments of volume	VOLUME	Average number of manual adjustments of volume by the part	Integer
Manual adjustments of program	PROGRAM	Average number of manual adjustments of programs (already loaded on the HA)by the participant	Integer

Table 5.4 Covariates—predictor variables for hearing loss

Covariates	Acronym	Description	Value type
Age	AGE	Years of age	Years
Age group	AGEGROUP	Per 5 years (65–70, 71–75, 76–80)	–
Biological gender	SEX	Female or male	F/M https://bit.ly/ 35jmbwQ
Ethnicity	ETHNOS	Predefined text for ethnic groups	–
Education level	EDU	Predefined text for education levels (categorical)	–
Living situation	LIVST	Predefined text for living status (categorical)	–
Diabetes (Mellitus)	DM	Predefined text for diabetes type (categorical)	–
Diabetes	DIABETES	Diagnosis or not of diabetes of any type	*YES/NO*
Hearing loss	HL	Diagnosis of hearing loss of any type	*YES/NO*
Fall over the last 12 months	FALL	Occurrence of fall during the last 12 months	*YES/NO*
Number of falls over the last 12 months	FALLS	Number of falls during the last	Integer
Weight Loss	WL	Unexplained significant weight loss during the last 12 months	*YES/NO*
Depression disorder	DPRSSN	Diagnosis of depressive disorder of any type/degree	*YES/NO*
Anxiety disorder	ANX	Diagnosis of anxiety disorder of any type/degree	*YES/NO*
Other medical history	MH	Diagnosis of any other comorbidity	*YES/NO*
Cognitive issues	CGNT	Diagnosis of cognitive issues of any type	*YES/NO*
CVD history	CVD	Diagnosis of CVD of any type	*YES/NO*
Score of geriatric depression scale [25]	GDS	Total score of GDS	Integer
Dexterity question (From HUI3 questionnaire)[26]	DXT	Score	Integer
MOCA questionnaire[27]	MOCA	Total score	Integer
MOCA—Alternating trail making	MOCA1	Alternating trail making relevant question score—Q1	Integer

According to the WHO global report, one out of three people older than 65 years old fall each year and this prevalence increases for people older than 70 years old. Falls are the second leading cause of accidental death after road traffic accidents. In the EU, an average of 35,848 older adults (65 and above) are reported to have died on an annual basis due to serious injuries caused by falls. This figure is expected to be an underestimation of the true deathly falls rate which probably is much higher. A recent study analyzing data from more than 200 hospitals from across Europe has estimated that every year within the EU, 3.8 million older people attend emergency

Table 5.5 Covariates—predictor variables for hearing loss

Covariates	Acronym	Description	Value type
MOCA visuoconstructional skills	MOCA2-3	Sum of visuoconstructional skills relevant questions score—Q1 and Q2	Integer
MOCA—naming	MOCA4	Naming related question score—Q4	Integer
MOCA—Memory 1st trial	MOCA51	Memory related question score—Q5 1st trial	Integer
MOCA—Memory 2nd trial	MOCA52	Memory related question score—Q5 2nd trial	Integer
MOCA—attention	MOCA6-8	Sum of attention-related questions score—Q6-8	Integer
MOCA—attention	MOCA9-10	Sum of language-related questions score—Q9-10	Integer
MOCA—abstraction	MOCA11	Abstraction-related question score—Q11	Integer
MOCA—delayed recall	MOCA12	Delayed recall-related question score—Q12	Integer
MOCA memory index score (MIS)	MIS	MIS score	Integer
MOCA—orientation	MOCA13	Orientation-related questions score—Q13	Integer
Drinking OH	OH	Average units per day (self-reported)	OH Units
Smoking habits	SMOKING	Pack of smoked cigarettes per day × years of active smoking	Pack years
PHQ-9 questionnaire [28]	PHQ9	Score	Integer
MDPQ questionnaire [29]	MDPQ	Score	Integer
EQ-5D questionnaire [30]	EQ5D	Score	Integer
FES-I questionnaire [31]	FESI	Score	Integer
EFS questionnaire [32]	EFS	Score	Integer
Godin leisure time questionnaire [33]	GLTQ GLTQ	Score score	Integer
Single item sleep scale [34]	SSQ	Score	Integer
IADL questionnaire [35]	IADL	Score	Integer
RGA questionnaire [36]	RGA	Score	Integer
FGA questionnaire [37]	FGA	Score	Integer
Mini BEST questionnaire [38]	MBEST	Score	Integer
RAPA questionnaire [39]	RAPA	Score	Integer
ABC questionnaire [40]	ABC	Score	Integer
MNA questionnaire [41]	MNA	Score	Integer
HEART score [42]	HEART	Score	Integer
Diastolic blood pressure	DIASTLC	mmHg	Integer
Systolic blood pressure	SYSTLC	mmHg	Integer
Heart pulse	PULSE	Number of heart beats per min	Integer
Irregular heart beat	IRR	Detection of irregularity in heart rate	Integer, 0= not present, 1=present
Number of episodes of irregular heart beat	IRRN	Number of episodes of irregularity of heart beat till that time point	Integer

Table 5.6 Covariates—predictor variables for hearing loss

Covariates	Acronym	Description	Value type
Body temperature	Tbody		°C, integer
Body weight	BW	Timestamped AND average body weight per week	kg, floating point
Body fat	BF	Timestamped AND average body fat per week	%, floating point
Body mass index (BMI) (advertised)	BMI	$weight/height^2$, Timestamped AND average per week	Floating point
Body water	BWATER	Timestamped AND average per week	%, floating point
Body lean mass (advertised)	BLM	Timestamped AND average per week	kg, floating point
Body muscle mass	BMM	Timestamped AND average per week	kg, floating point
Blood oxygen saturation	Bloodoxygen	Timestamped and average per day and per week	%, integer
No. desaturation episodes	DESATURATION	$SaO_2 < 92\%$ episodes	Integer
Active kcal (dietary cal.) burned through actual movement and activity during the monitoring per period	ActiveKilocalories	Average per day	kcal, integer
Cumulative duration of activities of moderate intensity, lasting at least	moderateIntensity DurationInSeconds 600 s at a time. Moderate intensity as activity with MET value range 3–6	Average per day	Seconds, integer
Minimum of heart rate values captured during the monitoring period, in beats per minute	minHeartRate InBeatsPerMinute	Per day	BPM, integer
Average of heart rate values captured during the last 7 days,in beats per minute	averageHeartRate InBeatsPerMinute	Per week	BPM, integer
Average heart rate at rest during the monitoring period, in beats per minute	restingHeartRate InBeatsPerMinute	Timestamped Timestamped	BPM, integer BPM, integer

departments (ED) with a fall-related injury; 1.4 million people need to be admitted to hospital for further treatment [46]. This fact makes falls the predominant cause (58%) of injury-related to ED attendances and costs to the EU at least 25 billion euros every year [46, 47]. As the population of the elderly in Europe is expected to grow by 60% by 2050, the number of fall-related deaths is expected to increase to almost 60,000 by 2050. This could result in annual fall-related expenditures exceeding 45 billion euros by the year 2050. Vestibular deficits are diagnosed in the majority of the fallers, since 80% of the adults with an unexpected fall suffer by an inner ear pathology affecting postural control [48]. Older adults with moderate cognitive impairment tend to fall twice as often as older adults with no cognitive decline [49].

The necessity to develop more efficient prevention strategies is widely recognized [50]. Worldwide interest has been focused on promotion of physical activity, muscle strengthening, gait and balance physiotherapy and cognitive training as the major pillars integrating to a multi-factorial, physical rehabilitation protocol, targeting falls prevention. Additionally, vision management, for the avoidance of further sensorial deprivation, concomitant medication for the identification of side effects or potential interactions, are functions that should be assessed in the context of an individualized multifactorial integrated solution [50].

A balance exercise regime, provided by a physiotherapy and/or a certified health professional, is an effective method for reducing the postural instability [51], symptoms arising from vestibular deficits [52], fear of falling and eventually falls [53] as well as for increasing functionality, physical activity and consequently social participation. Balance rehabilitation protocols are either personalized [54] and/or home-based [55] consisting of a multi-sensory set of exercises, having as a goal the re-weighting of sensory inputs, central nervous adaptation, coordination of the body segments, optimal selection of postural adjustments, strengthening and stretching used as appropriate. Both types of intervention are considered as a safe and effective treatment methods and minor side effects have reported.

Supervision promotes adherence to the program, ideally improving it, but its absence increases the withdrawal rates from rehabilitation protocols [56, 57]. Additionally, low levels of motivation [58], lack of information regarding on health benefits gained from targeted exercise [59], lack of specialized health care personnel and socio-economic factors [60] raise barriers to adherence.

Nowadays, most of the efficient falls prevention rehabilitation programs involve either a group-based practice or a home-based exercise regime [61] producing benefits in functional ability and mobility, without any reported clinically important difference [62]. The OTAGO exercise program (OEP) it is a well described falls prevention program, flexible in its implementation, which can be either home or community based. It consists of warm up and cool down phase, strengthening balance and gait exercises as the main pillars of the program, and can be performed either on a group or in personal [63–65]. It is a well-documented and structured tool, disseminated widely to the physiotherapy community as it offers a significant reduction of morbidity and mortality and falls for the participants in a one-year prevalence time [66]. Participants usually perform the exercises at least three times per week at home with each session last no more than 30 min. The closest supervision is performed by the clinician in the first 8 weeks of the program which is suggested to last in total 12 months. In order to promote more efficient outcomes, OEP is also given as an illustrated booklet in four different levels of difficulty (beginners, intermediate, advanced and experts). Several modified versions of OEP including augmented reality [67], extra exercise modules [68, 69] or a DVD [70] are targeting to increase efficiency through more customized approaches. As far as we know, there was not a solely personalized solution in order to overcome hazards arising during the assessment and /or intervention for people with Balance Disorders, that took into account all the aforementioned factors.

HOLOBalance is a beyond the state-of-the-art, virtual coaching platform for engaging patients with recorded falls and/or tendency to fall, into a multimodal balance and gait physiotherapy exercise protocol, including balance and gait exercises, gamified exercises, cognitive games, auditory training and a physical activity application designed and performed by a multidisciplinary consortium (otolaryngologists,
physiotherapists, neurologists, gerontologists) provides participants with individualized exercises according to their needs by displaying a 3d hologram reproducing a physiotherapist via an augmented reality environment. Data from motion capture sensors and wearable sensors (smart bracelet, smart glasses, pressure insoles) are feeding AI algorithms for exercise performance, behavioral analysis in terms of frustration, and a Decision Support System for progression of the exercise plan. These deep reinforcement learning models are continuously updating the patients' profiles with respect to their compliance to the exercises, their performance and their longitudinal progress, providing feedback to the clinicians through platform's dashboard. The HOLOBalance ecosystem through its multi-layer modules helps users comply with their treatment plan and coach them in order to achieve maximum effect [71].

On the SMART BEAR platform, Balance Disorders are monitored and discriminated through a six steps ruled-based screening procedure:

1. A history of previous falls
2. Medications intake
3. Presence of at least two of the following symptoms: unsteadiness, motion sickness, oscillopsia, difficulty walking on uneven surfaces, difficulty walking in the darkness, drunken feeling, lightheadedness, disorientation, tendency to fall
4. A score greater than 9 in the short form of Falls Efficacy Scale- International [72]
5. Abnormal score at least on the Timed Up and Go test [73] (AND/OR)
6. Abnormal score on the Romberg test on foam are the indications for a more detailed functional assessment of postural control.

SMART BEAR participants with confirmed balance disorders will be considered eligible for one of the two interventions offered during a multi-centre clinical study for balance rehabilitation, HOLOBalance intervention at home and OEP intervention via a mobile phone, lasting for eight consecutive weeks.

The OEP intervention is a fully automated modified version of the fall's prevention program described above. The training preparation procedure is defined in Algorithm 1. Specific scenarios were developed for addressing issues that may arise from the occurrence of yellow and red flags or CVDs-related and/or issues related to compliance and safe implementation of the OEP program (muscle soreness, persistent pain, chest pain, severe dizziness, shortness of breath, fall). These scenarios are addressed with messages in compliance to Algorithm 2. Predefined rules for progressing levels had been also established and are described in Algorithm 3.

The HOLOBalance has already been proved a safe, feasible and effective intervention. Its implementation to a larger sample size will give a better understanding

Table 5.7 The prediction models for HOLOBalance

Prediction models	Outcome variables	Description	Modelling tools	Expected impact relevant actions
PM1 HOLOBalance outcome measures improvement	HOLOBalance score	Average score for each performed exercise	Random Forest + SHAP (Explainability) instances: daily usage data	Patients with high expected outcome will be endorsed. Patients with low expected benefit will be considered for a more intensive training
PM2 HOLOBalance deviation in exercises performance	Number and degree of dedication in exercises, in terms of speed, range of movement and duration	Average number of reported symptoms for each performed exercise	Bayesian classifier+time series instances: dropout patients	Deviations which do not affect the outcome will be adapted. Exercises will be optimised and re-evaluated if the thresholds in speed, range and repetitions are effective
PM3 HOLOBalance technical issues	Technicians' involvement	Number of times technicians should be involved in HOLOBalance operation remotely	Random Forest + SHAP (Explainability) instances: daily usage data	Increased time and effort for education and explanation will be allocated during initial assessment
PM4 HOLOBalance occurrence of symptoms related to time	This model will predict the onset of symptoms during the exercises	Severity of symptoms provoked by the completion of the exercises (mild-moderate-severe) and recorded by the HOLOBalance platform with voice recognition	Bayesian classifier+generative models instances: dropout patients	Reduced time for particular exercises will be considered if symptom occurrence is predicted.HOLOBalance will stop an exercise a few seconds before any symptoms occur automatically. (generic time 1 min)

of parameters and patient profiles that could affect outcome on a beyond the-state-of-the-art balance rehabilitation program delivered in a mixed reality environment. The prediction models which will be developed are presented in Table 5.7. Following the same brainstorming procedure, clinical researchers developed prediction models for analyzing data collecting for the implementation of the OEP intervention in order to understand not only the factors that could affect outcome but also variables which will determine the profile of the people who will benefit the most as well as safety and Optimization.

Algorithm 1 OTAGO training preparation scenarios

---

if All features are within optimal range on daily average /weekly average / average of 2 consecutive days measurements **then**

    Practice is allowed - The following message will appear:

    Allow to practice. Please proceed.

end if

if BP values are outside the optimal range (yellow code in case of CVDs) in average daily /weekly average / average of 2 consecutive weeks measurements **then**

    Te following message will appear

    BP levels seems to be out of range. Ask for clinician's permission. Proceed with caution.

end if

if BP values are outside of optimal levels of CVDs at any time point **then**

    Red alert - Practice is not allowed - The following message will appear:

    Enter is not allowed. Please ask for help.

end if

if A fall has occurred on practice day **then**

    if The clinician has allowed the exercise **then**

        Practice is allowed with caution - The following message will appear:

        Exercise with caution. Do you have freed up the space where you will exercise? (YES/NO)

        if YES **then**

            Please have fully hand support despite the level of the platform.

            Set off the messages

        end if

    else

        Red alert - The following message will appear:

        Enter is not allowed. Please ask for help.

    end if

end if

if The user is experiencing a persistent pain OR severe shortness of breath OR significant unsteadiness on a scale 1-10 **then**

    Red alert - Practice is not allowed - The following message will appear:

    Enter is not allowed. Please ask for help.

else

    if Score 0-5 out of 10 **then**

        Access is allowed

    else

        if Score 6-7 out of 10 **then**

            Practice is allowed with caution - The following message will appear:

            Fully hand support despite the level of perform. Exercise with caution.

        end if

    end if

end if

Algorithm 2 Rules for Messages

---

while Doing exercises **do**
    Are you feeling well? (YES/NO)
    if no answer for $>$ 1 minute **then**
        Screen will switch off
        Recorded action will be $NOCOMPLIANCE$
    end if
    if answer = YES **then**
        Proceed
    end if
    if Answer = NO **then**
        The following messages will appear:
        Q1. Are you experiencing joints/muscles pain during exercises? (YES/NO)
        if Answer = NO **then**
            Proceed
        else
            if Answer = YES **then**
                Please check your position for proper performance
            end if
        end if
        if no answer for $>$ 1 minute **then**
            Screen will switch off
            Recorded action will be $NOCOMPLIANCE$
        end if
        Q2. Are you experiencing chest pain? (YES/NO)
        if Answer = NO **then**
            Proceed
        else
            if Answer = YES **then**
                The user has to ask for medical advice
            end if
        end if
        if no answer for $>$ 1 minute **then**
            Screen will switch off
            Recorded action will be $NOCOMPLIANCE$
        end if
        Q3. Are you experiencing severe dizziness? (YES/NO)
        if Answer = NO **then**
            Proceed
        else
            if Answer = YES **then**
                The user has to ask for medical advice
            end if
        end if
    end if
end while

Algorithm 3 Rules for Level Progression in the OTAGO training

---

if in 3 consecutive sessions question answer in A6 scenario < 2/10 **then**
    ADD the following message in same session:
    Do you feel that you could perform the balance exercises easily? (YES/NO)
end if
if *Y ES* **then**
    proceed to the next level
else
    if *N O* **then**
        Keep the same level, repeat the question above in the next session
    end if
end if

5.4   Initial Implementation and Testing

Five large-scale pilots, spanning across six different countries (Greece, Italy, Portugal, France, Spain, Romania), will be developed to demonstrate project achievements, recruiting 5100 elderly participants. The research project and its protocol are designed under the same philosophy in all involved pilot countries.

As said above, the Pilot of Pilots in Madeira, Portugal, is a smaller pilot that will include 100 patients to demonstrate, early in the project, the concept feasibility prior to the kick-off of the large-scale ones. It has the main objective to test the first release of the SMART BEAR technical infrastructure, and demonstrate the synergies implemented with other EU projects such as Smart4Health[24] and HOLOBalance, highlighting mutual cooperation and interaction between complementary solutions.

Concerning the synergies, Smart4Health aims to empower EU Citizens with an interoperable and exchangeable European Electronic Health Record (EHR) that will allow EU citizens to be active participants in managing their own health: in particular the synergy with Smart4Health focused on the Low Back Pain (LBP), which is included as additional condition [74].

The initial phases of the PoP were more of technical nature, configuring the necessary infrastructure for secure data collection from low-back pain and balance rehabilitation programs in the frame of the synergies. The selection and preparation of the wearable devices have been among the main activities, proving the initial sets of data for the SMART BEAR platform to provide early analytics and personalization strategies.

An initial demographics assessment of the target population was made to prepare the patient recruitment and a small-scale procurement has been done according to the estimates of comorbidities. At the time of writing, with a few months into the patient monitoring phase, 22 elderly participants were recruited and fully evaluated in the baseline assessment, providing individual medical background to the SMART BEAR platform.

---

[24] https://smart4health.eu/en/.

During the baseline assessment the candidates share their demographics information with the clinicians and they are visited by them based on their clinical history.

All the candidate participants must be of age between 65 and 80 years old and their clinical history including at least two of the following conditions: Hearing Loss, Cardio Vascular Diseases, Cognitive Impairments, Mental Health Issues, and Balance Disorders, as well as Frailty.

In order for the research to be compliant with the GDPR, the clinicians must provide clear information about the SMART BEAR project to the candidates, in particular concerning the data to be collected. An Informed Consent Form (ICF) signed by the candidates as a statement of the willingness to participate to the subsequent phases of the project.

Concerning the case of the Pilot of the Pilots all the patients have LBP in addition to two other comorbidities, 18 of them are already following the Smart4Health MedX physiotherapy sessions protocol, and three the HOLOBalance program, hence are sharing data between projects and demonstrating the technical synergies. In addition, over 18,000 observations have been collected from the wearable devices and more than 400 questionnaires are available in the data repository. Also two specific ICFs must be handed for the participants to express their willingness to participate respectively to the HOLOBalance and Smart4Health projects.

5.4.1   Data Insights on the Platform

The triggered clinical activities were enough to collect the first impressions from the clinical team. Data resulting from SMART BEAR will undoubtedly be promising, allowing a better understanding of the health of the elderly and helping in the future to establish predictive data associated with the comorbidities under study and their interaction with one another, creating personalized data for better and sustainable population aging. Thus, SMART BEAR could pave the way for new trends at the primary health care level allowing an early and predictive intervention within the comorbidities under analysis. Up to the moment, with the numbers involved, the analytic models provided in Sect. 5.3.1 is under development and the team is confident they will improve significantly during the project duration as it is possible to verify through the continuous updates to the platform being released on a periodic basis.

As described in Sect. 5.2.3.4, one of the key challenges of the project is to develop an easy-to-use Dashboard to provide clinicians access to all key capabilities of the platform, including data management or data analytics functionality, support decision making, and interventions, through different types of visualization techniques. The Dashboard is being used to register participants and upload assessments results and questionnaires and is providing some baseline descriptive analytics.

On the top left side of Fig. 5.5, one can see the navigation menu of the Dashboard, providing data directly taken from the first testing activities. The home page is the entry point for the clinician and displays a number of insights on the data being collected as well as some descriptive analytics.

On the top center of the figure, the clinicians have access to a simple pie chart where they can see the distribution of patients per comorbidity. For instance, at the moment 18 patients marked with LBP (33.96% of the sum of comorbidities in patients with data) are already sending data corresponding to back pain. This number corresponds to the patients that have initiated the MedX exercises.

Also, going into the detail of the observations being collected per device type per day, visible in the bottom left side of Fig. 5.5, the variation of the observations being taken by the patients becomes clear. As expected, the number of readings from the Smart Blood pressure monitor is higher than the ones from the smart scale, which according to the clinical protocol are expected to be taken once a week. Nevertheless, the numbers of the blood pressure readings are lower than expected. Each patient should take at least one measurement per day (the clinical protocol of SMART BEAR recommends two), and since the PoP has 17 patients with Cardiovascular Diseases that have already received a Blood pressure monitoring device, this figure highlights that not all patients are complying with the expected measurements and they should be contacted.

The Dashboard also provides a quick outlook on some health and well-being indicators (right side of Fig. 5.5). Indicators such as average body mass index, calculated using the initial assessment data and the collected weight from the smart scales use, physical activity, calculated using smartwatch data, or questionnaire results analysis per patient profile are already available. MoCA questionnaire results distributed by age group illustrate that in the group between 70 and 79 years old, MoCA results are lower, with zero questionnaires scoring above 26. Predictive analytics are currently being developed and not yet available for the PoP public use, which will allow automatic understanding and provision of interventions based on the collected data.

5.4.2 Data Insights on the SB@App

Discussions with the recruited participants reveal that they are overall satisfied with the technological solutions presented. They seem to have the general feeling of empowerment for their health and are effectively active on the path to healthy and independent living, seeking alternative solutions to monitor their health conditions. Participants recognize the innovative solution presented and the effectiveness of the equipment. They also note that the delivered devices are new-generation ones, making it possible to collect information that they would otherwise have no way of obtaining. On the downside, dealing with technology is often challenging for the elderly, and participants often struggle with uploading and updating data, device synchronization issues, and the number of tasks to perform daily with SMART BEAR that sometimes is overwhelming for them (e.g. too many devices and too many measurements). Fewer devices will probably produce better long-term results.

Through the SB@App, the patient has access to all the data being collected by the wearable devices and the SB@Home kit. As depicted in Fig. 5.7, it is possible to see live measurements as, for instance, the weight ("peso" in Portuguese) collected by the Smart scale, daily statistics such as sleep statistics ("estatisticas do sono" in

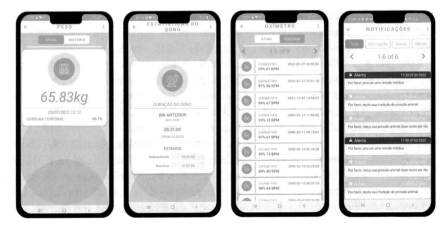

Fig. 5.7 SB app interface (Portuguese version)

Portuguese), collected by the smartwatch, or even historical data on oxygen levels collected by the oximeter ("oximetro"). All these data are interesting for the patients so that they can regularly check their health parameters. The values are then shared with the SMART BEAR platform and become part of the FHIR repository. Using such data, the BDA Engine component of the platform can send back notifications to the mobile app. As illustrated in Fig. 5.7 (right side), there are three types of notifications: information, warnings represented by the yellow color, and alerts represented by the red color. The warnings related to insufficient blood pressure monitoring, hence the message states that the user should take the blood pressure twice a day ("por favor, meça a sua pressão arterial duas vezes por dia") and requests to repeat the measurement ("por favor, repita a sua medição de pressão arterial"). The alerts are generated in this case due to an abnormal value of blood pressure and request the patient to seek a medical review ("por favor, procure uma revisão médica"). The more serious warnings (alerts) are also being displayed in the clinicians' message board on the Dashboard.

5.5 Data Analytics

Getting value from data implies understanding how to acquire knowledge from them. More generally, we can state Science is the process of organizing knowledge from the particular to the general and from the general to the particular. In SMART BEAR this process is realized according to the principles of the *Knowledge Uplift Model* (KUM) illustrated in Fig. 5.8. The data generated by the SB platform offer *descriptive knowledge* on the observed population or specific patients. For example, we can report about the dropouts, i.e. the number of participants who stopped using the provided devices. Besides, we can report on specific results obtained by a patient, e.g.

Fig. 5.8 The knowledge uplift model adopted in SB

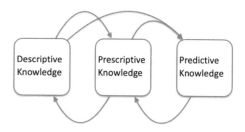

the `head turns per second` registered for a patient during a HOLOBalance physiotherapic exercise.

Descriptive knowledge can be turned to *prescriptive knowledge*. For example, triggering a notification to the case manager of the dropping out patients, or defining personalized exercise levels for a specific patient. Descriptive knowledge can be turned to *predictive knowledge* by using the collected data to verify specific hypotheses on the relationships between the observed factors. For example, creating predictive models to identify those factors that contribute to the prediction of the dropouts or to the number of tuning sections to set with the audiologist.

Predictive knowledge can also be exploited to generate prescriptive knowledge, for example defining a special communication plan for those patients with factors predicting dropout. Prescriptive knowledge also generates new descriptive knowledge when we observe the response to prescriptions. *Are the notified case managers able to reduce the dropout numbers? Is a patient with a personalized exercise level improving faster?* These examples clarify the KUM cycle can be continuously brought up.

In the context of medical research, the generic KUM of Fig. 5.8 can be further specified in terms of the data flow we have to support to drive it.

Even if in principle this process can significantly variate, depending on the needs, its concrete implementation in SMART BEAR follows the workflow described in Fig. 5.9. *Descriptive analytics* are initially identified to test the data quality. The SMART BEAR infrastructure acquires data from multiple sources such as device sensors and manually filled questionnaires. Sensors can have failures and send inaccurate data. A device can be disconnected or a user can refuse to fill a questionnaire. Data can be incomplete or not delivered in the appropriate time frame. Before including the records of a patient in data analytics a test is required to verify the required data quality level is achieved. Records not passing the test are excluded.

For example, Fig. 5.12 presents a dotted chart used to assess the completeness of sensor data. The collected observations are organized on a timeline, in our example with a periodicity of one day. Data imputation techniques can be considered to improve data completeness but supporting conditions must be verified. If we have a few missing observations we can apply multiple imputation if missing data are completely at random error on the effect size but not bias, if missing data are not at random the risk of bias is relevant [75].

A second assumption relates to the need of validating the feasibility of the prognostic models we want to verify based on the quality of the ML models we

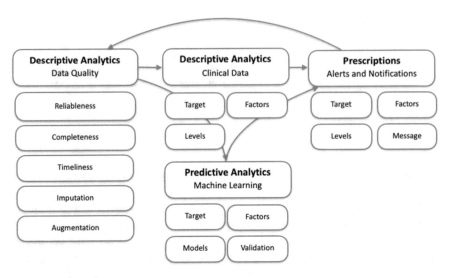

Fig. 5.9 The knowledge uplift model adopted in SB

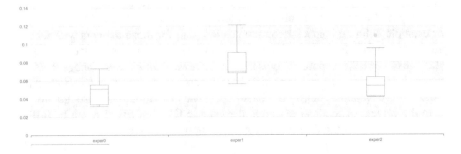

Fig. 5.10 Evaluating multiple predictive models

can expect given the data availability. The sample size must be evaluated with a temporal plan to define a credible timing for getting realistic volumes of data. We cannot plan using complex models if the data size is not appropriate. For example, experimental evidence from the literature [76] shows Random Forest is reliable with a sample size of 200 times the number of features in the feature space. This means once we know the sample size we can also identify the dimension of the feature space to be used and the modeling tool to select.

Figure 5.10, shows multiple predictive models on blood pressure evaluated using mean absolute percentage error (MAPE). More specifically, we tested an univariate model, a multivariable model, and a multivariable and multitarget model. Based on the best performance we obtained we can now select the model to be used in executing predictions. Figure 5.11, shows the predictive trend produced by the model for a specific patient (Fig. 5.12).

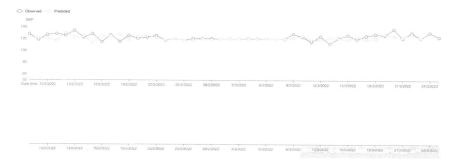

Fig. 5.11 Predicting the systolic blood pressure trend of a specific patient

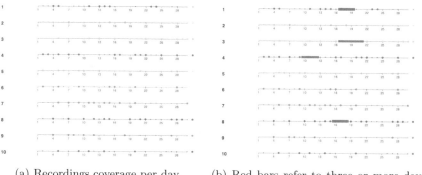

(a) Recordings coverage per day.   (b) Red bars refer to three or more days of missing values.

Fig. 5.12 Recordings coverage per day. The dimension of the dots refers to how many parts of the day are (i) recording in

5.6 Conclusion

Smart healthcare systems are based on wearable or IoT devices placed at the patients' homes. They are becoming more and more popular because the technology of such devices is mature enough and the costs are affordable. Moreover such systems are an attracting alternative to hospitalization of elderly people, especially those who need to be monitored for long-term non-acute diseases.

In this chapter, we have focused on the description of the e-Health platform provided by the SMART BEAR project, leading to a data-driven decision-making process supporting the creation of personalized interventions for the healthy ageing's sake. As described in Sect. 5.2, the SMART BEAR platform has been designed to collect data from a broad variety of devices handed to the patients, including smartphones, wearable devices and home sensors, and deliver interventions consisting of personalized notifications and alerts, in addition to specific training protocols, that are elaborated on the basis of the data collected.

The next step will be to implement the ML-based algorithms to provide and adjust the threshold values triggering the intervention delivery in the course of the monitoring, nonetheless some the rule-based interventions are already available for CVDs and are triggered if the collected data do not comply with the value or range to be set by the clinicians from the beginning.

Concerning the implementation of the clinical interventions according to the protocol, two examples have been envisaged in Sects. 5.3.1 and 5.3.2. The next step will be to implement the analytics for monitoring the Auditory Training and the training for Balance Disorders, in addition to all the other clinical scenarios.

Acknowledgements This work has been partly supported by the European Commission under the Horizon 2020 Framework Program, within the project SMART BEAR (Contract n. 852172).
Contributing Authors

Paolo Ceravolo (1), Fulvio Frati (1), Mattia Occhipinti (1), Christos Kloukinas (2), Konstantin Pozdniakov (2), Luigi Gallo (3), Ioannis Kouris (4), Eleftheria Iliadou (4), Dimitrios Kikidis (4), Christos Nikitas (4), Ioannis Basdekis (5), Carlos Agostinho (6), Alberto Acebes Martin (7) and Manuel Marcelino Perez- Perez (7).

(1) Computer Science Department, Universitá degli Studi di Milano, (2) Department of Computer Science, City, University of London, (3) ICAR, Consiglio Nazionale delle Ricerche (CNR), (4) National Kapodistrian University of Athens (NKUA), (5) SPHYNX, (6) UNINOVA, Center of Technology and Systems (CTS) and (7) Atos. These authors contributed equally to this work.

References

1. Bellandi, V., Basdekis, I., Ceravolo, P., Cesari, M., Damiani, E., Iliadou, E., M.D. Marzan, S. Maghool, Engineering continuous monitoring of intrinsic capacity for elderly people. In: Proceedings of 2021 IEEE International Conference on Digital Health (ICDH), 166–171 (2021)
2. Anisetti, M., Ardagna, C., Bellandi, V., Cremonini, M., Frati, F., Damiani, E.: Privacy-aware big data analytics as a service for public health policies in smart cities. Sustain. Urban Areas **39**, 68–77 (2018)
3. eHealth.: Electronic Health Record Sharing System: Protection of Data Privacy and System Security (2022). Available online: https://www.ehealth.gov.hk/en/whats-ehealth/security-and-privacy.html
4. European Commission, REGULATION (EU) 2016/679 on the protection of natural persons with regard to the processing of personal data and on the free movement of such data, and repealing Directive 95/46/EC (General Data Protection Regulation) (2022). Available online: https://eur-lex.europa.eu/eli/reg/2016/679/oj
5. ENISA.: Security and Resilience in eHealth Infrastructures and Services, 2015 (2021). Available online: https://www.enisa.europa.eu/publications/security-and-resilience-in-ehealth-infrastructures-and-services
6. NIST, 2020.: NIST Special Publication 800-175B Guideline for Using Cryptographic Standards in the Federal Government: Cryptographic Mechanisms (2022). Available online: https://nvlpubs.nist.gov/nistpubs/SpecialPublications/NIST.SP.800-175b.pdf
7. De Decker, B., Layouni, M., Vangheluwe, H., Verslype, K.: A privacy-preserving eHealth protocol compliant with the Belgian healthcare system. In: Proceedings of the 5th European PKI workshop on Public Key Infrastructure: Theory and Practice, pp. 118–133 (2008)

8. Loveless, M.: Understanding Bluetooth Security (2022). Available online: https://duo.com/decipher/understanding-bluetooth-security

9. Van Dijk, M., Juels, A.: On the impossibility of cryptography alone for privacy-preserving cloud computing. In: Proceeding of the 5th USENIX Conference on Hot Topics in Security, pp. 1–8 (2010)

10. Basdekis, I., Pozdniakov, K., Prasinos, M., Koloutsou, K.: Evidence based public health policy making: tool support. In: Proceedings of 2019 IEEE World Congress on Services, 272–277 (2019)

11. Anisetti, M., Ardagna, C.A., Braghin, C., Damiani, E., Polimeno, A., Balestrucci, A.: Dynamic and scalable enforcement of access control policies for big data. In: Proceedings of the 13th International Conference on Management of Digital EcoSystems, 71–78 (2021)

12. WHO.: Deafness and Hearing Loss (2022). Available online https://www.who.int/news-room/fact-sheets/detail/deafness-and-hearing-loss

13. Murray, C.J.L., Vos, T., Lopez, A.D.: Global, regional, and national incidence, prevalence, and years lived with disability for 310 diseases and injuries, 1990–2015: a systematic analysis for the global burden of disease study 2015. Lancet **388**(10053), 1545–1602 (2016)

14. Lin, F.R., Ferrucci, L., Metter, E.J., An, Y., Zonderman, A.B., Resnick, S.M.: Hearing loss and cognition in the Baltimore longitudinal study of aging. Neuropsychology **25**(6), 763–770 (2011)

15. Dawes, P., Emsley, R., Cruickshanks, K.J., Moore, D.R., Fortnum, H., Edmondson-Jones, M., McCormack, A., Munro, K.J.: Hearing loss and cognition: the role of hearing AIDS, social isolation and depression. PLoS ONE **10**(3), e0119616 (2015)

16. Li, L., Simonsick, E.M., Ferrucci, L., Lin, F.R.: Hearing loss and gait speed among older adults in the United States. Gait Posture **38**(1), 25–29 (2013)

17. McCormack, A., Fortnum, H.: Why do people fitted with hearing aids not wear them? Int. J. Audiol. **52**(5), 360–368 (2013)

18. Saunders, G.H., Dillard, L.K., Zobay, O., Cannon, J.B., Naylor, G.: Electronic health records as a platform for audiological research: data validity, patient characteristics, and hearing-aid use persistence among 731,213 U.S. Veterans. Ear Hear. **42**(4), 927–940 (2020)

19. Ferguson, M.A., Kitterick, P.T., Chong, L.Y., Edmondson-Jones, M., Barker, F., Hoare, D.J.: Hearing aids for mild to moderate hearing loss in adults. Cochrane Database Syst. Rev. **9** (2017)

20. Dillon, H.: Hearing Aids. Thieme Medical Publishers (2022). Available online: https://researchers.mq.edu.au/en/publications/hearing-aids

21. Timmer, B.H.B., Hickson, L., Laune, S.: Adults with mild hearing impairment: are we meeting the challenge? Int. J. Audiol. **54**(11), 786–795 (2015)

22. Ferguson, M.A., Henshaw, H.: Auditory training can improve working memory, attention, and communication in adverse conditions for adults with hearing loss. Front. Psychol. **6** (2015)

23. Gatehouse, S.: Glasgow hearing aid benefit profile: derivation and validation of a client-centered outcome measure for hearing aid services. J. Am. Acad. Audiol. **10**(2), 24 (1999)

24. Lawrence, B.J., Jayakody, D.M.P., Henshaw, H., Ferguson, M.A., Eikelboom, R.H., Loftus, A.M., Friedland, P.L.: Auditory and cognitive training for cognition in adults with hearing loss: a systematic review and meta-analysis. Trends Hear. **22**, 556 (2018)

25. Sheikh, J.I., Yesavage, J.A.: Geriatric depression scale (GDS): Recent evidence and development of a shorter version. In: Clinical Gerontology: A Guide to Assessment and Intervention, pp. 165–173 (1986)

26. Horsman, J., Furlong, W., Feeny, D., Torrance, G.: The health utilities index (HUI): concepts, measurement properties and applications. Health Qual. Life Outcomes **1**, 54 (2003)

27. Nasreddine, Z.S., Phillips, N.A., Bédirian, V., Charbonneau, S., Whitehead, V., Collin, I., Cummings, J.L., Chertkow, H.: The Montreal cognitive assessment, MoCA: a brief screening tool for mild cognitive impairment. J. Am. Geriatr. Soc. **53**, 695–699 (2005)

28. Kroenke, K., Spitzer, R.L., Williams, J.B.: The PHQ-9: validity of a brief depression severity measure. J. Gen. Intern. Med. **16**(9), 606–613 (2001)

29. Roque, N.A., Boot, W.R.: A new tool for assessing mobile device proficiency in older adults: the mobile device proficiency questionnaire. J. Appl. Gerontol. **37**(2), 131–156 (2018)

30. Nolan, C.M., Longworth, L., Lord, J., Canavan, J.L., Jones, S.E., Kon, S.S., Man, W.D.: The EQ-5D-5L health status questionnaire in COPD: validity, responsiveness and minimum important difference. Thorax **71**(6), 493–500 (2016)
31. Yardley, L., Beyer, N., Hauer, K., Kempen, G., Piot-Ziegle, C., Todd, C.: Development and initial validation of the falls efficacy scale-international (FES-I). Age Ageing **34**(6), 614–619 (2005)
32. Rolfson, D.B., Majumdar, S.R., Tsuyuki, R.T., Tahir, A., Rockwood, K.: Validity and reliability of the Edmonton frail scale. Age Ageing **35**(5), 526–529 (2006)
33. Godin, G.: The Godin-Shephard leisure-time physical activity questionnaire. Health Fitness J. Can. **4**(1), 18–22 (2011)
34. Snyder, E., Cai, B., DeMuro, C., Morrison, M.F., Ball, W.: A new single-item sleep quality scale: results of psychometric evaluation in patients with chronic primary insomnia and depression. J. Clin. Sleep Med. **14**(11), 1849–1857 (2018)
35. Lawton, M., Brody, E.: Assessment of older people: self-maintaining and instrumental activities of daily living. Gerontologist **9**(3), 179–186 (1969)
36. Little, M.O.: The rapid geriatric assessment: a quick screen for geriatric syndromes. Mo. Med. **114**(2), 101–104 (2017)
37. Walker, M.L., Austin, A.G., Banke, G.M., Foxx, S.R., Gaetano, L., Gardner, L.A., McElhiney, J., Morris, K., Penn, L.: Reference group data for the functional gait assessment. Phys. Ther. **87**(11), 1468–1477 (2007)
38. Löfgren, N., Lenholm, E., Conradsson, D., Ståhle, A., Franzén, E.: The Mini-BESTest-a clinically reproducible tool for balance evaluations in mild to moderate Parkinson's disease? BMC Neurol. **14**, 235 (2014)
39. Topolski, T.D., LoGerfo, J., Patrick, D.L., Williams, B., Walwick, J., Patrick, M.B.: The rapid assessment of physical activity (RAPA) among older adults. Prev. Chronic Dis. **3**(4), A118 (2006)
40. Powell, L.E., Myers, A.M.: The activities-specific balance confidence (ABC) scale. J. Gerontol. A Biol. Sci. Med. Sci. **50A**(1), M28-34 (1995)
41. Vellas, B., Villars, H., Abellan, G., Soto, M.E., Rolland, Y., Guigoz, Y., Morley, J.E., Chumlea, W., Salva, A., Rubenstein, L.Z., Garry, P.: Overview of the MNA-Its history and challenges. J. Nutr. Health Aging **10**(6), 456–463 (2006)
42. Six, A.J., Backus, B.E., Kelder, J.C.: Chest pain in the emergency room: value of the HEART score. Neth. Heart J. **16**(6), 191–196 (2008)
43. Rubenstein, L.Z.: Falls in older people: epidemiology, risk factors and strategies for prevention. Age Ageing 35 Suppl 2, ii37–ii41 (2006)
44. Thibaud, M., Bloch, F., Tournoux-Facon, C., Brèque, C., Rigaud, A.S., Dugue, B., Kemoun, G.: Impact of physical activity and sedentary behaviour on fall risks in older people: a systematic review and meta-analysis of observational studies. Eur. Rev. Aging Phys. Act. **9**, 5–15 (2012)
45. Ambrose, A.F., Paul, G., Hausdorff, J.M.: Risk factors for falls among older adults: a review of the literature. Maturitas **75**(1), 51–61 (2013)
46. WHO.: Falls (2022). Available online: https://www.who.int/news-room/fact-sheets/detail/falls
47. Stevens, J.A., Corso, P.S., Finkelstein, E.A., Miller, T.R.: The costs of fatal and non-fatal falls among older adults. Inj. Prev. **12**(5), 290–295 (2006)
48. Pothula, V.B., Chew, F., Lesser, T.H., Sharma, A.K.: Falls and vestibular impairment. Clin. Otolaryngol. Allied Sci. **29**(2), 179–182 (2004)
49. Tinetti, M.E., Speechley, M., Ginter, S.F.: Risk factors for falls among elderly persons living in the community. N. Engl. J. Med. **319**(26), 1701–1707 (1988)
50. NICE.: Falls in older people: assessing risk and prevention (2022). Available online: https://www.nice.org.uk/guidance/cg161/chapter/1-Recommendation/preventing-falls-in-older-people-2
51. Hu, M.H., Woollacott, M.H.: Multisensory training of standing balance in older adults: I. Postural stability and one-leg stance balance. J Gerontol. **49**(2) M52-61 (1994)
52. McDonnell, M.N., Hillier, S.L.: Vestibular rehabilitation for unilateral peripheral vestibular dysfunction. Cochrane Database Syst. Rev. **1**, CD005937 (2015)

53. Gillespie, L.D., Robertson, M.C., Gillespie, W.J., Sherrington, C., Gates, S., Clemson, L.M., Lamb, S.E.: Interventions for preventing falls in older people living in the community. Cochrane Database Syst. Rev. **9**, CD007146 (2012)

54. Badke, M.B., Shea, T.A., Miedaner, J.A., Grove, C.R.: Outcomes after rehabilitation for adults with balance dysfunction. Arch. Phys. Med. Rehabil. **85**(2), 227–233 (2004)

55. Skelton, D., Dinan, S., Campbell, M., Rutherford, O.: Tailored group exercise (Falls Management Exercise–FaME) reduces falls in community-dwelling older frequent fallers (an RCT). Age Ageing **34**(6), 636–639 (2005)

56. Hall, C.D., Herdman, S.J., Whitney, S.L., Cass, S.P., Clendaniel, R.A., Fife, T.D., Furman, J.M., Getchius, T.S., J. A, Goebel, N.T. Shepard, S.N. Woodhouse, Vestibular rehabilitation for peripheral vestibular hypofunction: an evidence-based clinical practice guideline. J. Neurol. Phys. Ther. **40**(2), 124–155 (2016)

57. Lilios, A., Chimona, T., Nikitas, C., Papadakis, C., Chatziioannou, I., Skoulakis, C.: The effect of supervision in vestibular rehabilitation in patients with acute or chronic unilateral vestibular dysfunction: a systematic review. Otol. Neurotol. **42**(1), e1422–e1431 (2021)

58. Hardage, J., Peel, C., Morris, D., Graham, C., Brown, C., Foushee, H.R., Braswell, J.: Adherence to Exercise Scale for Older Patients (AESOP): a measure for predicting exercise adherence in older adults after discharge from home health physical therapy. J. Geriatr. Phys. Ther. **30**(2), 69–78 (2007)

59. Schutzer, K.A., Graves, B.S.: Barriers and motivations to exercise in older adults. Prev. Med. **39**(5), 1056–1061 (2004)

60. Picorelli, A.M., Pereira, L.S., Pereira, D.S., Felício, D., Sherrington, C.: Adherence to exercise programs for older people is influenced by program characteristics and personal factors: a systematic review. J. Physiother. **60**(3), 151–156 (2014)

61. Winser, S.J., Chan, H.T.F., Ho, L., Chung, L.S., Ching, L.T., Felix, t.K.L., Kannan, P.: Dosage for cost-effective exercise-based falls prevention programs for older people: a systematic review of economic evaluations. Ann. Phys. Rehabil. Med. **63**(1), 69–80 (2020)

62. Sherrington, C., Michaleff, Z.A., Fairhall, N., Paul, S.S., Tiedemann, A., Whitney, J., Cumming, R.G., Herbert, R.D., Close, J.C.T., Lord, S.R.: Exercise to prevent falls in older adults: an updated systematic review and meta-analysis. Br. J. Sports Med. **51**(24), 1750–1758 (2017)

63. John Campbell, A., Clare Robertson, M.: Accident Compensation Corporation (ACC), University of Otago; New Zeland. Otago Excercise Programme to Prevent Falls in Older Adults (2022). Available online: https://www.livestronger.org.nz/assets/Uploads/acc1162-otago-exercise-manual.pdf

64. Bjerk, M., Brovold, T., Davis, J.C., Skelton, D.A., Bergland, A.: Health-related quality of life in home care recipients after a falls prevention intervention: a 6-month follow-up. Eur. J. Public Health **31**(1), 64–69 (2020)

65. Mansson, L., Lundin-Olsson, L., Skelton, D.A., Janols, R., Lindgren, H., Rosendahl, E., Sandlund, M.: Older adults' preferences for, adherence to and experiences of two self-management falls prevention home exercise programmes: a comparison between a digital programme and a paper booklet. BMC Geriatr. **20**(1), 209 (2020)

66. Thomas, S., Mackintosh, S., Halbert, J.: Does the 'Otago exercise programme' reduce mortality and falls in older adults?: a systematic review and meta-analysis. Age Ageing **39**(6), 681–687 (2010)

67. Yoo, H.-N., Chung, E., Lee, B.-H.: The effects of augmented reality-based Otago exercise on balance, gait, and falls efficacy of elderly women. J. Phys. Ther. Sci. **25**, 797–801 (2013)

68. Yang, X.J., Hill, K., Moore, K., Williams, S., Dowson, L., Borschmann, K., Simpson, J.A., Dharmage, S.C.: Effectiveness of a targeted exercise intervention in reversing older people's mild balance dysfunction: a randomized controlled trial. Phys. Ther. **92**(1), 24–37 (2012)

69. Liston, M.B., Alushi, L., Bamiou, D.E., Martin, F.C., Hopper, A., Pavlou, M.: Feasibility and effect of supplementing a modified OTAGO intervention with multisensory balance exercises in older people who fall: a pilot randomized controlled trial. Clin. Rehabil. **28**, 784–793 (2014)

70. Davis, J.C., Hsu, C.L., Cheung, W.: Can the Otago falls prevention program be delivered by video? A feasibility study. BMJ Open Sport Exerc. Med. **2**, e000059 (2016)

71. Gatsios, D., Georga, E.I., Kourou, K.K., Fotiadis, D.I., Kikidis, D., Bibas, A., Nikitas, C., Liston, M., Pavlou, M., Bamiou, D.E., Costafreda, S.: Achieving adherence in home-based rehabilitation with novel human machine interactions that stimulate community-dwelling older adults. In: Proceedings of the 12th ACM International Conference on PErvasive Technologies Related to Assistive Environments (PETRA 2019), pp. 616–619
72. Kempen, G.I., L. Yardley L, J.C. van Haastregt, G.A. Zijlstra, N. Beyer, K. Hauer, C. Todd, The Short FES-I: a shortened version of the falls efficacy scale-international to assess fear of falling. Age Ageing **37**(1), 45–50 (2008)
73. Shumway-Cook, A., Brauer, S., Woollacott, M.: Predicting the probability for falls in community-dwelling older adults using the Timed Up & Go Test. Phys. Ther. **80**(9), 896–903 (2000)
74. Marques, M., Lopes, F., Costa, R., Agostinho, C., Oliveira, P., Jardim-Goncalves, R.: Innovative product/service for personalized health management. In: Proceedings of the ASME 2019 International Mechanical Engineering Congress and Exposition (Volume 2B) V02BT02A029 (2019)
75. Jakobsen, J.C., Gluud, C., Wetterslev, J., Winkel, P.: When and how should multiple imputation be used for handling missing data in randomised clinical trials-a practical guide with flowcharts. BMC Med. Res. Methodol. **17**(1), 1–10 (2017)
76. Van der Ploeg, T., Austin, P.C., Steyerberg, E.W.: Modern modelling techniques are data hungry: a simulation study for predicting dichotomous endpoints. BMC Med. Res. Methodol. **14**(1), 1–13 (2014)

Chapter 6
Virtual Reality-Based Rehabilitation Gaming System

Vijay Jeyakumar, Prema Sundaram, Nithiya Ramapathiran, and Pradeep Kannan

Abstract Many human motor function impairments are caused due to a variety of neurodegenerative diseases, motor dysfunction disabilities and age-related issues. As the geriatric population progresses, the need for novel solutions to manage age-related diseases increases. To combat this, intensive rehabilitation treatment is instituted repetitively. However, the traditional rehabilitation treatment regimes, involving tedious and monotonous activity with numerous repetitions, lacking active patient participation are of boring and strenuous nature. This ultimately leads to suboptimal treatment outcomes necessitating long-term care. To overcome this, a range of interactive and easy measuring technology-based innovative solutions fused with the rehabilitation process is being investigated to ameliorate the effectiveness and productivity of rehabilitation programs and escalate the independence of patients and empower them to administer their treatment. Recently, game-based Virtual Reality (VR) rehabilitation protocol has turned out to be a promising therapeutic alternative, amalgamating Brain-Computer Interface (BCI) with VR to activate neuro-motor functions, sustain motivation and reach rehabilitation goals to improve the quality of life of patients. Virtual rehabilitation is a computer-generated interactive patient-centred simulation system combining computers, special interfaces, and simulation exercises that imitates reality and provides an artificial environment mimicking real-world experience. The architecture of the system is designed in such a way that it can remotely track the patients, obtain data, and tailor the rehabilitation sessions

V. Jeyakumar (✉)
Sri Sivasubramaniya Nadar College of Engineering, Chennai, India
e-mail: vijayj@ssn.edu.in

P. Sundaram
PSNA College of Engineering and Technology, Dindigul, India
e-mail: premas@psnacet.edu.in

N. Ramapathiran
Agni College of Technology, Chennai, India
e-mail: nithiya.bme@act.edu.in

P. Kannan
Chennai Institute of Technology, Chennai, India
e-mail: pradeepk@citchennai.net

© The Author(s), under exclusive license to Springer Nature Switzerland AG 2023
C. P. Lim et al. (eds.), *Artificial Intelligence and Machine Learning for Healthcare*,
Intelligent Systems Reference Library 229,
https://doi.org/10.1007/978-3-031-11170-9_6

according to the current needs of the patients. VR improves both motor skills and confidence for daily living and in numerous situations to enhance functional results, improving the clinical and social benefits of surgery. Thus, game-based VR is being developed to allow clinicians to create game-based VR tasks and this will serve to drive advances in rehabilitation interventions.

Keywords Exercise training · Game-based rehabilitation · Physiotherapy · Stroke rehabilitation · Virtual reality

Abbreviations

3D	3-Dimensional
AI	Artificial intelligence
ALP	Amyotrophic lateral sclerosis
AR	Augmented reality
ARAT	Action-research-arm-test
ASD	Autism disorder
BBT	Box-and-block-test
BWS	Body weight system
BCI	Brain-computer interface
CAREX	Cable-driven upper arm exoskeleton
CGBT	Computer game-based therapy
CIMT	Constraint-induced movement therapy
CP	Cerebral palsy
DALYs	Disability adjusted life years
ECG	Electrocardiograph
EEG	Electroencephalograph
EMG	Electromyograph
FES	Functional electrical stimulation
FIM	Functional-independence-measure score
FMA	Fugl-Meyer-assessment
GBD	Global burden of disease
HMD	Head mounted display
Hz	Hertz
IMU	Inertial measurement unit
IoT	Internet of things
IR	Infra-red
LED	Light emitting diode
LIS	Locked-in syndrome
MATLAB	Matrix Laboratory
MEG	Magnetoencephalography
MSD	Musculoskeletal Disorder
MSI	Musculoskeletal Injury

MVF	Mirror Visual Feedback
NASDAQ	National Association of Securities Dealers Automated Quotations
NEPSER	Neuroplasticity Principle-Based Sensory Rehabilitation
NLP	Natural Language Processing
NW	Nintendo Wii
OSD	Osgood schlatter disease
PPG	Photoplethysmography
RTP	Return to Play
SCI	Spinal Cord Injury
SMA	Shape Memory Alloy
SMR	Sensor Motor Rhythms
SSVEP	Somatosensory Visual Evoked Potentials
TIA	Transient Ischemic Attack
VR	Virtual Reality
VRC	Virtual Reality control
VRML	Virtual Reality Markup Language
WHO	World Health Organisation
WMFT	Wolf-Motor-Function-Test
XR	Extended Reality

6.1 Introduction

Rehabilitation works on the ideology that every person has got the fundamental policy to be a master in maintaining one's health. There is a marked difference between acute care and rehabilitation, where acute care refers to one's survival, while rehabilitation refers to personal care and autonomy. It is one of the prominent health care strategies which aids in the up-gradation, prevention, therapy and end-of-life care.

6.1.1 Rehabilitation

Rehabilitation is a set of interventions developed to advance optimal functioning and to minimize disability in people with impaired health conditions to improve a better interaction with their surroundings as defined according to the World Health Organization (WHO). The rehabilitation process is sketched to meet each one's definite needs to attain the maximum level of activity, autonomy and status of life but will not alter or revert the damage undergone due to an illness or trauma rather restores the well-being of an individual [1].

The general components for rehabilitation include the following:

- To treat disease and to prevent the problems associated with it

Table 6.1 Areas of rehabilitation

Patient requirements	Examples
Personal care skills	Eating, grooming
Physical health	Medication
Household support	Lifestyle and financial concerns and their adaptability
Emotional hold	Behavioral issues
Pain and stress relief	Medications to overcome pain
Job training	Vocational skills
Interaction skills	Socialising among others
Learning skills	Analytical skills
Oratory skills	Different methods of communication
Breathing care	Treatments to improve lung physiology
Portability skills	Mobility to different environments
Awareness and education	Family awareness and use of techniques to train

- To overcome disability by increasing activity
- To establish tools to adapt and alter the surroundings
- To create awareness among people to improve lifestyle.

Rehabilitation can extend its support in any one of the patient-centric areas and is depicted in Table 6.1.

6.1.1.1   Elements of Rehabilitation

The various elements of rehabilitation utilized to improve the lifestyle of people are

(A) Preventive rehabilitation

It is one of the common methods of rehabilitation occurring in people with chronic disease conditions aimed to ward off or slow down the onset of impairments and to improve self-management in cancer patients.

(B) Restorative rehabilitation

It concentrates on procedures to ameliorate impairments usually in people following a surgery or an acute disease namely stroke.

(C) Supportive rehabilitation

It is also termed adaptive rehabilitation where it can improve an individual's care features through the help of assistive technology.

(D) Palliative rehabilitation

It helps to improve functional autonomy and to relieve symptoms in people with life-threatening conditions to lead a good quality life with utmost comfort and dignity [2].

6.1.1.2 Objectives of Rehabilitation

The objectives outlined in rehabilitation are

- Preventing functional loss
- Retarding the rate of functional loss
- Restoring function to its maximum
- Compensating functional loss
- Conserving current functional ability

6.1.1.3 Outcomes of Rehabilitation

The various benefits rendered by rehabilitation overtime includes the following

- Reduced demand for health services out of hospitals
- Improved autonomy
- Increased self-care conditions
- Reduced independence
- Better recovery to working conditions
- Finally improved value of life and well-being.

6.1.1.4 Scope of Rehabilitation

It is an umbrella with a wide spectrum to support communication, improve health, well-being and combat acute illness like trauma and thus requires support in the following areas

(i)   Development of supplementary skills to overcome hurdles
(ii)   Establishment of independence in conditions like dementia
(iii)   Improves performance in athletes
(iv)   Retrieve from sudden acute illness like stroke
(v)   Recover from crucial shock to regain back the usual skills after an accident
(vi)   Govern chronic problems through rehabilitation interventions to maximise function
(vii)   Self-care to avoid secondary complications in people with depression
(viii) Acquire advocacy in vulnerable individuals [3].

6.1.1.5 Benefits of Rehabilitation

At the outset, the use of assistive technology and its various benefits are listed in Table 6.2.

Table 6.2 Benefits of rehabilitation

Physical benefits of rehabilitation	Enhances	• Strength and flexibility • Balance and coordination • Gait and posture
	Reduces	• Pain and risk of falls • Inflammation • Unexpected complications • Continuous support and dependence
Psychological benefits of rehabilitation	Enhances	• Self-esteem • Independence and wellbeing
	Reduces	• Complication rates
Lifestyle benefits of rehabilitation	Enhances	• Social participation • Return to working conditions • Quality of life
	Reduces	• Dependence
Economic benefits of rehabilitation	Enhances	• Earning ability • Potential of children
	Reduces	• Associated Hospital costs • Hospital Readmissions • Length of stay • Number of appointments

6.1.1.6 Types of Rehabilitation

1. Orthopaedic and musculoskeletal rehabilitation

   It follows therapeutic interventions to improve recovery and pain management in patients with musculoskeletal disorders by framing personalised therapy regimes to enhance physical strength and mobility. E.g. Aerobics and other exercises performed individually or in groups to strengthen muscles.
2. Neurological rehabilitation

   This approach involves simulation of the brain in patients with stroke. Along with pharmacological treatments, the use of assistive devices, physiotherapy, safety training and occupational therapy can strengthen muscles, overcome weakness, improve balance, coordination and cognition. These patients can recover in phases of early and late stages of the disease to carry out regular household chores [4]. E.g. Fitness exercise, physiotherapy.
3. Cardiac rehabilitation

   This is an advanced rehabilitation protocol to be adapted in patients with severe cardiovascular abnormalities like heart attack, which includes health education, simple physical exercises and management of stress to alleviate risk for sudden demise and control symptoms [5]. E.g. Hand exercise, breathing exercises.

4. Pulmonary rehabilitation

   Pulmonary rehabilitation practices procedures based on an assessment to optimize respiratory functions in patients having moderate to severe chronic pulmonary diseases.

5. Geriatric rehabilitation

   Older patients show chronic diseases and comorbidities making them carry out a sedentary lifestyle due to aging. Thus, improving their physical activity regularly can enhance their active life expectancy and bring down the risk of progressive chronic conditions. E.g. Home-based multimodal exercise and nutrition.

6. Renal rehabilitation

   This type of rehabilitation is found to be most efficient in people with chronic kidney diseases following dialysis and can improve the quality of life through increased cardiopulmonary functions and ventilation efficiency. Chronic kidney disease can end up in secondary sarcopenia which can also be managed with supervised rehabilitation and strengthening exercises. E.g. Intradialytic exercises.

7. Burn rehabilitation

   Various rehabilitation methods have assisted to improve pain management, anxiety, gait functions, limb movements, mental satisfaction and lessened muscle tension in patients who have sustained burn injuries [6]. E.g. Robotics, music therapy, behavioural therapy.

The global concept of rehabilitation explained that over 15% of the global population lives with some form of disability and according to a recent survey, 2.41 billion people live with impairments and need rehabilitation services to overcome their disease or injury. The life expectancy has gone above 60 years of age but, people living with chronic diseases experiencing disability are increasing leading to the need for rehabilitation regimes, especially amidst susceptible populations all over the world [7].

Though rehabilitation is a requisite health service crucial among children, adults and the elderly, the highest contributors to the global need for rehabilitation depends on stroke and musculoskeletal disorders.

6.1.2 Stroke

Stroke is a crucial medical emergency condition and needs prompt and early treatment action to avoid damage to brain tissues and related complications. Either a rupture or bleeding of a blood vessel in the brain or a block in the blood vessel to the brain causes a stroke. This is due to the poor blood flow resulting in reduced oxygen and nutrients supply to the brain tissue causing brain cells to die within minutes. People who have had strokes live less than a year and it predominantly affects people over 65 years of age. In 2020, according to the information from the Centre for Disease Control and Prevention, stroke was considered the leading cause of mortality behind neurological reasons and ranked 5th among all diseases in the world.

6.1.2.1 Signs and Symptoms

The onset of symptoms is very rapid over seconds to minutes and depends on the portion of the brain tissue affected. The right identification of a stroke episode can be found by detecting face weakness, a drift of one arm downward and slurred speech. The signs and symptoms appear very soon after the occurrence of stroke.

- Inability to move leading to loss of balance and coordination
- Numbness in one side of the body leading to unilateral paralysis
- Speaking trouble and slurred speech
- Dizziness
- Vision loss
- Altered consciousness
- Lack of responsiveness and understanding
- Increased agitation or seizures
- Sudden severe headache.

The other common chronic secondary complications include pneumonia and bladder control loss. Early and prompt treatment is required to reduce brain damage, long-term disability and mortality in stroke survivors [8].

6.1.2.2 Classification

(i) Ischemic stroke

It is the most common form of stroke and 87% of strokes are ischemic strokes due to a blocked artery either by a clot or a plague resulting in severe ischemia. Symptoms of this form of stroke usually last longer or sometimes become permanent. Hemorrhagic transformation can also occur when there is bleeding in the areas of ischemia.

Blood supply to brain tissue can be decreased due to obstruction by a blood clot or an embolus or when there is a total blood volume reduction. Sometimes the cause of stroke is unknown and termed cryptogenic and accounts for nearly 30 to 40%. Ischemic stroke can be treated if detected within 3–4 h using clot-dissolving medicines.

(ii) Hemorrhagic stroke

Hemorrhagic stroke results from bleeding of a blood vessel due to a leak or burst and blood seeps into the brain tissue. This may occur due to unregulated high blood pressure, overuse of anticoagulants, aneurysms, trauma or ischemic stroke. The two subtypes of hemorrhagic strokes are

- Intracerebral haemorrhage—It is the most common type of hemorrhagic stroke where bleeding occurs within brain tissue due to the burst of an artery flooding the neighbouring tissue which can be either intraparenchymal or intraventricular.
- Subarachnoid haemorrhage—It is the less common type of hemorrhagic stroke where bleeding occurs outside the brain tissue but within the skull exactly between the arachnoid and pia mater.

The most common symptom is a severe headache popularly termed thunderclap. Sometimes people may experience a Transient Ischemic Attack (TIA) referred to as a mini-stroke when there is a temporary reduction of blood supply to the brain tissue which reverses on its own. The symptom lasts for less than 1–2 h and it's not permanent. But people having a TIA have an increased risk for stroke later.

6.1.2.3   Causes

Stroke episodes can be due to any one of the following

- Thrombosis occurs either in a large or a small blood vessel
- Embolism in the artery
- Cerebral hypoperfusion is usually due to cardiac arrest
- Cerebral venous sinus thrombosis
- Intracerebral haemorrhage.

6.1.2.4   Risk Factors

The risk factors associated are

- Sedentary lifestyle
- Use of drugs and smoking
- Obesity
- Unhealthy diet
- Increased blood pressure
- Cardiovascular disease
- Elevated blood lipid profile
- Diabetes
- Kidney disease
- Family history of stroke
- COVID-19 disease.

Also, men and people aged 55 years are more prone to the risk of stroke attack.

6.1.3   Musculoskeletal Disorders (MSDs)

Musculoskeletal disorders constitute nearly 150 medical conditions affecting the human musculoskeletal system causing injury and pain which ranges from sudden and severe acute problems such as a fracture to irreversible chronic injuries such as arthritis. It can arise due to a sudden exertion, repetitive strain or continuous exposure to strain, vibration or wrong posture and can affect the spine, extremities, neck and shoulders. It constitutes the biggest category of workplace disorders [9].

According to the Global Burden of Disease (GBD), these disorders affect approximately 1.71 billion people worldwide and is ranked second among the various disabilities affecting mankind. The highest burden is due to low back pain which is prevalent among 568 million people. These conditions predominantly reduce movements and thereby cause early retirements, lower well-being and lessen societal participation [10].

The musculoskeletal disorder affects

- bones causing osteoporosis, fractures
- joints causing rheumatoid arthritis, spondylitis, stiffness, dislocation
- ligaments causing inflammation
- muscles causing spasms, cramps, sarcopenia
- tendons causing sprains, strains
- skeleton causing poor posture problems
- cartilage causing overuse injuries.

6.1.3.1   Causes

MSDs can arise due to the following factors

(i)   Biomechanical or ergonomic
(ii)   Physical
(iii) Psychological
(iv)   Occupational factors [11].

6.1.3.2   Symptoms

Common symptoms of MSDs include

- Severe ache on movements
- Stiffness of joints
- Muscle burning sensation
- Tiredness
- Muscle twitches
- Sleep disturbances [12].

Examples of MSDs include

- Carpal tunnel syndrome
- Epicondylitis
- Tendonitis
- Back Pain
- Tension neck syndrome
- Hand-arm vibration syndrome
- Ligament sprain
- Thoracic outlet compression
- Digital neuritis
- Dequervain's syndrome
- Mechanical back syndrome
- Degenerative disc disease
- Ruptured/Herniated Disc.

6.2   Classical Treatment Approaches

Thus with the increasing geriatric population, disabilities related to human motor dysfunction predominantly due to stroke and musculoskeletal disorders also progress eliciting the need for customized rehabilitation treatments to improve autonomy in stroke and disabled persons. The methods and procedures for treating stroke and musculoskeletal disorders are discussed in the following section.

6.2.1   Methods and Procedures for Stroke Treatment

In low and middle-income countries there is a steady increase in the number of new stroke cases recording more than one crore accounting for a mortality rate of 75% and 80% of disability-adjusted life years (DALYs). Among the stroke survivors only 5–20% show complete recovery while the majority possess Upper Limb functional deficits with no better protocol for therapy. The duration of practice, intensity and frequency of rehabilitation is directly related to the recovery rate after stroke [13].

1. Treatment of stroke follows three stages
2. Prevention

   This can be done by considering the risk factors like high blood pressure, cardiovascular disease, and diabetes and treating people to prevent the first or subsequent stroke episodes.
3. Acute stroke therapy

   Acute treatments are carried out to cease a stroke during the episode by either dissolving the clot or stopping the bleeding using drug therapy which is the most common treatment method.

4. Post-stroke rehabilitation

Rehabilitation after stroke provides novel ways for patients to regain and relearn skills that were lost due to brain damage. The main aim of stroke rehabilitation is to increase independence and to provide the best possible quality of life by improving physical, mental, social and spiritual health after a stroke to restore functional well-being. Research has shown that the functions associated with the specific area of damage earlier, restore to other parts of the brain after a stroke and hence practising can improve rewiring of neurons.

Post-stroke rehabilitation programs are customized to meet patient-specific needs which are carefully planned, well-focused, involve repetitive practice and should be initiated within 48 h after stroke in the hospital itself. Reaching the rehabilitation goal relies on various variables including the pathophysiology and severity of the stroke, type and extent of disability, general health of the patient and their family support.

6.2.1.1   Stroke Management

Stroke recovery focuses on various major areas including

- Upper Limb functional rehabilitation

  The latest research focus is on observation of action in enhancing the motor function and dependence of using upper limb activities in day-to-day living. This therapy improves better arm and hand coordination with fewer adverse effects. Constraint-Induced Movement Therapy (CIMT) and mirror therapy with repetitive practice was found to be effective in upper limb functionality [14].
- Cognitive rehabilitation
    To improve attention deficits in stroke patients, cognitive rehabilitation is found to be effective and research is going on to check for the sustained effects in daily tasks.
- Gait rehabilitation
    Research on improving motor functions and walking speed in patients encountered with stroke is in progress and seems to enhance walking endurance and personal assistance.
- Physical and occupational rehabilitation

  Physical therapy concentrates on improving joint motions and their strengthening through exercises and repeated learning of tasks namely bed mobility, walking and other motor functions, especially on the hemiplegic side employing CIMT [15].
- Speech and language rehabilitation

  This therapy is recommended as a part of post-stroke rehabilitation to improve communication impairments and speech production disorders thereby the overall

communication, writing practice, reading style and expressive language are improved over long periods.
• Physical fitness improvement

The general fitness and health of a person have usually reduced following a stroke which can also, in turn, affect the extent of rehabilitation. Thus physical exercises prove to be beneficial in improving permanent health status.
• Use of assistive devices

Assistive Technology can improve mobility in patients with the use of devices namely wheelchairs, canes, ankle–foot orthosis, Walkers, etc.
• Yoga

Practicing yoga can elevate stress-related anxiety by improving pain management, endurance mental health and overcoming disability to lead a peaceful life.

The different approaches to stroke rehabilitation depend on the body part affected or the type of impairment caused due to a stroke episode and includes.

(i)   Physical activities
(ii)   Motor skill exercise to rejuvenate muscle strength and coordination. E.g. During swallowing.
(iii)   Mobility training to better make use of mobility aids like a walker, wheelchairs or an ankle brace. E.g. During walking.
(iv)   Constraint-induced therapy also called forced-use therapy involves movement and functioning of the affected limb to its fullest without restraining the unaffected limb.
(v)   Range of motion therapy employs exercises to decrease spasticity and improve range of motion [16].

Technology augmented physical activities include

• Electrical stimulation to re-educate the muscular contraction
• Robotic technology to strengthen impaired limbs
• Wireless technology to monitor post-stroke tasks
• Virtual reality to make patients interact with the virtual real-time environment.

(ii)   Cognitive and emotional activities

• Cognitive therapy overcomes the lost abilities of cognition through occupational and speech therapy.
• Communication or speech therapy helps overcome communication disorders so that a patient could regain speaking and listening skills.
• Psychological therapy sets right the emotional disturbances and improves mental health through counselling and group participation activities.
• Drug therapy improves alertness and settles agitation with the prescription of antidepressants.

Experimental therapies namely non-invasive brain stimulation involving Transcranial Magnetic Stimulation, biological stem cell therapy and alternative medicine employing massage, herbal treatments and acupuncture are being investigated in post-stroke patients.

6.2.2   Treatment Approaches for Musculoskeletal Disorders

Maintaining good bone strength and joints is important for preventing musculoskeletal pain and this can be achieved by limiting repetitive movements, maintaining the right posture, practising the perfect lifting procedures and performing stretching exercises regularly. But in the worst case, the common treatment approaches for MSDs include:

- Drug therapies
- Use of orthopaedic devices
- Acupuncture
- Chiropractic medicine
- Rehabilitation therapies.

6.2.3   Limitations in Traditional Approaches

- Implementation of high-intensity training in a real-time setting
- The quick loss of interest in repetitive training and exercises
- Lack of motivation, feasibility and safety towards the tedious medical regime
- Lack of encouragement in patient skill upgradation
- Poor adherence and annoyance due to long hours of workouts
- Lack of availability of therapist and equipment
- Low level of commitment in-home rehabilitation regime
- Poor patient compliance and Long term care
- Suboptimal treatment outcomes
- No creativity and customized treatment methods
- Less interaction and non-availability of techniques to measure recovery rate
- Limited entertainment and less diversity of content in gaming.

Thus, to promote patient's compliance and activate neuro-motor activities to their fullest towards rehabilitation therapy lacking in traditional approaches, various modern rehabilitation technologies have come up as a tool to increase motivation and reach rehabilitation goals.

6.3   Modern Rehabilitation Technologies

Rehabilitation plays an important role among human beings from childhood till the end of their life. Both healthy and unhealthy people can also use this rehabilitation practice. Gait analysis helps us to study the issues in the kinematics of human motion. Rehabilitation supports the people in various ways as follows

- Fast recovery from an unexpected illness. E.g. Stroke, Trauma
- Speedy recovery from surgery. E.g. Knee replacement
- Aggressive people who need support. E.g. Mental Illness
- Reduce anxiety and depression in individuals. E.g. Psychosis.

Orthopaedic and neurological rehabilitation involves the use of orthotics and prosthetics to replace a limb or to maintain the anatomical position of the human body that is impaired or missing. As traditional prosthetics were too heavy, people couldn't wear them for long periods and were also not comfortable for children. Classical orthosis, namely hand-on-thigh gait devices used by polio-affected children were difficult to carry. It was then replaced by modern prosthetic technology namely knee ankle foot orthosis made up of thermoplastics or carbon fibre material to keep their knees from dragging [17]. Modern prosthetics are having a very huge growth and development so that people have started using advanced limbs nowadays. They offer a variety of advantages like lightweight, comfortability and high functioning which allows disabled persons to live an independent and normal life.

6.3.1   Physical Prosthetics

Over a decade, prosthetics have been made through plaster casting of the affected or missing limb. Depending on the comfort level of the individual, it is simple to incorporate into their everyday routines such as driving, walking, and so on. Recent prostheses designs have increased strength while reducing weight employing pioneer materials such as kevlar, titanium and carbon fibre, which are robust, durable and assist us in designing lightweight prostheses [18].

6.3.1.1   Classification of Prosthesis

(i)   Based on the level of amputation

    (a)   Upper Limb Prosthetics are mainly used during upper limb amputation or deficiency. One of the important prostheses in the upper limb is a myoelectric prosthesis which is based on the study of muscle activity of the hand using EMG pattern. In recent techniques, pattern recognition controlled myoelectric hands are in use which does multiple axis movements instead of opening and closing hands. E.g. Transradial, Transhumeral, shoulder disarticulation.

(b) Lower Limb Prosthetics are mainly used during lower limb amputation such as Transtibial which needs artificial foot, ankle and shank, whereas a transfemoral amputation needs replacement of the missing part of the thigh and artificial knee as a prosthetic [19]. E.g. Knee and Hip Disarticulation, Foot Amputation.

(ii) Based on the construction design

(a) Exoskeletal Prosthesis is the covering that is present outside, supporting the total body weight. Outer covering sockets are made up of resin over foam or wood as a filler material. E.g. People affected with Spinal Cord Injury (SCI), major trauma like stroke and cerebral palsy.

(b) Endoskeletal prostheses are present inside the skin layer called pylon, constructed using lightweight carbon fibre and metal. Endoskeletal prosthesis offers easy alignment and replacement of components. E.g. Transfemoral and Transtibial Prosthesis.

6.3.1.2 Components of Prosthesis

- Body of prosthesis-Outer structure made up of durable, lightweight material
- Socket-Holder in which residual limb is present.
- Control system-Signals from the sensor are converted into electrical signals.
- Harness/suspension system-Harnesses are made out of a socket fit attached to a residual limb and dacron straps.
- Terminal device-Bionic hand, Gloves, Hook.

Another key recent innovation in physical prosthetics is the development of targeted muscle reinnervation work on powerful prostheses that are resilient, integrated, self-determined and adaptable. Another cost-effective and low-budget physical prosthesis is a customized, hardware-specified 3D printing limb specially designed for kids. Customized 3D printing is an open-source platform and the user can design it by themselves in low-income families. Also, experts can design various implants and anatomical models using 3D prosthetics [20].

6.3.2 Sensory Prosthetics

Traditional prosthetic devices are unable to acquire general sensory information while a person is moving or interacting with an object. They are experiencing trouble while managing the force required to move the prosthetic hand, which could lead to medical complications. The feedback system can be utilized to collect sensory information from the prosthesis and convey it to the brain or neurological system which then sends a receptor signal to the skin, muscle and joint [21]. There are various sensory prosthetic devices used for a variety of rehabilitation purposes and are shown in Table 6.3.

Apart from the above said sensory prosthetics, there are still a few more to be addressed namely,

- 3D printed wearable module- Facial Rehabilitation (Impersonate and activate the facial muscle movement). E.g. facial paralysis.
- Hybrid vibrotactile stimulator -Sensor Rehabilitation (Parallel sensing streams delivered to a patient at one point). E.g. Upper extremities.
- Prosthetic leg—Natural sensation of touch and proprioception.
- Stroke sensory rehabilitation—Fast recovery due to sensory feedback.
- Sensory enabled neural prosthesis—Amputee for processing regular activities in-home. E.g. spinal cord injury and mental illness.

6.3.3   Robotics Rehabilitation

Robotics is the design and construction of machines to perform human tasks. As illustrated in Fig. 6.1, robotics are now used in various fields. Robotic precision and artificial intelligence (AI) techniques are used to perform repetitive tasks and to work in hazardous environments where humans are unable to work. It is capable of performing difficult tasks that humans are incapable of performing. They are becoming even smarter as AI advances. Overall, robots have the potential to be the ideal assistant for humans in resolving a wide range of problems in a variety of industries.

In recent years, incredible progress has been made in robotics applications such as moving objects or devices using multi-programmed software to complete tasks in bionic components. The ability to offer more dosage and higher-level instruction for patients with disorders such as stroke and tetraplegia (spinal cord abnormalities) is a major benefit of using robotics in rehabilitation.

6.3.3.1   Classification of Rehabilitation Robotics

(i) Therapeutic Robotics- Exoskeleton and Immunoregulatory type devices are utilized to provide user-defined training. Exoskeletons are more expensive to build than immunoregulatory devices. E.g., Direct control of joints by robots that can provide mechanical stress on the distal limbs.
(ii) Assistive Robotics—Utilized for compensatory purposes, such as treatment with the help of robots. E.g. Stroke rehabilitation [29].

Robotics systems based on the Internet of Things (IoT) are employed in upper limb prostheses, orthotics and people with motor disabilities such as stroke, tremor and brain injury and are depicted in Table 6.4. Patients, rehabilitation specialists and physiotherapists can all be found under one roof using IoT-based rehabilitation. The

Table 6.3 Various sensory prosthetics with their applications and limitations

S. No.	References	Methodology	Advantages and application	Limitations
1	Peripheral nerve stimulation [22]	• Sensory feedback • Revokes somatotopic and permits haptic feedback	• Enhanced high sensitivity during touching, vibration • Induce exhaustive feedback such as textures and so on. E.g., Prosthetic hand	• Less spatial resolution • The coupling of feedback with sensitivity is irresolvable due to the size of the stimulator
2	Myoelectric prosthetic hand [23]	• Vibration stimulator • Vibration sheets made up of shape memory actuators are used	• Low-cost • Efficient • Non-invasive sensory prosthetics • E.g., Hand, arm and knee controlled prosthetic hand	• Prolonged vibration and changes inaccuracy
3	Vibrotactile stimulator for gait analysis [24]	• Used for Lower prosthesis • Produces low-intensity vibrations when gait transitions change • The individual's gait phase can be maintained as a result of this training	• Low-cost gait analysis • Speed recovery without cognitive burn • E.g., an Elderly patient having a transfemoral amputation	• The sample size is very low • Follow-up time is very low • No possibility of extension
4	Wearable feedback prosthetics [25]	• Ambulation feedback • The gadget for lower extremity amputees stretches the skin on the lateral surface	• Optimal accuracy of 98% is achieved • E.g., Lower limb amputee due to trauma and congenital defect	• Conjunctival irritation on the skin surface
5	Waist wearable feedback prosthetics [26]	• The wearable feedback prosthetic device can emit mild vibrations in the wrist when there is a walking phase change	• The symmetry index of gait was increasing • E.g. Irregularities in the spatiotemporal gait phase	• Concurrent compression on the trunk and pelvis will increase
6	Neuroplasticity principle-based sensory rehabilitation (NEPSER) [27]	• Motor and sensory recovery-NEPSER • Significant training using sensory modalities such as visuoperceptual, motor functional task for 8 week	• Not only enhancing sensory recovery it also enhances the motor and functional recovery • E.g., Poststroke hemiparetic patients	• Heterogeneity in the study the brain activities • Modality of sensory defects

(continued)

Table 6.3 (continued)

S. No.	References	Methodology	Advantages and application	Limitations
7	Sensory attenuation in rehabilitation [28]	• Basal ganglia task-related sensory information has been studied	• Easy navigation and interaction with the environment • E.g., Parkinson"s disease	• Sensory input for exercise programs is not enough

Fig. 6.1 Application of robotics in various fields

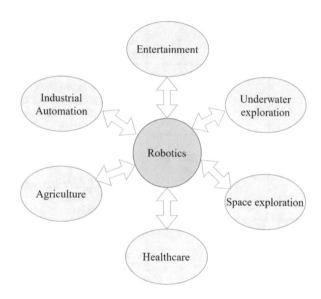

doctor can keep an eye on the patient from afar and patients can be trained in the comfort of their own homes, where they can undertake simple and repeated therapies [30]. The ROBIN is a rehabilitation robot that not only stabilizes body positions but also allows patients to perform simple hand movements including grasping and reaching for objects. This robot encourages individuals to exercise through video games, which can lead to more rehabilitation activities and improved motor function in the patient, resulting in a faster recovery. ROBIN is highly valuable for patients who are unable to visit their physician or therapist regularly [31]. It also incorporates artificial intelligence and results in breakthroughs in neurological rehabilitation. This brain rehabilitation program can teach a non-technical individual how to change the programming and neural robotics set up to ensure that the patient participates actively [32].

Key factors of Robotics Rehabilitation

- Self-executing systems make the user walk fast and also maintain their normal gait phase.

Table 6.4 Robotics applications in rehabilitation

S. No.	Prosthetics	Technology	Applications
1	Bionic glove	• Wearable robotic hand • SMA actuators assist pressure in the fingertip sensors • Information sent from robots to users	• Restore grip strength after stroke or accident
2	Robot-assisted gait analysis	• Joint trajectory to entire gait cycle and provide the stiffness • Replacement for wheelchair technology • Implantable therapies	• Stroke and spinal cord injury
3	Ankle Bot	• Exoskeleton robot • Apply the appropriate force to the ankle and train it to improve both walking style and balance	• Amputation • Muscular dystrophy • Cerebral palsy
4	CAREX (Cable-driven upper arm exoskeleton)	• Novel robots arm made up of robot-controlled prosthesis • 10 times lighter than arms • Assist the muscle and motor pattern	• Lightweight prosthetic hand
5	Genium Knee	• Microprocessor-controlled knee joint • Made up of the latest sensor and computer technology • Able to walk or stand on a slope • Able to optimize the wing phase	• Osgood schlatter disease (OSD)
6	MIT manus	• Simple video game for sensory-motor interfacing • People need to draw a shape or need to move along the point	• Post-stroke upper limb amputee
7	FLOAT	• Multidirectional overhead BWS (Body weight system) • Safe gait training for the person in a 3D environment • Computer-assisted robots	• Gait rehabilitation for paediatrics

- It is a mind-controlled device.
- It reduces physical stress as well as complications.
- High comfort and mobility in amputee life.

Limitations

- A complete report on the employment of robotics in rehabilitation has yet to be obtained.
- There is a substantial ethical and methodological constraint when robot-assisted rehabilitation is used for stroke victims.
- Simple movement patterns are utilized mainly for amusement, not for functional purposes.
- This therapy is out of reach for the poor or cannot be used by the general community due to its exorbitant cost.

6.3.4 Brain-Computer Interface (BCI)

For proper movement and motor control, neuronal interaction between the muscle and the brain is essential. If there is a medical issue, communication gets disrupted and the brain is unable to communicate, which may result in paralysis or neuronal damage. A Brain-Computer Interface can then be used to reawaken the brain that has been silenced by diseases such as amyotrophic lateral sclerosis (ALP), multiple sclerosis and brainstem stroke. BCI is a collection of basic software tools that employ an algorithm to convert brain impulses into actions. The operation of the BCI is shown in Fig. 6.2.

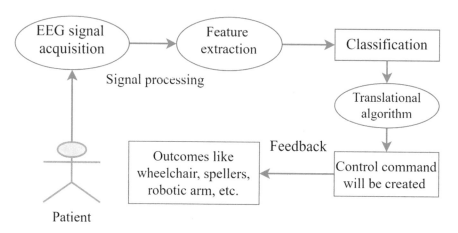

Fig. 6.2 Workflow diagram of brain-computer interface

Table 6.5 Physiological signals for BCI applications

S. No.	Physiological signals	Advantages	Limitations
1	Scalp EEG—scalp Recording of the electrical activity of the brain	• Easy • Safe • Less expensive	• Intracranial Information can't be gathered from the outside surface like the skull and scalp • Some information may be lost
2	Micro EEG—implantation of microarray in the cortex Individual neuron action potential is measured	• For a deep understanding of neurons and synapses	• Complex Neurosurgical procedure • The long-term functional stability is questionable
3	Intracortical BCI—microelectrode measurement from ventricles. Recording of intracranial scale pressure	• Larger area recording • More information can be acquired	• Neurosurgical implantation • Long-term electrode stability is unanswerable
4	Magnetoencephalography (MEG)—magnetic field generated due to an electrical activity from the cell axon Detection of (mu) rhythm	• Satisfactory control on BCI	• Difficult to conduct the experiment and obtain the result • Expensive
5	fMRI-functional MRI—various brain lobes Measures the activity level of oxygen	• Human brain-controlled robotic arm	• Cumbersome • Expensive

Dr J. Vidal discovered the brain-computer interface in 1970 while studying Electroencephalography (EEG) analysis and cerebral activity. BCI enables users to establish a direct link between their brain and external technologies which can lead to a variety of applications for disabled people, one of the most well-known of which is the human brain-controlled wheelchair. The analysis of brain signals utilising electrodes on the cortical surface, cortex and scalp is the most important aspect of the BCI interface and the technologies are named as follows in Table 6.5 [33].

6.3.4.1 BCI Components

As shown in Fig. 6.2, the following are the components of BCI:

• Signal acquisition unit—The EEG brain signal is obtained using scalp electrodes, then the electrical signals are transformed into digital signals and supplied to the computer.
• Signal processing unit- Utilizing captured EEG signal and a large amount of data, features such as alpha (8–12 Hz), beta (12–35 Hz), gamma (greater than 35 Hz),

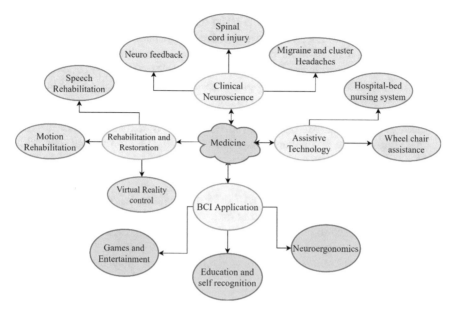

Fig. 6.3 BCI applications

delta (0.5–4 Hz), and Theta (4–8 Hz) waveforms can be extracted and can be converted into the control commands using translational techniques.

- Computer System- The algorithm's control command could be sent to output devices such as a wheelchair, robotic arm, spellers and cursor control.

BCI has applications in a variety of sectors as shown in Fig. 6.3 explained as follows [34].

The various applications of rehabilitation are

1. Rehabilitation and restoration—BCI has a wide range of applications in rehabilitation, as illustrated below

   a. Speech Rehabilitation—BCI is primarily used to help persons with speech disabilities, such as aphasia, improve communication. The disabled person selects one letter on a monitor and asks to build words to improve their speech capacity. E.g., Amyotrophic lateral sclerosis, locked-in syndrome (LIS).

   b. Motion Rehabilitation—The major goal of BCI is to improve the motor movement of impaired limbs, which will be categorized as.

   Lower limb-based on the frequency of visual stimuli from P300, determination movement direction can regulate wheelchair movement.

   Upper limb-major BCI's goal is to eliminate upper limb limitations by employing P300 or Somatosensory Visual Evoked Potentials (SSVEP). Using the above-mentioned potential, it can control the robotic arm's movement using a gripper. E.g. stroke rehabilitation and cerebral palsy.

c. Virtual Reality control (VRC)—The basic purpose of a BCI system is to improve communication between a disabled person and an external device. The person using brain patterns can move or touch the virtual object on the monitor, and the computer can then identify the event and communicate the elevated command prompt to the device. E.g. spinal cord injury and amyotrophic lateral sclerosis (ALS).

2. Clinical Neuroscience—The study of the nerve system is identified as clinical neuroscience and anyone can control the rehabilitation gadget using this. The following are some of the other applications of BCI-based rehabilitation in clinical neuroscience.

a. Neurofeedback—The use of BCI in Neurofeedback aids people in achieving a faster recovery and improving their overall quality of life. By employing neurofeedback to target brain activity, it is possible to increase brain performance. The expert can gather the individual's reaction by indulging in personal interaction with them. E.g. ALS, cerebral palsy, brainstem stroke.

b. Spinal cord injury—For examining the motor action improvement in spinal cord injury patients, Pfurtschellar combined multiple systems such as BCI, Functional Electric Stimulation (FES), and Sensor motor rhythms (SMR). This, in turn, improves peripheral nerve and motor neuron function. E.g. Spinal cord injury.

c. Migraine and cluster headaches—BCI is also utilized in the treatment of migraines, headaches, and depression. To detect migraines, EEG-based categorization methods are used. In the visual evoked potential environment, there is a general change in EEG complexity for migraine and head discomfort patients. Physical therapy can be provided by BCI to relieve tension in the cervical spine and muscular stiffness, hence reducing discomfort due to headaches and migraine.

3. Assistive technology—some examples of BCI's use in assistive devices include:

a. Hospital bed nursing system—LED stimulation is used to elicit the user's SSVEP as an input signal. The programmable gate array is then produced by the filter, amplifier circuit, and SSVEP processor to acquire and process the subject demand utilizing SSVEP. A specific drive circuit known as an H-bridge DC (Direct Current) motor is used to control the attitude of the hospital bed. E.g. spinal cord injury, muscular dystrophies, chronic peripheral neuropathies.

b. Wheelchair system—The P300 controlled wheelchair may receive direct commands from an EEG signal and deliver them to the wheelchair as control. The majority of disabled people are requesting this controlled wheelchair. E.g. Paralyzed and stroke rehabilitation.

- Neuroergonomics- The study of the human brain during daily activities and at work is known as neuroeconomics. Places of work, transportation, and home automation can all benefit from using a brain-computer interface to enhance safety, comfort, and physiological control over our daily activities. BCI has recently been integrated with IoT, which has enhanced the study and safety of individuals.

- Educational and self-recognition-using neurofeedback from functional MRI (fMRI), BCI can improve education and self-recognition in the following ways.

(i) It is used to offer training to combat depression and other psychiatric diseases.

(ii) It also helps to manage stress during sports competitions.

4. Games and Entertainment—Nonmedical BCI has a wide range of applications in gaming and entertainment, including the following:

(i) Brain Arena is a football game in which two BCIs are used. Goals can be scored by just moving your left or right hand.

(ii) The user simply needs to move the ball from side to side, which will relax the folks. The game's eventual result is a stress reduction.

6.4 Virtual-Reality (VR)

The user's interaction with the simulated environment is maintained with Virtual Reality (VR) where it allows users to interact with and experience real-world environments and may be utilised for both educational and entertaining purposes. Virtual reality in 3D portrays a physical and mental sense of being in the actual world.

6.4.1 Classification of Virtual Reality Based on Experience

- Fully Immersive simulations—It is capable of providing a fully immersive experience, including sound, vision and sense. Individuals have the impression that they are in the actual world. E.g. Gaming and Entertainment purposes like 3D filming.
- Semi-Immersive simulations- It provides a partial realistic experience where the complete vision of the virtual environment will be unavailable. It is used mainly for education and training purposes. E.g. aircraft simulators, medical surgery simulators.
- Non-Immersive simulations—No realistic experience in a virtual environment. A person knows we are in a physical place and interacting with the virtual one. E.g. Basic level of gaming.

The milestones in virtual reality are examined in Table 6.6.

Table 6.6 Milestones in virtual reality

Timeline	Scientist/inventor	Technology development	Applications
1838	Sir Charles Wheatstone	Mirror stereoscope	Photo or image gave the user a sense of immersion and depth
1890	Thomas Edison	Kinetoscope and kinetograph	Early motion picture
1935	Stanley Weinbaum	Fictional model for VR	Story over how, with the help of a pair of glasses, we can enter a fictional world
1929	Edwin link	Link trainer	Mechanical aeroplane simulator for training purposes
1956	Morton Heilig	Sensorama	First VR machine with Vibrating chair, smell and 3D screen
1961	C. Comeau & J. Bryan	Headsight	First head mount display used for motion tracking
1965	Sutherland	Sketchpad	Computer hardware for the interaction of the user in the virtual world
1965	Robert Mann	VR training environment for orthopaedics	Helps to learn various surgery techniques
1966	Thomas Furness	First flight stimulator	Military purpose
1968	Bob Sproull	Sword of damocles	Head mount display connected with a computer instead of a camera
1969	Myron Krueger	Artificial reality –Video place	It allows people who are thousands of miles apart to communicate with each other in a computer-generated environment
1975	Krueger's	Video place	Large room with big screen, Innovation of virtual communication
1977	Dan sandin	Sayre Glove	Light sensors with a light source on one side and a photocell on the other end of a flexible tube are used to measure finger flexon, lightweight and inexpensive
1979	Mc Donell-Douglas	Head tracker vital helmet	Military purpose
1980	Robert Mann	Wearable HMD	Visualization of medicine

(continued)

Table 6.6 (continued)

Timeline	Scientist/inventor	Technology development	Applications
1985	Jaron lanier and Thomas Zimmerman	Registered VR company	For selling VR goggles and data glove
1987	British aerospace	Virtual cockpit with the speech recognition system	Training simulator
1989	Scott foster	VIEW- astronaut stimulator	Astronaut stimulator
1991	Antonio Medina	Computer simulated teleoperation-from the Earth to mass robot rover design 3D gaming	3D gaming
1994	Dav Raggett	VRML (Virtual reality markup language)	File format for representing a 3D image
1997	Georgia Tech	Virtual Vietnam -VR based war zone	VR based war zone
2001	Maurice Benayoun	SAS cube	PC based cubic room
2007	Google	Street view map	Navigation purpose
2015	Wall street journal	VR roller coaster	For following the NASDAQ market
2021	Facebook	Horizon workroom	VR based conference rooms

6.4.2 Virtual Reality Devices

Virtual reality mostly deals with the sensory feedback of human beings and some of the common sensory-based devices used in virtual reality as shown in Fig. 6.4 are follows:

1. Head Mount Display

   - Pair of goggles over your eyes.
   - Provides 3D imaging virtual environment.
   - Includes headphones, sensors and blindfolds.
   - Very heavy, not able to use for long term.
   - The operation involves two screens with different stereoscopic images to create a 3D Effect.

2. Immersive Rooms

   - Due to discomfort in the head mount, an immersive room concept is introduced.
   - The changing stereoscopic image is displayed on the wall of the room.
   - This immersive room is helpful, especially in a simulation environment.

Fig. 6.4 Basic components
of virtual reality

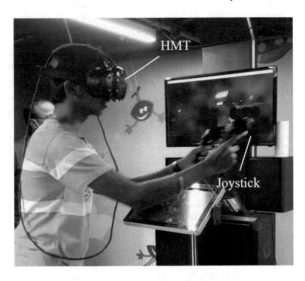

3. Hand Gloves

- It is a normal glove made up of various types of sensors for the detection of hand movements.
- Some of the sensors used in hand gloves are accelerometer (orientation of hand), hand bend sensors and gyros (Measuring the hand rotation).

VR is an emerging field with various types of applications in different fields is as shown in Fig. 6.5.

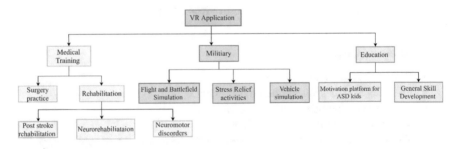

Fig. 6.5 Application of virtual reality in various fields

6.4.3 VR in Rehabilitation

The new method with improved intensity, frequency and time of the exercise without any stress is VR. It is a forefront technology ready to face recent therapeutic challenges, train people in a motivational way and boost the people's performance in a better way in a live environment. VR can work out real-life tasks as rehabilitation therapy [35].

Key Features of VR in Rehabilitation:

- It is easily adopted by all types of patients under therapy and the treatment is specific. E.g. Stroke survivors.
- VR provides a realistic environment so that the patient can take therapy in different scenarios and also in various phases.
- VR will make rehabilitation therapy an interesting and most interactive one with different types of games.
- VR will join hands with a human–computer interface for monitoring day-to-day life training activities and makes VR a safe and immersive training method which is not possible with other rehabilitation techniques. E.g. Autism patients.
- Interactive tools like tactile interfaces, mice, joypads make VR an entertaining and interactive one to track motions, especially for kids having Cerebral Palsy.

6.4.4 Game-Based VR Rehabilitation

No universal protocols are available to treat the upper limbs affected by stroke. The traditional treatment procedures are mostly repetitive training that is been given to motors causing a poor recovery rate. As discussed in Sect. 6.4, the VR based system is being used for various commercial applications and also as an assistive device for medical applications. For the past two decades, VR has been used in the healthcare ecosystem as a computer-interactive simulation that helps out disabled people to feel and practice the real-world experience in a virtual environment. If the post-therapy training is suggested through gaming than the conventional physiotherapy treatment plans, the patient's motor performance would exhibit greater improvement. Commercially available low-cost consoles have increased the attention of researchers and clinicians to recommend gaming-based therapy to patients. The observations by the clinicians after recommending VR based gaming rehabilitation has proved that there are significant improvements in movements, power and velocity. The most important elements of game-based interactive rehabilitation VR systems are illustrated in Fig. 6.6.

Some of the studies reveal that the treatment should be exciting, task-specific, interactive, encouraging, and intensive for neural disorders to recover at a faster rate. VR-based game therapy offers goal-oriented training to the patients to enhance motor, cognitive and learning skills. Many treatment plans recommend the patients to take up

Fig. 6.6 Elements of
game-based interactive
rehabilitation VR systems

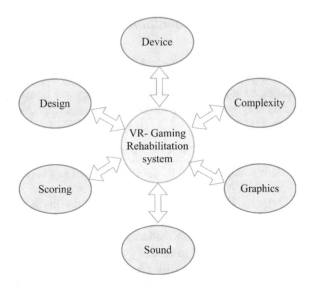

a task about an average of 30–45 min per day five times per week. Apart, constraint-induced movement therapy (CIMT) suggested for upper-limb rehabilitation for post-stroke requires 3–6 h of walking per day lasting up to 4–5 months. Such repetitive tasks lead to poor outcomes due to frustration among patients and caregivers. Though many gaming based systems are proposed by the researchers, still there are some limitations in them.

Limitations of Game-based rehabilitation without VR.

1. The integration of traditional rehabilitation treatment procedures into gaming-based systems.
2. Issues in solving neuromotor and cognitive disabilities simultaneously.
3. Lack of platform to integrate all game-based rehabilitation systems for various causes.
4. Lack of an alert system to avoid risky situations for the patients.
5. Lack of monitoring, controlling and evolution of patients using data observed.

As illustrated in Fig. 6.6, a tailor-made VR-Gaming rehabilitation system consisting of devices like accelerometers, gyroscopes, depth sensors, robotic gloves, VR head mounts, and other immersive components support the entire system. Many scoring methods have been proposed since January 2000. They are Fugl-Meyer-assessment (FMA), Wolf-motor-function-test (WMFT), Box-and-block-test (BBT), Action-research-arm-test (ARAT) and functional-independence-measure score (FIM). Based on the recent studies of rehabilitation, a gaming experience for the patients improves their interest and involvement in taking up long-duration training. Such approaches involve an intelligent system to get the feedback of the patients' response during the training, thereby optimal training is possible. To propose an approach for any treatment plans, two different approaches are followed. They are (i) user-centric approach and (ii) System-centric approach.

Fig. 6.7 User-centric
VR-gaming plan

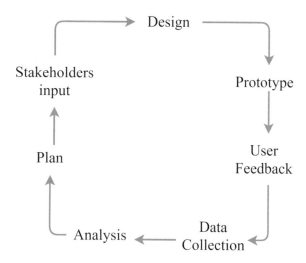

6.4.4.1   User-Centric VR-Gaming Rehabilitation System

User-centred gaming is an iterative process that is usually designed, based on the interviews with stakeholders and the results derived from other gaming activities carried out before the design plan. The interviews are made with various stakeholders who explain their conventional game-based rehabilitation experiences and detailed information is gathered based on the interaction. The challenges, opportunities, and possible risks are assessed from the questionnaire. Based on these inputs, a preliminary design plan is proposed. The essential resources like software and other hardware components are recommended for the prototype by the team in consultation with the expert members like game developers, clinicians, therapists and sports personalities. A brainstorming session is planned with the stakeholders to collect the issues that are faced. Till the team agrees to implement and validate the results, the process is repeated (brainstorming, expanding, and refining) as illustrated in Fig. 6.7.

6.4.4.2   System-Centric VR-Gaming Rehabilitation System

Many systems have been proposed to provide self-training to post-stroke patients at the chronic stage. Hardware-based solutions are used to estimate the patients' health status during joint movements. Goniometers or protractors are used to find the range of motion, joint velocity, torque, and reaching time. However, such instruments provide very low accuracy and are dependent on the evaluators.

6.4.5 System Requirements

Different hardware-based sensors are used to measure the conditions of the patients for physical rehabilitation. They are:

- Accelerometer—Patients' movements are observed by force sensors.
- Smart haptic gloves—Joint angle and grasping forces are measured.
- Xbox one—A Kinect camera to observe the gesture of the participants.
- Mirror—A mirror is placed in the patient's midsagittal plane with one limb behind the mirror. Mirror visual feedback (MVF) is a favourable technique to improve the performance of neurorehabilitation without training.
- Wearable sensors—To measure ECG, temperature, glucose, blood pressure, PPG, and respiration rate.
- Inertial sensors and force sensors—Gait analysis and measurements of knee angle, and foot planar pressure. An inertial measurement unit (IMU) is used to record the fall detection and posture monitoring for elderly.
- Leap motion sensor—Hand movements are tracked.

Fusion of multiple sensors like Kinect camera, bioelectric sensors, inertial sensors, pressure sensors, and motion sensors (IR, ultrasound, depth sensor, and camera with multi-array microphones) are used to observe the patients with upper and lower limb palsy, Parkinson's disease, stroke, multiple sclerosis, brain injury, and an autism spectrum disorder.

6.4.6 System Architecture

As mentioned in Sects. 6.4.4.1 and 6.4.4.2, the VR-based gaming rehabilitation system consists of two important interfacing components. They are (i) Patient interface and (ii) Therapists console. The patient interface has NLP interfacing elements to feel, hear and speak to the interactive rehabilitation system (Fig. 6.8).

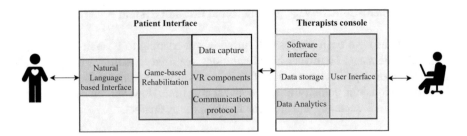

Fig. 6.8 System architecture

The various sensors and interactive elements (VR components) support the patients to train in a sporty environment with external commands towards a task-oriented ecosystem. Simultaneously, the vital parameters are also observed by the wearable systems. The primary objective of the system is to make the patients participate and be self-motivated. The therapists from the user interface observe and assess the patient's physiological and psychological parameters analysing large amounts of data that are being recorded. Such data is interpreted and visualised from different perspectives. This supports therapists in making well-defined decisions for futuristic exercise and rehabilitation training procedures.

6.5   VR Applications for Rehabilitation

In the past decade, the rehabilitation process helps to treat and slow down the disorder in various fields such as cardiology, oncology, neurology, and orthopaedics. Nowadays, it has witnessed burgeoning attention by implementing virtual reality (VR) technology for diagnosis and giving therapy for rehabilitation patients.

Importantly, VR presents an opportunity to assess various rehabilitation scenarios that are more challenging and are highly relevant to deal with real-world applications. Virtual reality is a key technology that provides feedback to patients during the rehabilitation process on a preferred schedule. In most of the VR applications outcome was delivered through sensory modalities including visual (eye) and auditory (ear) senses. Various real-world environment applications targeting various specific disorders like traumatic brain injury and learning disabilities are very useful for monitoring [36]. The simple structure of the VR system is designed in such a way that it can remotely track the patient's date, and initiate the rehabilitation sessions according to the current needs of the patients. Extended Reality (XR) is another science-based revolutionizing technology in Industry 4.0. It is more of mimicking real-life situations and scenarios.

This section covers different VR techniques in the field of mental rehabilitation for post-stroke treatments, cerebral palsy and autism disorders, also the role of VR in upper limb prosthetic training and the impact of sports rehabilitation. The two important categories of Virtual Reality in the healthcare field are simulation and interactive tools. Most doctors mainly prefer VR as a simulation tool before planning for surgery. The advantage of the technology is that surgeons can make mistakes during the process and learn from them without taking any risks to the patients.

6.5.1   Virtual Reality in Mental Rehabilitation

The virtual mode of the rehabilitation process for patients with mental disorders has been proven to be effective in modern-day healthcare delivery [37]. According to the authors, patients treated with virtual reality-based rehabilitation processes for mental health disorders, have reported to experience lower levels of depression, anxiety, and other negative symptoms than the standard treatment and also the recovery time is faster than the conventional method. VR in stroke rehabilitation helps patients to regain their muscle control [38]. Dementia is an abnormality with persons with loss of thinking and remembering ability can be addressed efficiently using VR technology. Psychiatric illness is termed as emotional and behavioural disorders in patients undergoing mental stress. VR treatment has the chance for patients with psychiatric illnesses to deal with a sudden changing phobia, anxiety, mental depression and cognition. Cerebral palsy (CP) is an abnormality that causes variations in the patient's tone of muscle, stance and limb movements, it requires rehabilitation techniques to support and cure the patient. The physicians face difficulties in performing physical and cognitive tasks using the VR technique for patients with CP. VR training is given to children affected by CP disorder to improve their interaction with other individuals. There are only a reduced number of randomized trials implemented using the VR technique, this is the key area that needs to be improved shortly.

6.5.1.1 Virtual Reality in Post-Stroke Treatments

According to statistics in India, the number of patients diagnosed with stroke is increasing in recent years. Recent research in the year 2022 suggests that the prevalence of stroke in countries like India ranges from 105 and 152 cases per 100,000 people per year [39]. Also according to the National Institutes of Health, there is a global alarm for increased cases of stroke patients annually. It is challenging to devise innovative rehabilitation programs for patients other than the conventional treatments. Hence, exploring VR in the rehabilitation process provides effective behavioural recovery and positive patient feedback.

6.5.1.2 The Computer-Based Desktop VR System

A VR system was designed with help of a computer for stroke patients with upper arm impairment by rehabilitating hand function. It consists of input–output gloves to make them suited for hand rehabilitation exercises. Input glove is a user glove with a pressure sensor and is advised to be worn on the patient's hand. Output glove is a feedback glove designed to be an exoskeleton biomechanical device used to measure force using implanted sensors in it.

User-glove is embedded with 18 pressure sensors, preferably strain-gauge sensors. It is designed to measure angles of the metacarpophalangeal joints and proximal interphalangeal of fingers. Each angle is calculated when the patient is allowed to do wrist flexion during rehabilitation exercises. During the VR rehabilitation process, every hand joint angle is converted into glove-sensor voltage as an output.

Feedback-glove is an output exoskeleton device that applies force to the user's fingertips. Pneumatic actuators with less weight are placed at the tips of each finger.

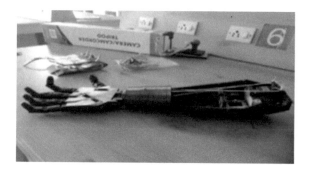

Fig. 6.9 Designed output exoskeleton system for VR rehabilitation system

An actuator is a sensor that converts applied energy in the form of force or pressure into mechanical motion. In the VR system around 16 N of force is slowly applied and displacement inside the glove (fingertip) is measured concerning their angle. The joint angles of all fingers are estimated as shown in Fig. 6.9.

Those two data are considered as sensor data and acquired data are filtered and taken for evaluation of patient's improvement in VR rehabilitation process in regular trials for a few weeks. The performance evaluation is very helpful for physiotherapists and patients to know their improvement in the post-stroke treatments.

The rehabilitation exercises with the implementation of the VR technique along with user and feedback gloves is illustrated in Fig. 6.10. The VR simulations tool needs to evaluate using four exercises for analyzing one particular parameter of the hand movement. The performance is calculated based on the range of hand movement, asking the patient to move one hand at a time, speed and strength of hand movement. During each trial, the patient is instructed to flex each finger one by one as much as possible and then open them to the maximum possible angle possible. The workout is performed separately for four fingers (ring, middle, index and thumb) excluding the little finger because of negligible movement from it. Different combinations of finger exercises are executed to obtain and evaluate all ranges of motion. The filtered data is stored in a database for future reference and for setting up a target for the next visit for rehabilitation. Based on the performance, a new target is calculated and assigned for a patient and taken as a new trial. Implementing target-based exercises in VR simulation requires a previous target to evaluate the patient's movement. Each time the same set of a VR rehabilitation process is continued and applied to the patient.

6.5.1.3 Application: Computer Game-Based Therapy for Post-stroke Therapy

In this section, the author identifies the various applications for post-stroke treatment both in VR and CGBT.

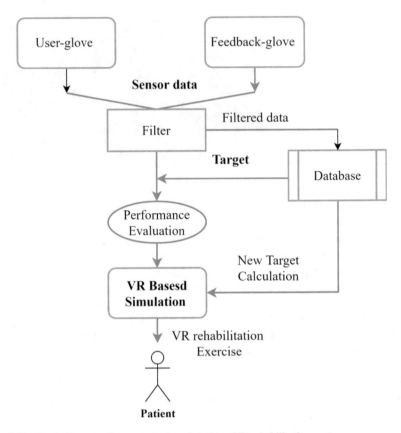

Fig. 6.10 Block diagram of a computer-based desktop VR rehabilitation system

- Virtual Underwater fire CGBT game was designed to study the patient's upper extremity movement and hand–eye coordination.
- Virtual Goalkeeper games is one of the CGBT games expected to analyze the upper extremity parameters like speed controlling, stamina, precision, and various motion range.
- Bug hunter is a CGBT game that efficiently improves upper limb impairments and studies the capability of the hand to react to all challenges given to patients in the stroke group.
- The rollercoaster virtual game was designed to increase the speed of upper Extremities and trunk movements.
- Nintendo Wii (NW)—Type of CGBT video games brings some fun for stroke patients in their post-treatment for the recovery process and help patients to regain the lost strength and core motor skills.
- XaviX Tennis Racket—Type of CGBT tennis in video games mode where the user can control the game using a tennis racket. It is very interactive and fun to

play. The user can play tennis action by putting serve, volley at baseline of court, charging the net and pitching the ball with wireless XaviX Technology.

- Sony Playstation MOVE—High-Velocity Bowling is one of the virtual games available in the playstation network developed by Sony Entertainment. The patients undergoing upper hand stroke treatment can use this CGBT tool for recovery.
- The other games available in the CGBT environment using the above tool are Nintendo Wii bowling, boxing, goalkeeper game, XaviX bowling, bird hunter, shooting, etc.

In the investigation done through these commercial video games for improving upper extremity function after stroke on 24 patients with first-time stroke, results are effective in CGBT based recovery process compared with conventional rehabilitating treatment. Assessment of motor function was done, results are efficient in XaviX tennis application compared to conventional physical exercise [33].

6.5.1.4 Limitations

The software interface used in various video games and system setup is in other languages like Japanese and it is not easy to understand by the users. The software response time of the game is too fast and not easy for patients to play. In some CGBT processes with haptic devices to control a non-immersive environment, some patients may have difficulty handling it. During the study, some patients felt that games were too difficult. The difficulty levels of the games may be increased/decreased considering the patient post-treatment process.

6.5.2 Autism

Autism is a neuro disorder identified for the patient with difficulty with social interaction, behavioural changes, and lack of communication and has restrictions without emotional ties. In the reported case, children with the autistic disorder will have noticeable stereotypical movements, such as coordinated hand clapping or arm flapping whenever the child is getting excited or upset. It is characterized by childhood. More cases are reported recently worldwide and identified as a developmental disabilities.

Very simple VR activity-based training practice was given to children like reading social signals helps them to express socially appropriate behaviours. Training in a virtual outdoor environment, children with autism disorder were seen interacting with faster recovery [40]. Various virtual reality systems are implemented to identify the moving and walking pattern of ASD children. One such VR-based system is discussed in this section to capture the acceleration speed and moving gestures of the children affected with autism. In this study, 5 children with autism have taken

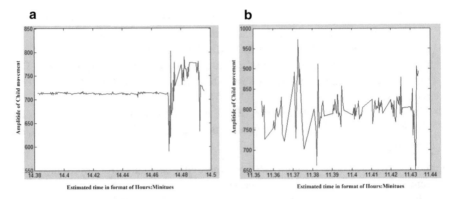

Fig. 6.11 Plotted graph of **a** normal child, **b** an autistic child

part in analysis and the average age of autistic children undergone in the study was 5–15. The VR task was to identify the various walking gestures and speed of the child. The obtained output is evaluated by plotting the graph (Time vs. Amplitude of child movement) using MATLAB software as shown in Fig. 6.11. The analysis using the VR system clearly shows the difference in the pattern of movement for normal children and autistic children. Each of the autistic children has different walking movements and speeds. The child affected with autism disorder's walking speed differs from a healthy person is monitored and evaluated by the physician and physiotherapist. This analysis will be very helpful for the doctors to analyze the walking speed and conclude the disorder to the children is hyper or hypo.

Results of the certain investigation by evaluating the capability of the VR system during the rehabilitation process are encouraging. But still, there are some restrictions of the current study to proceed with children with the disorder. Additionally, a fundamental challenge in designing VR and XR systems is the accuracy in interactions, and the need for a robust device in the VR platform.

6.5.3 Cerebral Palsy

Cerebral palsy (CP) is termed to be a disorder with the movement of any person due to muscle stiffness and reported in early childhood where the babies won't be able to crawl or sit, walk initially as other children of the same age group because of preterm birth or low weight during birth. According to recent statistics, one to nearly four per thousand children reported with cerebral palsy around the world. In a recent study conducted in the year 2010, 58.9% of CP-affected children can walk on their own, 7.8% of children need hand-held assistive devices to walk, and 33.3% of them cannot walk [41].

Giving early treatment to CP patients with the assistance of VR techniques is very helpful for paediatricians, neurologists and parents to handle them better during treatment procedures. Therapeutic tools were introduced by various physiotherapists and physicians with some virtual reality games, this ambience helps to cure neurological disorders in a faster and more interactive manner [42]. For CP patients, VR technology motivates the patients through the rehabilitation process by offering more security, flexibility exercises, attracting patients towards given tasks and increasing social interface.

6.5.3.1 Application: Virtual Game System for Cerebral Palsy

According to the studies and surveys of authors, one of the most popular VR gaming is the 'Wii game' is a motion-detecting video game platform bringing physical activity into gameplay. It provides good results for CP patients by helping children to improve hand function. Players are CP patients, they swing a handheld remote device that interacts with on-screen activities to deliver a more productive physical gaming experience. According to the author [43] the CP patients were separated into two groups:

- The first group received a standard conventional method of neurodevelopmental rehabilitation treatment for patients with cerebral palsy.
- The second group of CP patients was given VR therapy by allowing them to play 3 games of virtual tennis, boxing and baseball using a Wii game-pad and treatment was given to the patients continuously for 6 weeks.

Check Limit Game: In this game-based VR system, two methods are followed. The first one is by connecting the Kinect sensor used for motion capture by attaching it to the patient's body and the second method of motion capture is done using the touchscreen. The response through these interfaces to the game is recorded. The game-based analysis system was established by the Information Systems Laboratory at the University of Sao Paulo [44]. After the analysis of motion capture in two systems of VR games, the Kinect system gives better performance than the Touchscreen method [45].

6.5.3.2 Outcomes and Limitations

The physician then evaluated the independence of each patient and the arm-hand mobility of each child. As expected, the second group that had been playing video games in VR systems for several weeks scored ominously higher in tests that measured for identifying the abilities of a patient's arm movement. Wii-fit VR video games system for CP patients is a promising sign by giving better evaluation results in both static and performance parameters when combined with regular treatment in children with mild CP [46]. Although there are still very few clinical trials and real-time studies are carried out, there are still more unaddressed problems while implementing virtual reality on humans.

6.5.4   Upper Limb Prosthetic Training

Nowadays amputation cases have increased drastically because of road accidents and in severe cases, they have to face the fate of amputation. Upper arm training is considered one of the therapeutic procedures in neuro-rehabilitation for patients with paralyzed upper extremities. Artificial prosthetic hands are the best possible choice if the patient loses their upper limb. In recent years 3D printing has become a handy tool to design and print artificial upper limbs. CURA is popular software used to design the prosthetic model named Bionic arm and output is uploaded in the 3D printer for printing artificial limbs [47].

To provide training to the prosthetic upper limb, micro servo motors are connected using fishing lines. An electromyogram (EMG) signal is acquired to train the Bionic arm as shown in Fig. 6.12 using a clamp electrode attached with micro servo motors. The EMG signal for both muscle contraction and relaxation is obtained and transmitted to the Arduino board for training purposes. After receiving the signal from the EMG regarding muscle contraction and relaxation of the Bionic arm, evaluation is made to observe the performance of the upper prosthetic limb. Based on the evaluation, the real-time prosthetic arm is designed and used for amputee patients.

6.5.4.1   Application: Serious Gaming VR System

Serious gaming is a VR tool used recently in clinical practice that has gained more attention in treating motor dysfunctions in the upper extremity.

- Various categories of game types are incorporated in serious gaming tools like virtual reality (VR), augmented reality (AR), video games, e-board games, and mobile health games [48].
- Serious gaming is simulated in the real world in 3D virtual environments using computer graphics.

a   **b**

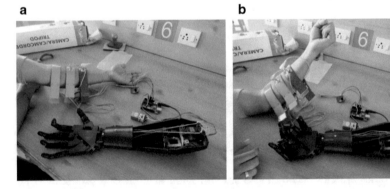

Fig. 6.12   a During contraction and **b** relaxation of Bionic arm

- Kinect depth sensors are used to capture body parts and follow their movements in VR systems and analyze the performance of the upper extremity. It can be combined with EMG and other biosignals during gaming.
- The Kinect sensors were positioned on upper limb measuring areas to track the coordinates of the arm movement and hand movement.
- IDLE RACING GO is a gaming platform using video gaming techniques that bring a unique idle clicking experience for the user and can be analysed based on their performance in the gaming levels.

6.5.5 Sports Rehabilitation Exercises

In sports, many indoor and outdoor athletes are prone to physical or internal injuries due to various reasons like an increase in athlete's workload. Because of the demands of competitive sport, the inability to manage player workload results in excessive wear and tear of muscle/bone. An immediate and effective rehabilitation exercise program helps the players to regain their physical strength, flexibility, and stamina quickly after an injury, empowering them to resume their athletic activities. Sports Rehabilitation is a key process for a player's sports life that helps to decide the return of injured players safely to practice or competition. Physiotherapists in the healthcare field work closely with injured players to undergo the rehabilitation phase for recovery by giving wide-ranging training, especially in the musculoskeletal system.

6.5.5.1 Case Study: The Pattern of Common Musculoskeletal Injuries in Male Basketball Players

Musculoskeletal Injury (MSI) is the possible sports injury commonly registered in any person participating in sports like basketball and volleyball. In these types of sports, heavy complex movement was given to muscles and joints like jumps, sudden turns and rapid changes in direction of the person. According to the muscle study conducted [49], the injury site at the right knee is in high danger with 40.17% because of the heavy workload compared to the left knee. The lowest possible injury site in basketball is the right thigh with an injury range of 0.71–0.87%.

6.5.5.2 Sports Rehabilitation Protocol Findings

The most common injury in the musculoskeletal system of any sportsperson is hamstring injury and it is considered complex for any individual. The occurrence of hamstring injury is widely seen in athletes involving fast sprinting, hurdling and water-skiing. Hamstring muscles are stabilized in the hip and knee joint region during an excessive contraction while playing and doing exercises. According to recent literature, severe hamstring injuries should undergo surgery and be followed by rehabilitation protocols to slow return of play (RTP). The sportsperson diagnosed with this type of injury is very challenging because of the complexity in anatomy surrounding the tissue. The VR based assistive devices support sportspersons with a lower extremity injury to stabilise both the foot and ankle.

During COVID–19 pandemic, many sports personalities have been affected by continuous lockdowns. The global sports calendar has been impacted, so lack of sports activities in lockdown time results in loss of performance for a player in their respective field [50]. Globally, most athletes are almost stuck indoors due to this novel disease affecting their mental health and overcoming this situation is a major challenge for any player and the physiotherapist. VR based gaming solution is an alternate and best approach to make them be in practice forever.

6.5.5.3 Guidelines for Sports Rehabilitation

Various guidelines to be followed during VR rehabilitation are-

- Based on the medical needs and resources, sports rehabilitation programs are to be modified and customised to access VR devices.
- Keeping patients interested while attending the program and undergoing a gaming system.
- Robust gaming platform: gaming tool to be user friendly and it should be used at any time and any place, especially in the comfort zone of the patient.
- Utmost care is to be taken to ensure the privacy of patients attending the rehabilitation program.
- Ability to record and communicate the progress of patients during rehabilitation games to the caretakers and patients. Patient gaming profile should be maintained properly.

6.6 Summary and Conclusion

The aim of this chapter proposed by the authors expressed their views on the use of modern rehabilitation technologies in terms of VR techniques. The role of Virtual Reality and its application discussed in this chapter have significant potential and positive impact on individual lives and in the healthcare field. The challenges behind the conventional rehabilitation processes were explored and a user-centric VR-Gaming rehabilitation system for the comfort zone of the patient during post-treatment has been proposed. Implementation of a VR-gaming rehabilitation system recommended to patients with stroke, cerebral palsy and autism disorders employing upper limb prosthetics and sports rehabilitation can have a major role to be played by engineers and physiotherapists. There is a wide range of virtual reality applications in modern rehabilitation treatments that were summarized in this chapter. The VR system not only helps for better therapy for patients but keeps them interested while performing the rehabilitation program in a robust environment. The use of VR in association with post-therapy patients has shown encouraging results. In this chapter, the role of virtual games in faster recovery during post-therapy was discussed. The various applications of the rehabilitation process were illustrated in all sections for better quality patient care with faster recovery time. Case studies on sports rehabilitation exercises provided a systematic review for various musculoskeletal injuries to athletes and guidelines for them to return to play (RTP).

Acknowledgements The authors would like to sincerely thank reviewers for thoughtful comments and efforts towards improving this chapter. Also, they would like to extend their gratitude to the editors for considering this chapter and including in the book.

References

1. Cieza, A., Causey, K., Kamenov, K., Hanson, S.W., Chatterji, S., Vos, T.: Global estimates of the need for rehabilitation based on the Global Burden of disease study 2019: a systematic analysis for the global burden of disease study 2019. Lancet **396**(10267), 2006–2017 (2020)
2. Parola, V., Coelho, A., Neves, H., Cardoso, D., Almeida, M., Cruz, A., Apóstolo, J.: Palliative rehabilitation interventions in palliative care: a scoping review protocol. JBI Evid. Synth. **18**(11), 2349–56 (2020)
3. Mauk, K.L.: Overview of rehabilitation. Rehabilitation Nursing: A Contemporary Approach to Practice. Jones & Bartlett Learning, LLC (2011)
4. Proffitt, R.: Home exercise programs for adults with neurological injuries: a survey. Am. J. Occup. Ther. **70**(3), 7003290020p1–7003290020p8 (2016). https://doi.org/10.5014/ajot.2016. 019729
5. Virani, S.S., Alonso, A., Aparicio, H.J., Benjamin, E.J., Bittencourt, M.S., Callaway, C.W., et al.: Heart disease and stroke statistics—2021 update: a report from the American Heart Association external icon. Circulation **143**, e254-743 (2021)
6. Joo, S.Y., Lee, S.Y., Cho, Y.S., Lee, K.J., Kim, S.H., Seo, C.H.: Effectiveness of robot-assisted gait training on patients with burns: a preliminary study. Comput. Methods Biomech. Biomed. Eng. **23**(12), 888–893 (2020)
7. Murray, C.J. L., Vos, T., et al.: Disability adjusted life years (DALYs) for 291 diseases and injuries in 21 regions, 1990–2010: a systematic analysis for the global burden of disease study 2010. Lancet **380**(9859), 2197–223 (2012)
8. Allman, C., Amadi, U., Winkler, A.M., Wilkins, L., Filippini, N., Kischka, U., Stagg, C.J., Johansen-Berg, H.: Ipsilesional anodal tDCS enhances the functional benefits of rehabilitation in patients after stroke. Sci. Ttransl. Med. **8**(330), 330 (2016)
9. Barbe, M.F., Gallagher, S., Massicotte, V.S; Tytell, M., Popoff, S.N., Barr-Gillespie, A.E.: The interaction of force and repetition on musculoskeletal and neural tissue responses and sensorimotor behavior in a rat model of work-related musculoskeletal disorders. BMC Musculoskelet. Disord. 14 303 (2013). https://doi.org/10.1186/1471-2474-14-303.PMC3924406.PMID24156755
10. Mishra, S.D., Sarkar, K.: Work-related musculoskeletal disorders and associated risk factors among urban metropolitan hairdressers in India. J. Occup. Health **63**(1), e12200 (2021). https://doi.org/10.1002/1348-9585.12200.PMC7883474.PMID33586840
11. Lowe, B.D., Weir, P.L., Andrews, D.M. Cincinnati.: Observation-based posture assessment: review of current practice and recommendations for improvement. DHHS (NIOSH) Publication No. 2014–131 (2014)

12. Gallagher, S., Heberger, J.R.: Examining the interaction of force and repetition on musculoskeletal disorder risk: a systematic literature review. Hum. Factors J. Hum. Factors Ergon. Soc. **55**(1), 108–124 (2013). https://doi.org/10.1177/0018720812449648.PMC4495348.PMID23516797

13. Dobkin, B.H.: Rehabilitation after Stroke. N Engl J Med. **352**(16), 1677–1684 (2005). https://doi.org/10.1056/NEJMcp043511

14. Kwakkel, G., Veerbeek, J.M., van Weegen, E.E., Wolf, S.L.: Constraint-induced movement therapy after stroke. Lancet Neurol. **14**(2), 224–34 (2015)

15. Gandhi, D.B.C., Sterba, A., Kate, M.P., Khatter, H., Pandian, J.D.: Computer game-based rehabilitation for poststroke upper limb deficits- systematic review and meta-analysis. Int. J. Physiotherapy, **7**(1), 47–53 (2020). https://doi.org/10.15621/ijphy/2020/v7i1/193674

16. Tamayo-Serrano, P., Garbaya, S., Blazevic, P.: Gamified in-home rehabilitation for stroke survivors: analytical review. Int. J. Serious Games **5**(1), 1–26 (2018). https://doi.org/10.17083/ijsg.v5i1.224

17. Andregård, E., Magnusson, L.: Experiences of attitudes in Sierra Leone from the perspective of people with poliomyelitis and amputations using orthotics and prosthetics. Disabil. Rehabil. **39**(26), 2619–2625 (2017)

18. Mamalis, A.G., Ramsden, J.J., Grabchenko, A.I., Lytvynov, L.A., Filipenko, V.A., Lavrynenko, S.N.: A novel concept for the manufacture of individual sapphire-metallic hip joint endoprostheses. J. Biol. Phys. Chem. **6**(3), 113–117 (2006). https://doi.org/10.4024/30601.jbpc.06.03

19. Windrich, M., Grimmer, M., Christ, O., Rinderknecht, S., Beckerle, P.: Active lower limb prosthetics: a systematic review of design issues and solutions. Biomed. Eng. Online **15**(3), 5–19 (2016)

20. Manero, A., Smith, P., Sparkman, J., Dombrowski, M., Courbin, D., Kester, A., Womack, I., Chi, A.: Implementation of 3D printing technology in the field of prosthetics: past, present, and future. Int. J. Environ. Res. Public Health **16**(9), 1641 (2019)

21. Raspopovic, S., Valle, G., Petrini, F.M.: Sensory feedback for limb prostheses in amputees. Nat. Mater. **20**(7), 925–939 (2021)

22. Kim, K.: A review of haptic feedback through peripheral nerve stimulation for upper extremity prosthetics. Curr. Opin. Biomed. Eng., 100368 (2022)

23. Miyahara, Y., Kato, R.: Development of thin vibration sheets using a shape memory alloy actuator for the tactile feedback of myoelectric prosthetic hands. In: 2021 43rd Annual International Conference of the IEEE Engineering in Medicine & Biology Society (EMBC) pp. 6255–6258. IEEE (2021)

24. Crea, S., Edin, B., Knaepen, K., Meeusen, R., Vitiello, N.: Time-discrete vibrotactile feedback contributes to improved gait symmetry in patients with lower-limb amputations: a case series. Phys. Ther. **97** (2016). https://doi.org/10.2522/ptj.20150441

25. Husman, M.A.B., Maqbool, H.F., Awad, M.I., Abouhossein, A., Dehghani-Sanij, A.A.: A wearable skin stretch haptic feedback device: towards improving balance control in lower limb amputees. In: 2016 38th Annual International Conference of the IEEE Engineering in Medicine and Biology Society (EMBC), pp. 2120–2123 (2016). https://doi.org/10.1109/EMBC.2016.7591147.

26. Martini, E., et al.: Increased symmetry of lower-limb amputees walking with concurrent bilateral vibrotactile feedback. IEEE Trans. Neural Syst. Rehabil. Eng. **29**, 74–84 (2021). https://doi.org/10.1109/TNSRE.2020.3034521

27. Arya, K.N., Pandian, S., Agarwal, G.G., Chaudhary, N., Joshi, A.K.: Effect of neuroplasticity-principles-based SEnsory-rehabilitation (NEPSER) on sensori-motor recovery in stroke: study protocol for a randomized controlled trial. Neurol. Res. Pract. **3**(1), 1–9 (2021)

28. Kearney, J., Brittain, J.S.: Sensory attenuation in sport and rehabilitation: a perspective from research in Parkinson's disease. Brain Sci. **11**(5), 580 (2021)

29. Chang, W.H., Kim, Y.H.: Robot-assisted therapy in stroke rehabilitation. J. Stroke **15**(3), 174 (2013)

30. Pradhan, B., Bharti, D., Chakravarty, S., Ray, S.S., Voinova, V.V., Bonartsev, A.P., Pal, K.: Internet of things and robotics in transforming current-day healthcare services. J. Healthc. Eng. |Article ID 9999504 (2021). https://doi.org/10.1155/2021/9999504
31. Loureiro, R.C., Smith, T.A.: Design of the ROBIN system: a whole-arm multi-model sensorimotor environment for the rehabilitation of brain injuries while sitting or standing. In: Proceedings of the 2011 IEEE International Conference on Rehabilitation Robotics, pp. 1–6, IEEE, Zurich, Switzerland, June 2011 (2011)
32. Nizamis, K., Athanasiou, A., Almpani, S., Dimitrousis, C., Astaras, A.: Converging robotic technologies in targeted neural rehabilitation: a review of emerging solutions and challenges. Sensors 21(6), 2084 (2021)
33. Shin, J.H., Ryu, H., Jang, S.H.: A task-specific interactive game-based virtual reality rehabilitation system for patients with stroke: a usability test and two clinical experiments. J. Neuroeng. Rehabil. 11, 32 (2014)
34. Bamdad, M., Zarshenas, H., Auais, M.A.: Application of BCI systems in neurorehabilitation: a scoping review. Disabil. Rehabil. Assist. Technol. 10(5), 355–364 (2015)
35. Boedecker, C., Huettl, F., Saalfeld, P., Paschold, M., Kneist, W., Baumgart, J., Preim, B., Hansen, C., Lang, H., Huber, T.: Using virtual 3D models in surgical planning: workflow of an immersive virtual reality application in liver surgery. Langenbecks Arch. Surg. 406(3), 911–915 (2021)
36. Rizzo, A., Schultheis, M., Kerns, K., Mateer, C.: Analysis of assets for virtual reality applications in neuropsychology. Neuropsychol. Rehabil. Neuropsychol Rehabil. 14, 207–239 (2004). https://doi.org/10.1080/09602010343000183
37. Krebs, H.I., Hogan, N., Aisen, M.L., Volpe, B.T.: Robot-aided neurorehabilitation. IEEE Trans Rehabil. Eng. 6(1), 75–87 (1998). https://doi.org/10.1109/86.662623
38. Jack, D., et al.: Virtual reality-enhanced stroke rehabilitation. IEEE Trans. Neural Syst. Rehabil. Eng. 9(3), 308–318 (2001). https://doi.org/10.1109/7333.948460
39. Jones, S.P., Baqai, K., Clegg, A., Georgiou, R., Harris, C., Holland, E.J., Kalkonde, Y., Lightbody, C.E., Maulik, P.K., Srivastava, P.M., Pandian, J.D., Kulsum, P., Sylaja, P.N., Watkins, C.L., Hackett, M.L.: Stroke in India: a systematic review of the incidence, prevalence, and case fatality. Int. J. Stroke 17(2), 132–140 (2022)
40. Park M.J., Kim D.L., Unjoo, Na, E.J., Jeon, H.J.: A literature overview of virtual reality (VR) in treatment of psychiatric disorders: recent advances and limitations. Front. Psychiatry (2019)
41. Chen, Y.P., Kang, L.J., Chuang, T.Y., Doong, J.L., Lee, S.J., Tsai, M.W., Jeng, S.F., Sung, W.H.: Use of virtual reality to improve upper-extremity control in children with cerebral palsy: a single-subject design. Phys. Ther. 87(11), 1441–1457 (2007)
42. Tarakci, D., Ersoz Huseyinsinoglu, B., Tarakci, E., Razak, O.A.: (2016) Effects of Nintendo Wii-Fit® video games on balance in children with mild cerebral palsy. Pediatr. Int. 58(10), 1042–1050 (2016)
43. Machado, F.C., Antunes, P., Souza, J., Levandowski, D., Oliveira, A.: Virtual reality technology for rehabilitation of cerebral palsy: a literature review. Temas em Psicol. 22, 565–577 (2014) https://doi.org/10.9788/TP2014.3-03
44. Koutsiana, E., Ladakis, I., Fotopoulos, D., Chytas, A., Kilintzis, V., Chouvarda, I.: Serious gaming technology in upper extremity rehabilitation: scoping review. JMIR Serious Games 8(4), e19071 (2020). https://doi.org/10.2196/1907
45. Okonkwo, C.A., Okereke, E.C., Umunnah, J.O., Ibikunle, P.O., Egwuonwu, V., et al.: Pattern of Musculoskeletal injuries amongst male amateur basketball players in Anambra State. Nigeria. Int. J. Sports Exerc. Med. 8, 212 (2022). https://doi.org/10.23937/2469-5718/1510212
46. Molina, C.S., Faulk, J.B.: Lower Extremity Amputation. (Updated 2021 Aug 25). In: Stat Pearls (Internet). Treasure Island (FL): Stat Pearls Publishing (2022)
47. Kalra, S.S., Mallick, A., Dande, J.: Sports medicine practice during COVID-19 pandemic—a "New Normal." Int. J. Sports Exerc. Med. 6, 174 (2020). https://doi.org/10.23937/2469-5718/1510174

48. Durkin, M.S., Benedict, R.E., Christensen, D., Dubois, L.A., Fitzgerald, R.T., Kirby, R.S., Maenner, M.J., Van Naarden, B.K., Wingate, M.S., Yeargin-Allsopp, M.: Prevalence of cerebral palsy among 8-year-old children in 2010 and preliminary evidence of trends in its relationship to low birthweight. Paediatr. Perinat. Epidemiol. **30**(5), 496–510 (2016)
49. Chen, M.H., Huang, L.L., Lee, C.F., Hsieh, C.L., Lin, Y.C., Liu, H., Chen, M.I., Lu, W.S.: (2015) A controlled pilot trial of two commercial video games for rehabilitation of arm function after stroke. Clin. Rehabil. **29**(7), 674–682 (2015). https://doi.org/10.1177/0269215514554115
50. Leal, A.F., da Silva, T.D., Lopes, P.B., et al.: (2020) The use of a task through virtual reality in cerebral palsy using two different interaction devices (concrete and abstract)—a cross-sectional randomized study. J. Neuro Eng. Rehabil. **17**, 59 (2020). https://doi.org/10.1186/s12984-020-00689-z

Chapter 7
The Use of Serious Games for Developing Social and Communication Skills in Children with Autism Spectrum Disorders—Review

Polina Mihova, Margarita Stankova, Filip Andonov, and Stanislav Stoyanov

Abstract The rate of Autism Spectrum Disorder (ASD) diagnoses has peaked in recent years—2000 study found ASD birth-year prevalence of one in 150 eight-year-olds, or 0.67%—which at the time was considerably higher than previous findings. In 2021, the U.S. Centers for Disease Control issued alarming new data indicating that the rate of autism among American eight-year-old children had risen again, this time to 1 in 44, or about 2.3% (American Psychiatric Association in Diagnostic and statistical manual of mental disorders. Arlington [1]). Many studies prove the effectiveness and positive impact of using smart telephones, mobile apps, and computer games to practice skills as therapy for children with ASD (Meghan et al. in Pediatrics 141:335–345 [2]). This review summarizes some of the most interesting and accessible serious games described in the scientific literature and designed to improve the social and communication skills of infants and toddlers with ASD. Learning and playing games are fundamental to the development of children's social skills allowing them to form independent relationships with peers (Simonoff et al. in J Am Acad Child Adolesc Psychiatry 47(8):921–929 [3]). As autistic children often have difficulty with peer relationships (Gordon-Lipkin et al. in Pediatrics 141(4) [4]), developing game-based skills through computer-assisted solutions could be an essential tool for autistic children to improve their social performance. The results were identified through extensive literature search conducted in the Central and Eastern European Online Library (CEEOL), EBSCO: Academic Search Complete, EBSCO: eBook Academic Collection and ScienceDirect, Academic Search Complete, Health Source: Consumer Edition, ScienceDirect, Scopus, Web of Science and Wiley Online Library for a time period between 2006 and 2021 by using a combination of the following free-text terms: autism, ASD, social skills, serious games, computer games, education, communication, software, portable, computer-based. The search was limited

P. Mihova (✉) · M. Stankova · F. Andonov · S. Stoyanov
New Bulgarian University, Sofia, Bulgaria
e-mail: pmihova@nbu.bg

S. Stoyanov
Department of Natural and Computing Science, University of Aberdeen, Aberdeen, UK

© The Author(s), under exclusive license to Springer Nature Switzerland AG 2023
C. P. Lim et al. (eds.), *Artificial Intelligence and Machine Learning for Healthcare*,
Intelligent Systems Reference Library 229,
https://doi.org/10.1007/978-3-031-11170-9_7

to papers published in the English language. We finally highlight current common limitations and address new challenging research directions.

Keywords Autism spectrum disorder · Serious games · Computer technology · Social skills

Abbreviations

ASD	Autism Spectrum Disorder
ADHD	Attention Deficit Hyperactivity Disorder
ICT	Information and Communication Technologies
GPU	Graphics Processing Unit
SG	Serious Games
USB	Universal Serial Bus
SEN	Special Educational Needs
AR	Augmented Reality
SLT	Speech and Language Therapist
TUI	Tangible User Interface

7.1 Introduction

The inclusion of technology to aid work with children with special educational needs has become increasingly popular in recent years. In general, technology allows for variety, attracts children's attention, increases their motivation, provides visual presentation of stimuli, helps develop additional skills that cannot be enhanced using conventional approaches. In addition, children are constantly immersed in technology and its use for skills development provides opportunities for indirect interventions.

Educational computer games—web based, for mobile devices, for desktop computers and even for the emerging fields of augmented and virtual reality can be successfully introduced in the assessment and therapy of children with autism spectrum disorders (ASD). These technologies are indispensable tools for aiding children with ASD acquire both academic and social skills.

7.2   Background

7.2.1   Autism Spectrum Disorder (ASD)

Autism spectrum disorder (ASD) is a set of neurodevelopmental conditions characterized by problems in the following two domains: (1) deficits in social communication and social reciprocity and (2) restricted and repetitive patterns of behavior, interests, or activities (American Psychiatric Association). The conditions included in the specter are characterized by the problems in these two domains, but the group is generally heterogeneous in terms of additional symptoms and their severity as well as in terms of etiology and the need for treatment. Usually, children with ASD receive treatment and support from a professional, sometimes from a team of professionals, more often individually, less often in a group. If the methods used are evidence-based practices for ASD therapy, this is often difficult to provide and, in many cases, too expensive, so the focus is on additional supportive strategies that can help achieve the results of the treatment without replacing it. These additional strategies may be aimed at the main symptoms or at additional, concomitant disorders such as anxiety, depression [2]; oppositional behavior [3], ADHD [4], language and speech disorders [5, 6].

7.2.2   Application of Information and Communication Technologies in Therapy

In recent decades, the use of Information and Communication Technologies (ICT) has grown exponentially and is now ubiquitous. Not only are personal computers a common household item but personal mobile devices have reached all corners of the world. Furthermore, smart gadgets are being developed thanks to cheap and easily accessible integrated electronic modules like ESP-8266 and ESP 32.

This opens new possibilities to help children and adults diagnosed with ASD to learn skills in a new way, tailored to their special needs.

There are several objectives for the use of ICT for ASD assessment and treatment:

- to help with the sensory and cognitive difficulties of the patients.
- to provide new ways for therapy and training.
- to provide educational tools for the acquisition of academic skills.
- to give the patient the opportunity to control her focus on a certain goal.
- to entertain and provide fun.

More specifically, modern technologies can help improve the following skills:

- learning
- memory
- attention

- language and communication
- reading and writing
- problem solving
- mathematical skills
- cooperating with others/social behavior
- first aid
- working abilities
- motor functions
- skills to overcome frustration
- self-control
- social skills
- understanding of social rules.

A benefit of using those technologies is that they can be designed in such a way as to adapt to the specific needs of a specific user. This includes not only customization, but also intelligent adaption during their use.

It is also important to note that the use of ICT is not limited to patients, but can also facilitate parents/guardians, caregivers, and professionals in the field of medicine, psychology, speech and language pathology, occupational therapy, and social work.

7.2.3 Types of Technologies

Various types or classes of technologies have been shown beneficial to children with ASD:

- Websites—their main advantage is their accessibility. Browser-based text-based, 2D and 3D games as well as a variety of multimedia content can be developed and using responsive design played on an entire range of devices—from laptops to mobile phones or smart TVs.
- Desktop applications—with the current dominance of the MS Windows operating system, desktop computers and laptops present a large, unified target for developing software. Several powerful 3D game engines like Unity and Unreal allow for the relatively easy creation of virtual worlds with impressive realism.
- Mobile apps—the last decade has seen smartphones accessible to almost everybody. Touch screens, powerful processors and integrated GPUs allow for the development of any type of game or application. The market is dominated by just two operational systems: Apple's iOS and Google's Android.
- Augmented/virtual reality devices—although still more expensive and less popular than the above-mentioned technologies, augmented or virtual reality devices are becoming more accessible with big companies, including Facebook, investing in such technologies.
- Serious games—any type of game, including those listed here, whose primary goal is not 'fun' per se, but the gamification of an existing process.

- Physical devices, robots, etc.—tangible objects that provide more than audio-visual experience and are a desired tool when dealing with children with ASD.

7.2.4 Serious Games

Probably one of the largest types of applications are the Serious Games (SG). Games are a form of entertainment that broadens our horizons beyond what is immediately conceived. All games share common characteristics such as established rules, rivalry, place and time, elements of fiction, elements of chance, pre-set goals and last but not least—gaining pleasure. Social games date back five millennia but it was the year 1974 that was marked as the most important year in the history of modern gaming as it was then that Dungeons and Dragons hit the market [7].

Presumably, the most common definition of serious games is "games that do not have entertainment, enjoyment, or fun as their primary purpose" [8]. Following this definition, serious games can be distinguished from video games by their design goals, because serious games have a main design goal other than entertainment. This means that the player is exposed to an environment that offers content based on know-how or experience. This experience relates to the specific context of serious games such as welfare, education, and health. Therefore, the authors [9] define serious gaming as an application with three components: experience, entertainment, and multimedia. The SG are also called learning or educational games and are a virtual simulation with a video-game structure whose purpose is to promote the development of important skills and strategies in order to increase the cognitive and intellectual abilities of the users [10]. These types of games are gaining popularity and have a share of the global game market [11]. Games can be used to promote thinking, visual attention, hand–eye coordination, visual spatial behavior, motor skills [12], social skill training [13]. Children respond positively to the introduction of gaming in learning and the majority of parents and experts have a similar attitude [14, 15]. Games can help children learn how to win and lose, to start from scratch, and to find various coping strategies. Multiplayer games teach children to take turns, wait for their turn, observe, and analyze other players' behavior.

Studies have researched the application of SG for children with ASD [16]. Video games can be used to reduce the symptoms of ASD and although their effect is not significant, their help creates a positive attitude and adherence to treatment [17]. When working with autistic children, computer games can be beneficial for reducing anxiety [18], improving face recognition skills, [19] and teaching new skills, including social skills and emotion regulation [20].

In general, serious games are usually 2D, mobile based, iOS or Android games, fewer are web-based, and their primary function is a Picture Exchange Communication System (PECS)—where the users communicate their needs by exchanging pictures with their communicative partners [21–23], some specific social skill learning games like catching the bus or a general skill practicing application like drawing and playing music [24]. A key aspect of serious games is their ability to use personalization [25] and that could be greatly beneficial for children with ASD [26]. For example, mathematical tasks can be adapted to the needs of a specific user [27] and the adaptation of the content is beneficial to the learning process [28, 29].

Interactive robots in ASD research and treatment are still an area that is in its infancy. There have been a few attempts in this direction. The authors [30] initially developed a robot to mimic autism-like behaviors in order to better understand autism spectrum disorder. Their idea evolved and they subsequently researched its potential use in therapy sessions. They used an ADOS-2 diagnostic tool to program the robot to display ASD-type behavior when interacting with humans. The set of external stimuli was predefined.

Bartneck et al. [31] took a different approach. They studied the effects of integrating a powerful 3D game engine (Unity 3D) with sensors and actuators. The benefit of this approach is that the body of the robot can be made in many different ways. For their first prototype they used a Lego set, servomotors, and a USB webcam to make the robot "see." They continued the experiments with a 3D-printable open-source robot called inMoov.

Augmented reality has still not gained much popularity but some early attempts at providing this technology to children with ASD showed it has potential [32]. They developed games targeting children aged 8–15. Even though they used a technology that was being phased out (Adobe Flash), the results were promising. For example, the user had to control an animated character by tilting a blue colored object left or right. With the current state of cameras, processing power, optimized for AI tasks, the potential of augmented reality is almost limitless.

Microsoft's Kinect sensor combines multiple technologies for depth sensing and provides immersive gaming experiences [33]. A robot described by [34] used a Kinect sensor to imitate autistic children. Other uses of the Kinect sensor include games that allow children to play in teams [33].

Several attempts to use augmented reality (AR) for games have been made. A game called Augmented Reality Gamebook [35] contains several scenarios for stories that are audio-visually presented. In the newer versions of the iPhone mobile phone platform there are built-in sensors similar in principle to the Kinect sensor that allows for AR applications.

7.3   Aim of the Study

The aim of the study is to present the use of serious games for the development of social and communication skills in children with ASD by reviewing articles in this area that describe the development of such games and their use in working with children with autism. Given the diversity of technologies used and their different applications for children with ASD in terms of assessment, treatment, relaxation and entertainment, learning and mastering new skills, we want to emphasize technologies and games that have been tested and their authors present the positive impact on the development of social and communication skills, which are key to the overall functioning of children with ASD and to draw some conclusions on the use of serious games.

The review of the selected technologies does not claim to be a comprehensive and complete presentation of all the technologies in the field, but it highlights the contributions that could guide readers to embark upon including technology in their work, research, or practice.

7.4   Material and Methods

The results were identified through literature searches conducted in Central and Eastern European Online Library (CEEOL), EBSCO: Academic Search Complete, EBSCO: eBook Academic Collection and ScienceDirect, Academic Search Complete, Health Source: Consumer Edition, ScienceDirect, Scopus, Web of Science and Wiley Online Library for a time period between 2006 and 2021.

We searched those four major online databases, using the search terms ("autism" OR "ASD") AND "social skills" AND ("serious games" OR "computer games" OR "computer-based" OR "mobile app" OR "portable" OR "software") AND "education" AND "communication." The search and selection of the results were conducted in January 2022. Forty studies of over 150 results were selected, part of these proving the need for and the benefits of adopting games for treatment of children with ASD. Eleven of the analyzed publications were selected as they present original technologies and developments by the authors. A brief summary of each of these publications is presented below.

7.4.1   Relevant Research

Play therapy is a method of treatment commonly used for children with ASD and other special educational needs (SEN). This technique allows children to optimize and improve their social and communication skills while playing in their own way [36]. Taking into account the facts that play is an essential part of all aspects of child development, and educational computer games are an effective support tool in teaching children without developmental disabilities, the authors [37] believe that games can also be used effectively in the education of children with autism. They analyze and describe the characteristics that dedicated educational computer games should have in teaching children with autism. The researchers [38] summarize articles with research results published over a period of 20 years and discuss appropriate theoretical models for designing serious games to improve the social behavior in people with ASD. The analysis of the pre-selected forty articles shows that a considerable number of studies in this area are aimed at children with high-functioning ASD or Asperger's syndrome. In addition to the general aspects of social behavior, more attention is paid to the recognition/naming and selection of emotions. The authors note a number of shortcomings in the design of existing serious games, offering improvements that can increase the effectiveness of games designed for people with ASD.

A survey among Bulgarian SLT specialists on the use of educational computer games in teaching practice involved 103 respondents who answered twenty-six questionnaires. The study shows the wide availability of games, which are not used excessively, as well as a clear need for structured policies, standards, rules, and methods for developing specialized educational computer and mobile game applications to support the work of SLT specialists in Bulgaria [14, 39].

Without claiming to be exhaustive, below we have listed some examples of games applicable to children with ASD resulting from our review of the literature on the usability of games and the results of their application.

Examples of games to help children with ASD.

The presented games were selected on the following criteria:

1. Games aimed at developing communication and social skills
2. Presentation of the technology
3. Year of development—after 2011
4. Tested on patients.

Example 1. ECHOES

The serious game ECHOES helps learning and communication in children with ASD. Children with ASD interact with a virtual character in specially designed social situations through a multitouch display and eye-gaze tracking. The interactions between the child and the agent include everyday situations at school and in the community that are part of the child's environment. The established social partner can act as a peer and as a tutor for children with ASD by supporting their communication skills and helping them to understand other people's language and interpret their nonverbal behavior. The training activities are organized according to the established principles for working with children with ASD [40].

Example 2. Emotiplay.

Serious games have shown to be able to produce simplified versions of the social and emotional world around us. A study by Fridenson-Hayo and Lassalle [41], conducted an intercultural evaluation of Emotiplay, with the following participants: 15 children from the United Kingdom, 38 from Israel and 36 from Sweden, respectively. The game aims to teach emotion recognition (ER) in a fun and intrinsically motivating way to six- to nine-year-olds with high functioning ASD for a period of 8–12 weeks. Researchers report a significant improvement in participants' performance in ER body language and integrative tasks. Thanks to Emotiplay, children acquire the ability to recognize faces with their emotions, voices, body language and their integration in the context of their social presentation in an effective, motivating and psycho-educational way. Parents also report that their children have improved their adaptive socialization, and that they show reduced symptoms of autism after using the SG.

Example 3. Lego Therapy.

Levy et al. [42] study the impact of school-based Lego Therapy groups for adolescents diagnosed with ASD. The therapeutic program is based on the work of pre-trained school staff working with five adolescents with

ASD, analyzing the intervention and its results on the duration of social engagement and the frequency of social initiations, reactions, and positive social behavior for five out of six participants. The results suggest that Lego Therapy groups may be an effective intervention at school to optimize social skills for adolescents with ASD.

Example 4. Learning emotions. The educational computer game developed by the Bulgarian scientific team: Stankova et al. [43], as an output of scientific project Pedagogical and Technological Issues of Educational Computer Games was introduced in the e-learning platform Moodle. It is based on the emotional intelligence development model and its main goal is to develop skills for recognizing, understanding, and naming emotions in children with ASD using storyboards and emoticons. The game consists of seven modules mainly based on plot pictures depicting emotions, distinguishing these emotions as well as working with emoticons and comparing them with emotion-related situations depicted in images. The game offers participants a specific combination of visual presentation and auditory perception of named emotions, which integrates the ability to upgrade emotion recognition skills by reporting errors, searching for additional information, right and wrong attempts in different modules of the game, as well as time for completing the tasks. To further evaluate the results, a survey for parents was used collecting information about the child's behavior, his/her interest in play and his/her motivation [44].

Example 5. SG Lego-like building blocks prototype. Barajas et al. [45] develop a serious game which, in the form of a game therapy tool, aims to improve social and cognitive skills for children with autism spectrum disorder. It consists of 2 components: a tangible user interface (TUI) and a graphical user interface (GUI). The TUI is made up of tangible Lego-like building blocks, complemented by electronic modules and representing a 3D virtual view of the board and the blocks. A total of nine children aged 6–15 participated in the preliminary experimental study. The proposed system showed an improvement in their social interaction through their joint play and exercise, and a reduction in solitary play was observed.

Example 6. ComFiM app—the developer team Ceccon et al. [46] of the ComFiM app aims to promote communication between people with autism spectrum disorders and to model it in an interactive and dynamic process. The game has several stages: first the player's knowledge is built while interacting with a virtual character, then at a later stage communication with another real participant in the game is stimulated using the skills gained so far. The results prove that the aesthetic experiences in ComFiM are in line with multigamers' media, as the architecture of the game successfully realizes situations of communication between players.

Example 7. An SG prototype for emotional skills. The tool offered by Dantas et al. [47] is a free software developed using HTML ver. 5.2, JavaScript and Python 3, and aims to improve emotional skills by recognizing and interpreting facial expressions in children with ASD aged 6–13. The user's facial expressions are captured by a webcam on a computer or smartphone, and the application monitors and stores the level of attention, number of hits, number of errors and the time required to express an emotion. The app contains animations, 2900 videos and a set of images of 75 people expressing each of the six emotions based on the FACS theory.

Example 8. Multiplayer PAR game—the game, developed on the ideology of Silva-Calpa et al. [48] comprises four models of cooperation to contribute to the skills of social interaction of people with autism spectrum disorders. The collaboration models used in the application are specifically tailored for users with High-Functioning Autism and is itself assessed by criteria for the social interaction actions achieved by users during their joint play. There were 51 test sessions recorded with audio and video (17 sessions for each phase of the game) with five young people with autism who took turns as teams in the games where their roles changed. The results prove and confirm that each model of cooperation motivates the need for cooperation and encourages the creation of situations for social interaction between users.

Example 9. FILL ME APP—The mobile game application designed by the team of authors—Armas, et al. [49] and a therapist considered the needs of the specialist and based the solution on a technology platform so that the game results can be validated. The application contains four game modules for children aged 3–10 which stimulate emotions through different visualizations: (1) Emotion Bubbles: animated bubbles containing basic and mixed emotions. The player must release the bubbles that contain the desired emotion, which is visualized through text or audio. (2) Logical Sequence: Two consecutive images appear on the screen for a few seconds. Three new images are then presented to the player. The player must choose which image completes the sequence. When they choose the right answer, the image becomes a puzzle they have to solve. (3) Emotion Sudoku: A traditional sudoku game that uses cartoon images of emotions instead of numbers. (4) Humpty Dumpty: A game that allows the therapist to play with his/her patients. The results showing that 67% of patients improved their emotion recognition skills were achieved over a period of two weeks of using the mobile game application in every therapy session with each child.

Example 10. FaceSay™—The game FaceSay, developed by Tsai et al. [50], was initially tested on 25 children with autism who played it and achieved an average score of 14.8 on a facial recognition test, and a control group—an average of 12.8. The children with Asperger's syndrome—24 in total, achieved a much higher score with an average of 18.4 compared to 15.4 in the control group, all in the ages between 6 and 15. The sex distribution was forty-four boys to five girls. In an emotion recognition test, children with autism who played FaceSay™ scored an average of 6.53, while the average score in the control group was 5.2. The children with Asperger syndrome had an average test score of 8.7 compared to the control group score of 6.79. The computer tests were conducted twice a week for a minimum of six weeks for an average of 20 min each session.

Example 11. LIFEisGAME iPad prototype—the prototype game LIFEisGAME developed by a team of Portuguese scientists—Alves et al. [51], was tested during 15-min game sessions by 11 children with RAS, aged 5–15, 91% male and 9% female, 82% verbal with ASD and 18% nonverbal with ASD. All participants had experience in playing computer games, and among the most challenging emotions to recognize were fear, disgust, and surprise. A particularly popular and highly satisfying part of the game is the application Sketch Mee. Its high degree of interactivity gives players the opportunity to create their own facial expressions, with the ability to change eyes, eyebrows, mouth, and nose, and subsequently this becomes their avatar in the game. Parents offer enriching the prototype with musical stimuli, and therapists add a recommendation to include instructions for visual games.

7.5 Discussion

The analysis of the literature in the field of using serious games for children with ASD the following conclusions may be drawn:

- The heterogeneous group of children with ASD is a challenge in terms of diagnosis, planning of therapeutic interventions, treatment, and inclusion in peer groups. In this sense, the application of technologies that are in themselves truly diverse would be an even greater challenge in terms of applicability, compliance with cognitive development levels, age, cultural and linguistic environment. Respectively, a personalized approach would be useful in the preparation and design of games to overcome at least some of these difficulties. This approach is already being applied and tested by some researchers who suggest the use of personalized elements like avatars and specific audio effects [26]. Each game developed for therapeutic purposes must be adapted to the potential, capabilities, needs and interests of the individual player, i.e., the content of the game should allow precise filtering on a number of parameters, such as age, gender, psychological state, disorder, etc.
- Games are often applicable to children with good cognitive functioning. On the one hand, the group of children with ASD is heterogeneous in terms of the level of functioning, and on the other hand, given the good applicability of games for learning specific knowledge and skills, they would be a good approach to support children with lower functioning. More effort into developing games suitable for children with intellectual disabilities is needed [52].
- Very often, in testing the effect of a game, single cases or small samples of children with ASD were used, which further complicates the statistical processing and conclusions. Particular attention in these studies should be paid to the heterogeneous nature of ASD and the selection of children who test the game should take into account many factors—age, level of cognitive development, level of social functioning, language, and cultural environment, if the game has such elements, the level of computer literacy of the children.
- A serious challenge specialists who develop or use such technologies face is to devise reliable methods for assessing their effect. Also, it would be necessary to assess the content validity and reliability of these methods so that they can gradually enter the regular programs to support children with ASD, but only after checking their compliance with the goals of treatment. As mobile technology evolves, a new concept called "mobile learning" gets acknowledged. To effectively achieve their goals of helping people with disabilities, mobile applications need to be assessed in a structured way [53].

- It is necessary to develop special methods for measuring the usability of games, and to develop and validate additional testing of the final effect of their application. In these methods, special attention should be paid to the satisfaction of children with ASD and their parents, as well as the possibility of using technologies for learning through fun and enjoyable experiences.
- Standardization and verification of the assessment: at present there are no validated standardized tools to prove that a game is really "serious" or to measure how "serious" it is. Game authors and creators, together with software engineers, need to build a scientifically based game model from the point of view of user experience. What are the elements that make up a "fun" design and how can its effectiveness be measured? Currently, many developers/researchers offer several types of serious games. However, there is great difficulty in evaluating a game for clinical or classroom use.
- Apart from being an additional therapeutic tool, serious games can also be used to teach basic skills in children with ASD—e.g., language, speech, reading, writing and math skills, as well as general knowledge. For this teaching to be successful, the games created should correspond to children's learning schedules and be made available to teachers and special educators, who will be able to supplement learning with games or replace basic learning approaches with serious games. This would be especially useful if the child experiences difficulties with concentrating, memorizing, or sustaining interest to what is taught in school.
- Serious games for learning specific skills should be accompanied by instructions for use and short guidelines for their application in order to be easy to use by professionals and teachers.
- Game developers should offer advice on the use of games and their capabilities.
- Teachers and professionals working with children with ASD should be provided easily accessible training courses in the application of serious games and the opportunities they offer.
- Balance: for the successful and purposeful creation of a game, a particularly crucial element is for the designer to achieve a balance between the fun element and the main goal of the game, which by no means should be just having fun. On the one hand, this means that the entertainment element of the game should be available, but it should not be predominant. Also, its exclusion in an attempt to achieve the main goal of the game is not justified, whether the latter is for training or treatment, or a combination of both, etc. The game should stimulate engagement, but it should definitely not deprive the player of the pleasure of playing the game itself, which is a means by which a specific goal can be achieved.
- The parents of children with ASD and the users themselves should also be involved in the game development in order to check their expectations in terms of content, elements of entertainment, types of rewards and incentives for correct answers/actions, level of language complexity in the instructions, etc.
- When testing serious games for assessment and treatment in children with ASD as well as for training in basic knowledge and skills, a greater emphasis should be placed on the subjective assessment by parents and children of the usability of the game, its complexity, entertainment value and emotional effect.

- In developing games oriented towards social skills training in order to compensate for some of the difficulties children with ASD face, more attention should be paid to the specificity of the symptoms of ASD and professionals who are familiar with the functioning of children with ASD should be involved in the development of such games.
- One should remember that when using therapeutic interventions, the main element is positive stimulation, providing fun and a pleasant experience. Games should bring not only positive results in terms of training and compensation of symptoms, but also a fun and enjoyable experiences for children and their parents

7.6 Conclusion

This article reviews previous studies, as well as developed and published serious games for children with ASD over the period 2006–2021. In order to avoid certain cognitive and behavioral stereotypes of players, such as repeated behavior patterns, parents, therapists, and instructors must be able to customize serious games for children with ASD. In addition, these specialized games provide tools for data analysis or visualization, taking into account the progress and development of the child's skills based on pre-set traceable parameters. Asperger [54] noted that the special interests and skills of people with ASD can reveal much about the nature of their condition as well as their potential achievements. He shared his observations that the conventional approach to learning is not applicable to them, as they create their knowledge and understanding through their own experience, accumulating practical knowledge and reflections. In this sense, video games are extremely attractive to many young people with ASD, who feel comfortable and at ease in the game reality. Previous research has shown the effectiveness of games in helping children with ASD to express their feelings, recognize their partner's emotions, and improve their level of engagement with others. Of course, games should not be considered a substitute for standard interventions, nor are they expected to be a panacea, but their presence in the daily lives of children with ASD certainly contributes to overcoming some of the many difficulties these children face.

The main purpose of the review was to assist the reader in understanding the various aspects of the possible positive impacts of using smart telephones, mobile apps, and computer games to practice different social skills as a therapy tool for youngsters with ASD. There has been much research and discussion on the development of skills of youngsters with ASD, including their ability for independent social interaction and performance. More research and testing are required to achieve an improved understanding of the use of technology in improving the social skills of children with ASD.

Acknowledgements In appreciation of the reviewers' careful suggestions and attempts to improve our article, we would like to express our gratitude.

References

1. American Psychiatric Association: Diagnostic and Statistical Manual of Mental Disorders, 5th edn. Arlington (2013)
2. Meghan, N., Qian, Y., Massolo, M., Croen, L.A.: Psychiatric and medical conditions in transition-aged individuals with ASD. Pediatrics **141**(Suppl. 4), 335–345 (2018)
3. Simonoff, E., Pickles, A., Charmanand T., et al.: Psychiatric disorders in children with autism spectrum disorders: prevalence, comorbidity, and associated factors in a population-derived sample. J. Am. Acad. Child Adolesc. Psychiatry **47**(8), 921–929 (2008)
4. Gordon-Lipkin, E., Alison, R., Marvin, J., Law, K., Lipkin, P.H.: Anxiety and mood disorder in children with autism spectrum disorder and ADHD. Pediatrics **141**(4) (2018)
5. Chawarska, K., Klin, A., Paul, R., Volkmar, F.: Autism spectrum disorder in the second year: stability and change in syndrome expression. J. Child. Psychol. Psychiatry **48**(2), 128–138 (2007)
6. Eigsti, M., Schuh, J.M.: Language acquisition in ASD: beyond standardized language measures. In: Naigles, L.R. (ed.) Innovative Investigations of Language in Autism Spectrum Disorder. Language and the Human Lifespan Series, pp. 183–200. American Psychological Association (2017)
7. Huizinga, J.: Homo Ludens: A Study of the Play-Element of Culture. Martino Publishing, Mansfield Centre, CT. ISBN 978-1-61427-706-4 (2014)
8. Michael, D.R., Chen, S.L.: Serious Games: Games That Educate, Train, and Inform, Muska & Lipman/Premier-Trade (2005)
9. Laamarti, F., Eid, M., El Saddik, A.: An overview of serious games. Int. J. Comput. Games Technol. **2014**, 15p (2014), Article ID 358152. https://doi.org/10.1155/2014/358152
10. Botte, B., Matera, C.M., Sponsiello, M.: Serious Games tra simulazione e gioco. Una proposta di tassonomia, J. e-Learning Knowl. Soc. **5**, 11–22 (2009)
11. Alvarez, J., Alvarez, A., Djaouti, D., Michaud, L.: Serious Games: Training & Teaching-Healthcare-Defence & Security-Information & Communication. IDATE (2010)
12. Mitchell, A., Savill-Smith, C.: The Use of Computer and Video Games for Learning: A Review of the Literature. Learning and Skills Development Agency (2004). Last accessed 21 Sept 2020. https://dera.ioe.ac.uk/5270/
13. Ahmad, M., Shahid, S.: Design and evaluation of mobile learning applications for autistic children in Pakistan. In: 15th Human-Computer Interaction (INTERACT), pp. 436–444, Bamberg, Germany (2015). ff10.1007/978-3-319-22701-6_32ff.ffhal-01599627
14. Stankova, M., Ivanova, V., Kamenski, T.: Use of educational computer games in the initial assessment and therapy of children with special educational needs in Bulgaria. TEM J. **7**, 488–494 (2018). https://doi.org/10.18421/TEM73-03
15. Tuparova, D., Veleva, V., Tuparov, G.: About some barriers in usage of educational computer games by teachers in STEM. In: 42nd International Convention on Information and Communication Technology, Electronics and Microelectronics, MIPRO 2019—Proceedings, 2019, pp. 727–730, 8756999 (2019)
16. Zakari, H.M, Ma, M., Simmons, D.: A review of serious games for children with autism spectrum disorders (ASD). In: Ma, M., Oliveira M.F., Baalsrud Hauge, J. (eds.) SGDA, vol. 8778, pp. 93–106. Springer, Heidelberg (2014)
17. Jiménez-Muñoz, L., Peñuelas-Calvo, I., Calvo-Rivera, P., et al.: Video games for the treatment of autism spectrum disorder: a systematic review. J. Autism Dev. Disord. **52**, 169–188 (2022). https://doi.org/10.1007/s10803-021-04934-9
18. Chen, J., Wang, G., Zhang, K., Wang, G., Liu, L.: A pilot study on evaluating children with autism spectrum disorder using computer games. Comput. Hum. Behav. **90**, 204–214, ISSN 0747-5632 (2019). https://doi.org/10.1016/j.chb.2018.08.057
19. Tanaka, J.W., Wolf, J.M., Klaiman, C., Koenig, K., Cockburn, J., Herlihy, L., Brown, C., Stahl, S., Kaiser, M.D., Schultz, R.T.: Using computerized games to teach face recognition skills to children with autism spectrum disorder: the let us face it! Program. J. Child Psychol. Psychiatry **51**(8), 944–952 (2010). https://doi.org/10.1111/j.1469-7610.2010.02258.x

20. Grossard, C., Grynspan, O., Serret, S., Jouen, A. L., Bailly, K., Cohen, D.: Serious games to teach social interactions and emotions to individuals with autism spectrum disorders (ASD), Comput. Educ. **113**, 195–211, ISSN 0360-1315 (2017). https://doi.org/10.1016/j.compedu.2017.05.002

21. Chien, M.E., Jheng, C.M., Lin, N.M., et al.: iCAN: a tablet-based pedagogical system for improving communication skills of children with autism. Int. J. Hum. Comput. Stud. **73**, 79–90 (2015)

22. King, M.L., Takeguchi, K., Barry, S.E., et al.: Evaluation of the iPad in the acquisition of requesting skills for children with autism spectrum disorder. Res. Autism Spectr. Disord. **8**(9), 1107–1120 (2014)

23. Ganz, J.B., Hong, E.R., Goodwyn, F.D.: Effectiveness of the PECS Phase III app and choice between the app and traditional PECS among preschoolers with ASD. Res. Autism Spectr. Disord. **7**(8), 973–983 (2013)

24. Hourcade, J.P., Bullock-Rest, N.E., Hansen, T.E.: Multitouch tablet applications and activities to enhance the social skills of children with autism spectrum disorders. Pers. Ubiquit. Comput. **16**, 157–168 (2012). https://doi.org/10.1007/s00779-011-0383-3

25. Bakkes, S., Tan, C.T., Pisan, Y.: Personalised gaming. J.: Creative Technol. (2012). Beaumont, R., Sofronoff, K.: A multi-component social skills intervention for children with Asperger syndrome: the junior detective training program. J. Child Psychol. Psychiatry **49**(7), 743–53 (2008)

26. Vallefuoco, E., Bravaccio, C., Pepino, A.: Serious Games in Autism Spectrum Disorder—An Example of Personalised Design, pp. 567–572 (2017). https://doi.org/10.5220/0006384905670572

27. Kallo, V., Kinshuk, Mohan, P.: Personalized game based mobile learning to assist high school students with mathematics. In: ICALT'10, 10th International Conference on Advanced Learning Technologies. IEE (2010)

28. Brisson, A., Pereira, G., Prada, R., Paiva, A., Louchart, S., Suttie, N., Lim, T., Lopes, R., Bidarra, R., Bellotti, F., Kravcik, M., Oliveira. M.: Artificial intelligence and personalization opportunities for serious games. In: Proceedings of AAAI Workshop on Human Computation in Digital Entertainment and Artificial Intelligence for Serious Games, Co-located with AIIDE 2012—8th Conference on Artificial Intelligence and Interactive Digital Entertainment

29. Zarraonandía, T., Díaz, P., Aedo, I.: Modeling games for adaptive and personalized learning. In: Gros, B., Kinshuk, K., Maina, M. (eds.) The Future of Ubiquitous Learning, pp. 217–239. Springer, Berlin (2015)

30. Baraka, K., Melo, F.S., Veloso, M.: Interactive robots with model-based "autism-like" behaviors: assessing validity and potential benefits. Paladyn **10**(1), 103–116 (2019). https://doi.org/10.1515/pjbr-2019-0011

31. Bartneck, C., Soucy, M., Fleuret, K., Sandoval, E.B.: The robot engine—making the unity 3D game engine work for HRI. In: Proceedings—IEEE International Workshop on Robot and Human Interactive Communication, 2015-Nov, pp. 431–437 (2015)

32. Bhatt, S.K., De Leon, N.I., Al-Jumaily, A.: Augmented reality game therapy for children with autism spectrum disorder. Int. J. Smart Sens. Intell. Syst. **7**(2), 519–536 (2014)

33. Boutsika, E.: Kinect in education: a proposal for children with autism. Procedia Comput. Sci. **27** (2014). https://doi.org/10.1016/j.procs.2014.02.015

34. Taheri, A.R., Alemi, M., Meghdari, A., PourEtemad, H.R., Holderread, S.L.: Comput. Sci. (2015). https://doi.org/10.1016/j.procs.2014.02.015

35. Brandão, J., Cunha, P., Vasconcelos, J., Carvalho, V., & Soares, F.: An augmented reality game book for children with autism spectrum disorders. In: The International Conference on E-Learning in the Workplace 2015

36. Morgenthal, A.H., Child-Centered Play Therapy for children with autism: a case study, Ph.D. dissertation, Clinical Psychology, Antioch University New England, Keene, New Hampshire (2015)

37. Cankaya, S., Kuzu, A.: Investigating the characteristics of educational computer games developed for children with autism: a project proposal. Procedia—Soc. Behav. Sci. **9**, 825–830, ISSN 1877-0428

38. Hassan, A., Pinkwart, N., Shafi, M. (2021) Serious games to improve social and emotional intelligence in children with autism. Entertainment Comput. **38**, 00417
39. Stankova, M., Tuparova, D., Tuparov, G., Mihova, P.: Barriers to the use of serious computer games in the prcatical work with children with educational difficulties. TEM J. **10**(3), 1175–1183 (2021)
40. Bernardini, S., Porayska-Pomsta, K., Smith, T.J.: ECHOES: an intelligent serious game for fostering social communication in children with autism. Inf. Sci. **264**, 41–60 (2014)
41. Fridenson-Hayo, S.B., Lassalle, S., Emotiplay', A.: a serious game for learning about emotions in children with autism: results of a cross-cultural evaluation. Eur. Child Adolesc. Psychiatry **26**(8), 979–992 (2017)
42. Levy, J., Dunsmuir S.: Lego therapy: building social skills for adolescents with an autism spectrum disorder. Educ. Child Psychol. **37**(1), 58–83 (2020), ISSN 0267-1611
43. Stankova M., Mihova, P., Kamenski, T., Mehandjiiska, K.: Emotional understanding skills training using educational computer game in children with autism spectrum disorder (ASD)—case study. In: 2021 44th International Convention on Information, Communication and Electronic Technology, MIPRO 2021, pp. 724–729, ISSN 1847-3946
44. Stankova M., Tuparova, D., Mihova, P., Kamenski, T., Tuparov, G., Mehandzhiyska, K.: Educational computer games and social skills training. Handbook of Intelligent Techniques in Educational process, Springer (in print) (a)
45. Barajas, A., Al Osman, H., Shirmohammadi, S.: A Serious Game for children with autism spectrum disorder as a tool for play therapy, pp. 1–7 (2017). https://doi.org/10.1109/SeGAH. 2017.7939266
46. Ceccon, P., de Araujo, B.B.P.L., Raposo, A.: ComFiM: a cooperative serious game to encourage the development of communicative skills between children with autism. In: Brazilian Symposium on Games and Digital Entertainment, SBGAMES. (2014). https://doi.org/10.1109/SBG AMES.2014.19
47. Dantas, A., Zanchetta do Nascimento, M.: Recognition of emotions for people with autism: an approach to improve skills. Int. J. Comput. Games Technol. **2022**, 1–21 (2022). https://doi. org/10.1155/2022/6738068
48. Silva-Calpa, G., Raposo, A., Suplino, M.: PAR: A collaborative game for multitouch tabletop to support social interaction of users with autism. Procedia Comput. Sci. **27**, 84–93 (2014). https://doi.org/10.1016/j.procs.2014.02.011
49. Armas, J., Pedreschi, V., Gonzalez, P., Díaz, D.: A technological platform using serious game for children with autism spectrum disorder (ASD) in Peru (2019). https://doi.org/10.18687/ LACCEI2019.1.1.278
50. Tsai, T.-W. Lin, M.-Y.: An application of interactive game for facial expression of the autisms. 204–211 (2011). https://doi.org/10.1007/978-3-642-23456-9_37
51. Alves, S., Marques, A., Queirós, C., Orvalho, V.: LIFEisGAME prototype: a serious game about emotions for children with autism spectrum disorders. PsychNology J. **11**(3), 191–211 (2013)
52. Grossard, Ch., Grynszpan, O., Serret, S., Jouen, A., Bailly. K.: Serious games to teach social interactions and emotions to individuals with autism spectrum disorders (ASD). Comput. Educ. **113**, pp. 195–211 (2017). ff10.1016/j.compedu.2017.05.002ff. ffhal01525828
53. Sanromà-Giménez, M., Lázaro Cantabrana, J.L., Usart Rodríguez, M., Gisbert-Cervera, M.: Design and validation of an assessment tool for educational mobile applications used with autistic learners. J. New Approaches Educ. Res. **10**(1), 101–121 (2021). https://doi.org/10. 7821/naer.2021.1.574
54. Asperger, H.: Autistic personality disorders in childhood. In: Frith, U. (ed.) Autism and Asperger Syndrome, pp. 147–183. Cambridge University Press, London (1944)

Chapter 8
Deep Learning-based Coronary Stenosis Detection in X-ray Angiography Images: Overview and Future Trends

Emmanuel Ovalle-Magallanes, Dora E. Alvarado-Carrillo, Juan Gabriel Avina-Cervantes, Ivan Cruz-Aceves, Jose Ruiz-Pinales, and Rodrigo Correa

Abstract Deep learning methods, particularly Convolutional Neural Networks, have been successfully applied in medical imaging. Robust stenosis detection in X-ray coronary angiography images is challenging because of the limited availability of rich medical data. Besides, due to the high mortality rates related to stenosis, it is paramount for a robust computer-aided diagnosis system. This study presents a succinct overview of state-of-the-art stenosis detection based on deep learning methods. Besides, a comprehensive overview of the main fundamentals for convolutional neural networks, attention modules, vision transformers, and quantum computing is presented. ybrid networks, including quantum models, can boost classical deep learning methods by providing a remarkable classification accuracy boost. hallenges and future directions for stenosis detection methods are discussed as a starting point for future research to improve the stenosis detection task.

E. Ovalle-Magallanes · J. G. Avina-Cervantes (✉) · J. Ruiz-Pinales
Telematics and Digital Signal Processing Research Groups (CAs), Engineering Division, Campus Irapuato-Salamanca, University of Guanajuato, Carretera Salamanca-Valle de Santiago km 3.5 + 1.8 km, Comunidad de Palo Blanco, Salamanca 36885, Mexico
e-mail: avina@ugto.mx

E. Ovalle-Magallanes
e-mail: e.ovallemagallanes@ugto.mx

J. Ruiz-Pinales
e-mail: pinales@ugto.mx

D. E. Alvarado-Carrillo · I. Cruz-Aceves
Center for Research in Mathematics (CIMAT), A.C. Jalisco S/N, Col. Valenciana, Guanajuato 36000, Mexico
e-mail: dora.alvarado@cimat.mx

I. Cruz-Aceves
e-mail: ivan.cruz@cimat.mx

R. Correa
Escuela de Ingenierías Eléctrica, Electrónica y de Telecomunicaciones, Facultad de Ingenierías Físico-Mecánicas, Universidad Industrial de Santander, Carrera 27 Calle 9, Bucaramanga 680002, Colombia
e-mail: crcorrea@uis.edu.co

© The Author(s), under exclusive license to Springer Nature Switzerland AG 2023
C. P. Lim et al. (eds.), *Artificial Intelligence and Machine Learning for Healthcare*,
Intelligent Systems Reference Library 229,
https://doi.org/10.1007/978-3-031-11170-9_8

Keywords Coronary stenosis · X-ray imaging · Deep learning · Quantum computing

Acronyms

AttFPN	Attention feature pyramid network
BiLSTM	Bi-directional long-short-term memory
CADx	Computer-aided diagnosis
CBAM	Convolutional block attention module
CCN	Convolutional neural networks
CHD	Coronary heart decease
CQ	Classical to quantum
CT	Computed tomography
CTA	Computed tomography angiography
DenseNets	Densely connected convolutional networks
DL	Deep learning
ECA	Efficient channel attention
Faster-RCNN	Faster-region based convolutional neural networks
GE	Gather-excite
Grad-CAM	Gradient-class activation map
LN	Layer-normalization
MIL	Multiple instance learning
MLP	Multilayer perception
MRA	Magnetic resonance angiography
MSA	Multi-head self-attention
NASNet	Neural architecture search network
NLP	Natural language processing
QC	Quantum to classical
QML	Quantum machine learning
R-FCN	Region-based fully convolutional networks
ReLU	Rectified linear unit
ResNet	Residual network
SA	Self-attention
SACSM	Second-order attention-based channel selection module
SCAM	Spatial and channel attention module
scSE	Spatial and channel SE
SE	Squeeze-and-excitation
SSD	Single shot multi-box detector
US	Ultrasound
VGG	Visual geometry group
ViT	Vision transformer
VQC	Variational quantum circuit
XCA	X-ray coronary angiography

8.1 Introduction

Coronary Heart Disease (CHD) has high morbidity, disability, and mortality rates, seriously affecting people's life quality and survival time [59]. A deficient supply of oxygen-rich blood characterizes the primary pathological feature of CHD to the heart muscle due to a partial narrowing or complete blocking of a coronary artery by adipose plaque formation [9, 35]. X-ray Coronary Angiography (XCA) remains the gold standard for CHD diagnosis to analyze this issue. It is due to the accurate definition of the coronary anatomy, obtaining high-resolution images of the main coronary arteries and their corresponding branches [27].

Although a variety of imaging technologies exists, such as Computed Tomography Angiography (CTA) and other less invasive procedures such as Magnetic Resonance Angiography (MRA) and Ultrasound (US) imaging, XCA is preferred by the experts. This choice is because, in the case of coronary artery bypass surgery, it is performed almost exclusively through the XCA screening test [6].

Figure 8.1 shows a coronary artery affected by stenosis using XCA imaging. In clinical practice, a cardiologist identifies coronary stenosis and other related anomalies on the coronary angiograms during an exhaustive examination of the images. Moreover, this process can be affected by intra- and inter-observer variability and some image artifacts, e.g., low contrast vessels and large intensity gradients. For such a reason, Computer-Aided Diagnosis (CADx) systems play a vital role in obtaining efficient and accurate stenosis detection to support and reduce the workloads of the medical expert diagnosis.

CADx systems based on machine learning techniques have become major research subjects in medical imaging during the last few decades. Even though such classical tools have shown enormous potential new algorithms have appeared, such as Deep Learning (DL). Now, the design of handcrafted features (e.g., kernel-based and morphological operators) is automatized and internally learned during the DL optimization process, as shown in Fig. 8.2.

Fig. 8.1 Visualization of a coronary artery under the XCA procedure. A cardiologist has labeled the two stenosis cases, shown in the left side's zoomed rectangles

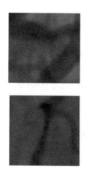
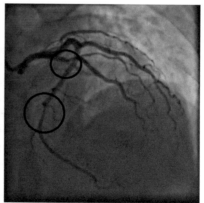

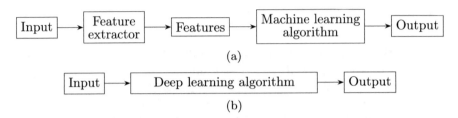

(a)

(b)

Fig. 8.2 Automatic recognition systems **a** handcrafted and **b** deep Learning feature extraction and classification pipeline

However, these DL methods manifest a trade-off between the final performance and the quality and quantity of the input training data. In medical imaging, generating annotated/labeled data is costly and time-consuming for physicians. Therefore, a limited amount of data exists, representing one of the main drawbacks of the state-of-the-art DL methods.

This chapter overviews the more recent state-of-the-art deep learning techniques applied in XCA images for stenosis detection and their drawbacks. Future trends are introduced, where new DL methods have already been explored in the medical image domain, but for different image modalities and tasks. These future research directions include attention mechanisms that automatically focus on specific objects in the image. Also, Vision Transformers is a convolution-free network that treats an image as a sequence of patches, taking advantage of each patch's position information. Moreover, hybrid models exploit Quantum Machine Learning (QML) as pre-processing step or as a feature enhancing at the top of a Convolutional Neural Network [8, 36]. Hence, QML offers innovative and powerful algorithms that can efficiently solve computational problems believed to be intractable for classical methods.

8.2 Convolutional Neural Networks

Convolutional Neural Networks (CNN) learn complex features through multiple scales in an automated fashion and then perform a classification task. Basic CNNs are typically built of four main layers: convolutional, pooling, activation functions (e.g., Rectified Linear Unit (ReLU)), and fully connected layers.

Figure 8.3 illustrates a typical CNN focused on image classification, where a sequence of layers transforms the 2D-input data into a class probability score.

Videlicet, a *convolutional layer*, is a set of multiple filters focused on extracting local features automatically. The convolution function receives an image $\mathbf{x}^{(l-1)}$, computing a new image, also known as feature map $\mathbf{x}^{(l)}$, denoted by

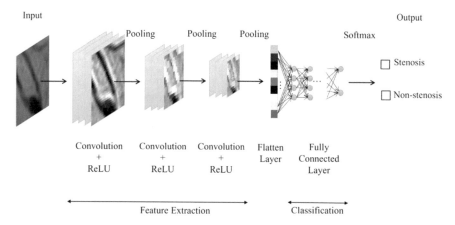

Fig. 8.3 The core building blocks of CNN: convolutional, pooling, fully-connected layers, and activation functions

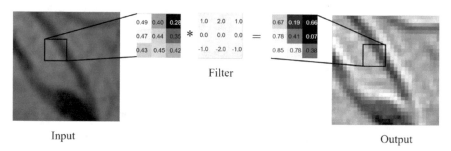

Fig. 8.4 Convolution operation with a given kernel size 3 × 3 and no bias term. A convolutional layer is conformed of a set of c filters, producing c-feature maps

$$\mathbf{x}(j)^{(l)} = \sum_{l=1}^{n} \left[\mathbf{x}(i)^{(l-1)} * k(i, j)^{(l-1)} + b(j)^{(l)} \right], \tag{8.1}$$

where $*$ is the 2D convolution operator, $k(i, j)^{(l-1)}$ is the kernel or convolutional filter being updated within network training, and $b(j)^{(l)}$ is the bias parameter. Figure 8.4 shows a graphical example of a single convolution operation.

Activation functions provide the nonlinear transformation capability required by CNNs. Some aim to solve the vanishing and exploding gradients problem by clipping the output of a given feature map in a range of values. Setting an activation function $f(x)$ after a convolutional layer is quite common, such as

- Sigmoid: This activation function is S-shaped with real numbers as input and output values in the range [0, 1],

$$f(x)_{\text{sigm}} = \frac{1}{1 + e^{-x}}. \tag{8.2}$$

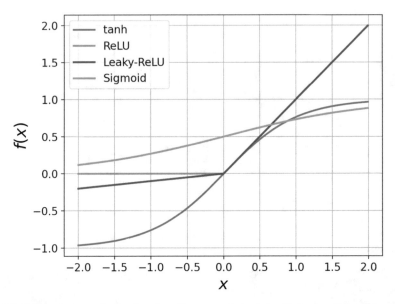

Fig. 8.5 More common activation function after a convolution layer. Notice how the positive values of ReLU and Leaky-ReLU overlap

- Tanh: Like the sigmoid function, its input is real numbers, but the output is restricted to $[-1, 1]$,

$$f(x)_{\text{tanh}} = \frac{e^x - e^{-x}}{e^x + e^{-x}}, \tag{8.3}$$

- ReLU: Maps the real input numbers to positive numbers,

$$f(x)_{\text{ReLU}} = \max(0, x). \tag{8.4}$$

- Leaky ReLU: This type of activation function based on a ReLU includes a slight slope, such as $\alpha = 0.1$ for negative values, ensuring that these inputs are never ignored,

$$f(x)_{\text{Leaky-ReLU}} = \begin{cases} x, & \text{if } x > 0 \\ \alpha x, & \text{otherwise.} \end{cases} \tag{8.5}$$

Figure 8.5 shows that the most popular activation functions are focused on different nonlinear transformations.

The *pooling layer* serves as a feature sub-sampler, reducing the spatial size of the feature map. Max- and average-pooling are the most used pooling methods. In a typical CNN setting, the pooling consists of a window Ω^k of size $k \times k$ and a stride s to downsample the image by $1/s$. A value of $k = 3$ and $s = 2$ is often employed. As such, in each pooling step, the feature maps are scaled by a factor of $1/2$. The

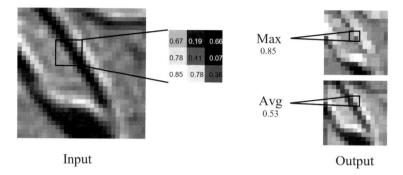

Input   Output

Fig. 8.6 Max- and average-pooling applied after a convolution operation within an activation function. One stride and window size of $s = 2$ and $k = 3$ are applied, respectively

Max-pooling can be defined as

$$f_{\max}(x) = \max_i x_i, \quad x \in \Omega^k, \tag{8.6}$$

and for the average-pooling:

$$f_{\text{avg}}(x) = \frac{1}{k} \sum_{i=1}^{k} x_i, \quad x \in \Omega^k. \tag{8.7}$$

This layer is generally used just after a block of convolutional layers. Figure 8.6 exemplifies these two common pooling operations.

After feature extraction performed by the convolutional layers, *fully-connected layers* learn nonlinear combinations given a flattened version of these features to accomplish the classification task. Figure 8.7 illustrates a fully-connected layer for a single feature map as input.

Building deeper networks meets the vanishing gradient problem. The gradient decreases exponentially during the backpropagation step as it propagates down from top to bottom layers. *Skip Connections* were introduced to solve this problem in different plain architectures. There are two main types of skip connections: *Addition and Concatenation*. He et al. propose a *Residual Network* (ResNet) that adopts residual learning to every few stacked layers [20]. In this way, the input from initial layers is passed to deeper layers by matrix addition such as

$$\mathbf{x}^{(l)} = \mathcal{F}(\mathbf{x}^{(l-1)}) + \mathbf{x}^{(l-1)}, \tag{8.8}$$

where $\mathbf{x}^{(l-1)}$ and $\mathbf{x}^{(l)}$ are input and output vectors of the layers, and $\mathcal{F}(\cdot)$ stands for the residual mapping function to be learned. Similarly, Huang et al. [24] introduce the *Densely Connected Convolutional Networks* (DenseNets) where the l-th layer receives the feature maps of all preceding layers, $\mathbf{x}^{(0)}, \ldots, \mathbf{x}^{(l-1)}$, as an input given

Fig. 8.7 The
fully-connected layer
operates on a flattened input
where each element is
connected to all neurons.
The flattened input is
typically obtained from
global pooled features

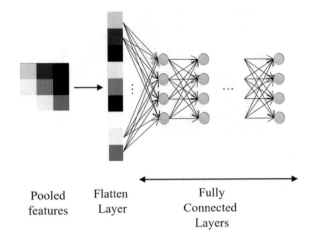

Pooled   Flatten   Fully
features   Layer   Connected
                                        Layers

by

$$\mathbf{x}^{(l)} = \mathcal{F}([\mathbf{x}^{(0)}; \ldots ; \mathbf{x}^{(l-1)}]). \qquad (8.9)$$

DenseNets concatenate the output feature maps of the previous layer with the next
layer rather than a matrix addition as ResNets.

8.3 Attention Mechanisms

The human visual system selectively focuses on salient structures to capture and
process specific objects. Therefore, attention mechanisms have been designed to
improve the representation power of CNN by automatically learning where to focus
on target structures.

The *Squeeze-and-Excitation* (SE) block enables the network to perform a dynamic
channel-wise feature recalibration [23]. The SE block has input the feature maps
$\mathbf{x}^{(l)} \in \mathbb{R}^{C \times H \times W}$ (obtained by a convolutional block operation). Each channel is
squeezed into a single numeric value using average pooling. Thus, a channel-wise
descriptor $\mathbf{z} \in \mathbb{R}^C$, such as,

$$z_c = \frac{1}{H \times W} \sum_{i=1}^{H} \sum_{j=1}^{W} x_c(i, j). \qquad (8.10)$$

A gating mechanism is introduced to control model complexity and aid generalization,
forming a bottleneck with two fully connected layers around the nonlinearity, i.e., a
dimensionality-reduction layer with a reduction ratio r,

$$\mathbf{s} = \sigma(\mathbf{W}_2 \delta(\mathbf{W}_1 \mathbf{z})), \qquad (8.11)$$

where δ and σ refer to the ReLU and sigmoid functions, respectively, $\mathbf{W}_1 \in \mathbb{R}^{C \times (\frac{C}{r})}$ and $\mathbf{W}_2 \in \mathbb{R}^{(\frac{C}{r}) \times C}$ are the parameters to be learned on the gating mechanism. Finally, each feature map of the convolutional block is weighted with the activations $\mathbf{s}$ as follows,

$$\hat{\mathbf{x}}^{(l)} = \mathbf{x}^{(l)} \otimes \mathbf{s}, \tag{8.12}$$

where $\otimes$ denotes channel-wise multiplication.

Subsequently, the *Efficient Channel Attention* (ECA) [56] architectural unit is introduced, based on SE blocks without dimensionality reduction. Given the channel-wise descriptor $\mathbf{z} \in \mathbb{R}^C$ after channel-wise global average pooling, the ECA efficiently captures local cross-channel interaction by considering every channel and neighbors by a 1D-convolution operation (f^k) of kernel size k. The kernel size captures the local cross-channel interaction.

$$\mathbf{s} = \sigma\left(f^k(\mathbf{z})\right). \tag{8.13}$$

Convolutional Block Attention Module (CBAM) [58] employs a combination of channel and spatial attention to aggregate fine informative features. Specifically, it employs global average pooling and max pooling. In such a way, given an intermediate feature map $\mathbf{x}^{(l)} \in \mathbb{R}^{C \times H \times W}$ as input, CBAM sequentially infers a 1D channel attention map $\mathbf{M}_c \in \mathbb{R}^{C \times 1 \times 1}$ and a 2D spatial attention map $\mathbf{M}_s \in \mathbb{R}^{1 \times H \times W}$ to generate a refined feature map, such as,

$$\mathbf{x}'^{(l)} = \mathbf{M}_c(\mathbf{x}^{(l)}) \otimes \mathbf{x}^{(l)}, \tag{8.14}$$

$$\hat{\mathbf{x}}^{(l)} = \mathbf{M}_s(\mathbf{x}'^{(l)}) \otimes \mathbf{x}'^{(l)}, \tag{8.15}$$

where $\otimes$ denotes element-wise multiplication. Like SE blocks, the channel attention module uses average pooling and max pooling on each channel feature, obtaining two vector descriptors $\mathbf{z}_{avg}^c$ and $\mathbf{z}_{max}^c$. Both descriptors go through a bottleneck dense layer network with shared weights:

$$\mathbf{M}_c(\mathbf{x}^{(l)}) = \sigma\left(\mathbf{W}_2 \, \delta(\mathbf{W}_1 \mathbf{z}_{avg}^c) + \mathbf{W}_2 \, \delta(\mathbf{W}_1 \mathbf{z}_{max}^c)\right), \tag{8.16}$$

with σ as a sigmoid function and δ a ReLU function. The spatial attention module captures the inter-spatial relationship of features. In this module, the pooling operations are computed along the channel axis generating two 2D maps: $\mathbf{z}_{avg}^s, \mathbf{z}_{max}^s \in \mathbb{R}^{1 \times H \times W}$. Those 2D maps are concatenated and convolved by a 2D kernel of 7×7. Thus, the spatial attention map is computed as:

$$\mathbf{M}_s(\mathbf{x}'^{(l)}) = \sigma\left(f^{7 \times 7}([\mathbf{z}_{avg}^s; \mathbf{z}_{max}^s])\right), \tag{8.17}$$

Table 8.1 Attention module parameters

Attention module	Attention type	Additional parameters
SE [23]	Channel attention	$2\dfrac{C^2}{r}$
ECA [56]	Channel attention	k
CBAM [58]	Channel and spatial attention	$2\left(\dfrac{C^2}{r}+k^2\right)$

The attention module requires additional learning parameters while intermediate feature maps with C channels are included

where σ is the sigmoid function, and $f^{7\times7}$ represents the 2D-convolution operation with a 7×7 kernel size. To sum up, Table 8.1 shows the number of parameters required in each attention module.

Other attention modules based on channel and spatial attention have been introduced, preserving satisfactory performance while decreasing the complexity. Common examples include the Gather-Excite (GE) [22], Spatial and Channel SE (scSE) [45] blocks, and Second-order Attention-based Channel Selection Module (SACSM) [29].

8.4 Vision Transformers

The breakthroughs from *transformer* networks [53] in Natural Language Processing (NLP) domain have inspired many research interests in the computer vision domain. Transformers use attention and self-attention mechanisms as the core module to replace the CNN backbone with a convolution-free deep network. The standard *transformer* receives as input a 1D sequence of token embeddings. To handle 2D images, Dosovitskiy et al. [17] introduced the *Vision Transformer* (ViT) for image classification. The main components of the transformer include Self-attention (SA), Multi-head Self-attention (MSA), and Multilayer Perception (MLP), as illustrated in Fig. 8.8.

ViT treats an image as a sequence of patches. First, the image $\mathbf{x} \in \mathbb{R}^{H \times W \times C}$ is divided into $N = HW/P^2$, not overlapping patches of size $P \times P$. Now, each patch is a matrix $\mathbf{x}_p \in \mathbb{R}^{P \times P \times C}$. Then the patches are flattened such that $\mathbf{x}_p \in \mathbb{R}^{P^2 \cdot C}$. Secondly, each flattened patch is mapped to a latent vector with hidden size D through a trainable linear projection. The output of this projection is known as *patch embeddings*.

Position embedding vectors $\mathbf{E}_{\text{pos}} \in \mathbb{R}^{(N+1) \times D}$ are added to the patch embedding vector to make position-aware. The position embedding vectors learn distance within the image, such that neighboring ones have high similarity. A learnable *class token* $\mathbf{x}_{\text{class}}$ is pre-appended to the patch embedding vectors as the 0th vector. The resulting sequence of embedding vectors serves as input to the encoder, which is formally defined as

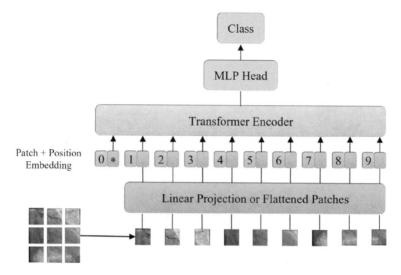

Fig. 8.8 Visual transformer. The ∗ symbol denotes an extra learnable (class) embedding

$$\mathbf{z}_0 = [\mathbf{x}_{\text{class}}; \mathbf{x}_p^1 \mathbf{E}; \mathbf{x}_p^2 \mathbf{E}; \dots; \mathbf{x}_p^N \mathbf{E}] + \mathbf{E}_{\text{pos}}, \quad \mathbf{E} \in \mathbb{R}^{(P^2 \cdot C) \times D}. \tag{8.18}$$

Next, the transformer encoder operated on the embedding vectors using alternating MSA layers and MLP blocks. The MSA consists of several *attention layers* or *heads* running in parallel. In standard **qkv** *self-attention*, a triplet containing queries **q**, keys **k** with associated values **v** for the input sequence $\mathbf{z} \in \mathbb{R}^{N \times D}$ is computed as

$$[\mathbf{q}, \mathbf{k}, \mathbf{v}] = \mathbf{z}\mathbf{U}_{qkv}, \quad \mathbf{U}_{qkv} \in \mathbb{R}^{D \times 3d_k}. \tag{8.19}$$

Thus, the self-attention is defined as follows,

$$\text{Attention}(\mathbf{q}, \mathbf{k}, \mathbf{v}) = \text{SoftMax}\left(\frac{\mathbf{q}\mathbf{k}^{\mathsf{T}}}{\sqrt{d_k}}\right)\mathbf{v}, \tag{8.20}$$

where $\frac{1}{\sqrt{d_k}}$ is a scaling factor, and d_k is the keys' dimension. *Multi-head self-attention* is the concatenation of the h parallel heads, such as

$$\text{MSA}(\mathbf{z}) = [\text{head}_1; \text{head}_2; \cdots; \text{head}_h]\mathbf{U}_{msa}, \quad \mathbf{U}_{msa} \in \mathbb{R}^{k \cdot d_k \times D}, \tag{8.21}$$

$$\text{head}_i = \text{Attention}(\mathbf{q}, \mathbf{k}, \mathbf{v}). \tag{8.22}$$

Notice that learned linear projections from keys, values, and queries are the input to the attention module. By reducing each head's dimensionality, $d_k = d_v = D/h$, the total computational cost is like that of single-head attention with full dimensionality.

Layer-normalization (LN) is applied before every block and residual connections after every block.

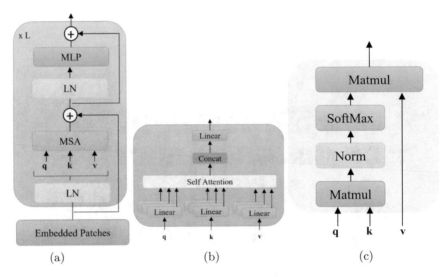

(a)   (b)   (c)

Fig. 8.9 The core elements of the ViT. **a** Transformer encoder. **b** Multi-head self-attention. **c** Self-attention

$$z'_l = \text{MSA}(\text{LN}(z_{l-1})) + z_{l-1}, \quad l = 1, \dots L. \tag{8.23}$$

Then, an MLP and an LN are added at the top of the MSA layer.

$$z_l = \text{MLP}(\text{LN}(z'_l)) + z'_l, \quad l = 1, \dots L. \tag{8.24}$$

A total of L blocks describes the transformer encoder, such that the output of the Transformer encoder at 0th position z_L^0 serves as the image representation **y**.

$$y = \text{LN}(z_L^0). \tag{8.25}$$

Figure 8.9 describes the ViT main elements: the transformer encoder, the multi-head self-attention, and the self-attention mechanisms. Bears in mind that the transformer encoder contains an MSA module, which holds the attention module.

8.5 Quantum Computing

From a literature review, the constant evolution of classical machine learning methods can be observed, particularly in the last decade, deep learning. This effect is due to the emergence of new problems that generate a large amount of data in a brief time. Therefore, new approaches are required to recognize patterns and classify such data. Recently, Quantum Machine Learning techniques have been demonstrated to be a powerful tool and, in some cases, more effective alternatives than their classical counterparts. This perception is particularly true because of the inherent advantages of quantum computing (including superposition and entanglement) to improve the performance of classical machine learning algorithms. Nowadays, a quantum neural network with multi-neuron interactions is available by a combination of extended classic Hopfield network and adiabatic quantum computation. Fard et al. proposed an associative memory to retrieve partial patterns with any number of unknown bits [19].

Especially, Quantum computing exploits the fact that quantum bits (*qubits*) can be in any possible linear combination of the two classical bit states (0 and 1). This unique phenomenon is called *superposition*. The two basic qubit states, analogs of classical bits state, are expressed as

$$|0\rangle = \begin{pmatrix} 1 \\ 0 \end{pmatrix}, |1\rangle = \begin{pmatrix} 0 \\ 1 \end{pmatrix}, \tag{8.26}$$

following the *Dirac BraKet notation*. Hence, the state $\psi \in \mathcal{H}^2$ of a qubit in superposition is defined as

$$|\psi\rangle = \alpha |0\rangle + \beta |1\rangle \quad \forall \alpha, \beta \in \mathbb{C}, \tag{8.27}$$

where $|\alpha|^2 + |\beta|^2 = 1$. So, any vector decomposed in the form

$$\begin{pmatrix} \alpha \\ \beta \end{pmatrix} = \alpha \begin{pmatrix} 1 \\ 0 \end{pmatrix} + \beta \begin{pmatrix} 0 \\ 1 \end{pmatrix}, \tag{8.28}$$

represents a quantum state. The Born rule states that the *measurement* of a qubit will get $|0\rangle$ with probability $|\alpha|^2$ and $|1\rangle$ with probability $|\beta|^2$. Notice that the outcome of the measurement is classical data.

Quantum states are manipulated using *quantum gates*, represented as a Hilbert space's rotation operation. These quantum gates can be represented by matrices and should satisfy the linearity and reversibility conditions such as

$$\mathbf{U}\mathbf{U}^\dagger = \mathbf{I}, \tag{8.29}$$

where $\mathbf{I}$ is the $n \times n$ identity matrix and $\mathbf{U}^\dagger$ indicates the complex conjugate of $\mathbf{U}^\mathsf{T}$. For a single-qubit operation, $n = 2$. As such, a vector $|\psi\rangle$ produces another vector $|\psi'\rangle$,

$$|\psi'\rangle = \mathbf{U} |\psi\rangle. \tag{8.30}$$

The most straightforward quantum operation is the NOT or bit flip gate, having the following matrix representation,

$$X = \begin{pmatrix} 0 & 1 \\ 1 & 0 \end{pmatrix}. \tag{8.31}$$

Fig. 8.10 Spherical
representation of the state of
a single qubit. θ is
inclination angle from $+z$
direction and ϕ is azimuth
from $+x$ direction

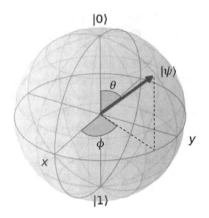

Meanwhile, the phase flip gate or Z gate negate the $|1\rangle$ state,

$$Z = \begin{pmatrix} 1 & 0 \\ 0 & -1 \end{pmatrix}. \qquad (8.32)$$

The Hadamard gate creates a uniform superposition of the two quantum basic states,

$$H = \frac{1}{\sqrt{2}} \begin{pmatrix} 1 & 1 \\ 1 & -1 \end{pmatrix}. \qquad (8.33)$$

By writing a quantum state in polar form, i.e., $\alpha = a e^{i\theta}$ and $\beta = b e^{i\varphi}$, 8.27 can be written as follows,

$$|\psi\rangle = e^{i\theta}\left(a\,|0\rangle + b\,e^{i(\varphi-\theta)}\,|1\rangle \right). \qquad (8.34)$$

The complex term $e^{i\theta}$ (global phase) does not affect the measurement (can be omitted), and $\phi = (\varphi - \theta)$, thus

$$|\psi\rangle = a\,|0\rangle + b\,e^{i\phi}\,|1\rangle, \qquad (8.35)$$

where $a, b \in \mathbb{R}$, and $e^{i\phi}$ is the relative phase. Since $a^2 + b^2 = 1$ needs to be fulfilled, $a = \cos\left(\frac{\theta}{2}\right)$ and $b = \sin\left(\frac{\theta}{2}\right)$ have the same relationship. In such a way, a single-qubit state is parametrized by two angles (θ and ϕ) as follows,

$$|\psi\rangle = \cos(\frac{\theta}{2})\,|0\rangle + \sin(\frac{\theta}{2})e^{i\phi}\,|1\rangle. \qquad (8.36)$$

Therefore, each qubit state vector and operations can be represented in 3-dimensional space (Bloch sphere), as illustrated in Fig. 8.10.

The RX, RY, and RZ gates rotate the state vector of a qubit about the axis x, y, z, respectively. They are defined as

$$RX(\omega) = \begin{pmatrix} \cos(\frac{\omega}{2}) & -i\sin(\frac{\omega}{2}) \\ -i\sin(\frac{\omega}{2}) & \cos(\frac{\omega}{2}) \end{pmatrix}. \qquad (8.37)$$

$$RY(\omega) = \begin{pmatrix} \cos(\frac{\omega}{2}) & -\sin(\frac{\omega}{2}) \\ \sin(\frac{\omega}{2}) & \cos(\frac{\omega}{2}) \end{pmatrix}. \qquad (8.38)$$

$$RZ(\omega) = \begin{pmatrix} e^{-i\frac{\omega}{2}} & 0 \\ 0 & e^{i\frac{\omega}{2}} \end{pmatrix}. \qquad (8.39)$$

Rather than obtaining measurements of outcome probabilities, *observables* allow computing a measurable quantity related to some physical property of the system. Mathematically, observables correspond to Hermitian matrices, i.e., $B = B^\dagger$ whose eigenvalues represent the possible values of the measurement outcome. However, since the measurement is probabilistic, the expectation value of an observable needs to be calculated as follows,

$$\langle B \rangle = \langle \psi | \mathbf{U}^\dagger B \mathbf{U} | \psi \rangle . \qquad (8.40)$$

For instance, the Z gate is Hermitian and has eigenvalues ± 1 with $|0\rangle , |1\rangle$ as eigenvectors.

The quantum state consisting of n *unentangled* qubits can be represented as the tensor product of the states of the individual qubits. Then, the state space of the system $\Psi \in \mathcal{H}^{2^n}$ is given by

$$|\Psi\rangle = |\psi_1\rangle \otimes |\psi_2\rangle \otimes \cdots \otimes |\psi_n\rangle . \qquad (8.41)$$

Multiple-qubit states can be written using a bit-string representation. For instance, the 3-qubit state $|1\rangle \otimes |0\rangle \otimes |1\rangle$ is $|101\rangle$.

Notwithstanding, if the n qubit state cannot be decomposed into the tensor product ($\otimes$) of individual states, the qubits are considered *entangled*. If a pair of qubits are entangled, the measurement on one qubit instantaneously affects the other qubit.

A sequence of quantum gates can be applied to single or multiple qubits. *Quantum circuits* are a common visual representation of these operations. Quantum circuits start with a set of qubits (wires) in an initial state, followed by a set of operations (gates), and end with a measurement of one or more qubits.

Figure 8.11 shows a 3-qubit quantum circuit where the first step is to apply a rotation gate to each circuit. Then, a Hadamard, NOT, and Hadamard gates are applied. It corresponds to obtaining the output state

Fig. 8.11 3-qubit quantum circuit. The qubit is indexed from left to right. Therefore, the state $|101\rangle$ represents that the first and third qubits are in state $|1\rangle$, and the second in state $|0\rangle$

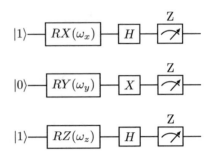

$$|\Psi'\rangle = (H \otimes X \otimes H)(RX(\omega_x) \otimes RY(\omega_y) \otimes RZ(\omega_z)) |\Psi\rangle .$$

Finally, a measurement over the Z observable is computed for each qubit.

Variational Quantum Circuit (VQC) is a quantum circuit modeled by learnable parameters that can be trained during an optimization process, i.e., a VQC can be seen as a convolutional layer in a CNN. Now, the measurement over and observable B is defined as

$$\langle B \rangle = \langle \psi | \, U(\theta)^\dagger B U(\theta) \, | \psi \rangle , \tag{8.42}$$

where $\theta = [\theta_1, \theta_2, \cdots, \theta_n]^\mathsf{T}$ is the set of free parameters for the quantum circuit U.

8.6 Stenosis Detection Methods Based on Deep Learning

Stenosis detection based on traditional machine learning techniques can be summarized in three steps: features' extraction, selection, and classification [28, 46, 54]. However, the deep learning paradigm can perform these three steps end-to-end during the optimization procedure. In particular, Convolutional Neural Networks (CNNs) have enabled outstanding performance gains in the medical image domain. While working on X-ray video sequences, it is necessary to filter the whole video, keeping only the frames with a visible artery tree to detect the stenosis. The classification process is conducted from the candidate frames by an object-based framework or image classification task. Image classification involves computing class labels probabilities to an image. In contrast, object localization and classification involve drawing a bounding box around objects of interest in an image and assigning them a class label. Figure 8.12 illustrates the broad pipeline of these two classification approaches.

8.6.1 Object-based Classification

In the medical image domain, object-based classification refers to identifying the location of lesions and classifying them. Accordingly, the candidate boxes are

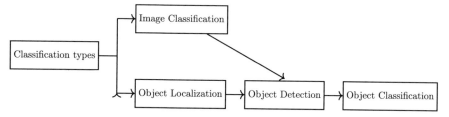

Fig. 8.12 Image and object-based classification approaches. Notice that object detection and object classification can be performed after image classification

generated surrounding the object detection proposals. The boxes close to each other will be grouped in a single cluster. Then, only clusters containing the most candidate boxes remain. Finally, a single bounding box is obtained for each object to assign a label. Different strategies have been proposed to solve the stenosis detection problem, where the feature extraction of the image relies on a CNN automatically. Wu et al. proposed to extract the candidate frame employing a UNet [44] where only segmented images with high responses are selected [60]. Subsequently, a DL-based object detection network provides potential stenosis regions refined by a sequence-non-maximum suppression algorithm to remove false positives stenosis cases. A VGG (Visual Geometry Group) network is used as a backbone model [49].

Pang et al. introduce the Stenosis-DetNet, an end-to-end network to select candidate frames from the raw X-ray angiography video [39]. Then, the candidate object bounding boxes containing stenotic regions are detected, optimizing them using prior coronary artery displacement information and image features. In this case, a Residual Network (ResNet) acts as a backbone model to extract the features [20].

Danilov et al. examine eight different object detection CNN architectures configurations to detect the location of a single stenotic lesion [16]. The object detector network configurations include a Single Shot multi-box Detector (SSD) [30], Faster-Region Based Convolutional Neural Networks (Faster-RCNN) [41], and Region-based Fully Convolutional Networks (R-FCN) [14]. So, some architectures have been efficiently employed as backbone networks: the MobileNet-v2 [47], ResNet50, ResNet101, Inception-v4 [50], and Neural Architecture Search Network (NASNet) [62]. The R-FCN + ResNet101 configuration has shown an optimal trade-off between accuracy and speed.

Figure 8.13 illustrates the stenosis detection workflow, taking the full screening test as input.

8.6.2 Image-Based Classification

Medical image datasets need much professional expertise to label them. Instead of detecting and classifying each object in an image, it can be more suitable to

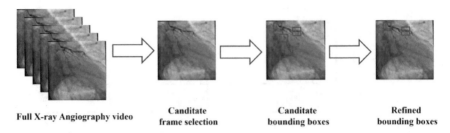

Fig. 8.13 From a whole sequence of X-ray angiography images, candidate images are selected, such that the full artery tree is visible. Then, the localization and detection of stenosis cases are performed

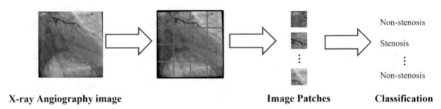

Fig. 8.14 Patch-based classification approach. Each image patch is classified as stenosis or non-stenosis

classify the whole image as a single class. Moreover, suppose a refined classification is required. In that case, a patch-based classification can be performed, assigning a class for each patch in the image. This patch-based approach can be seen as each patch representing a labeled object. In this context, Cong et al. put forward a previous step to separate the images by the angle view [13]. Then, the candidate frame selection is performed by a CNN composed of a pre-trained Inception-v3 [51] as a feature extractor feeding a Bi-directional Long-Short-Term Memory (BiLSTM). Consequently, an independent pre-trained Inception-v3 network classified these filtered images into the stenosis and non-stenosis classes.

Moon et al. propose a two-step method for automatic stenosis recognition from coronary angiography [34]. Firstly, a keyframe detection selects only images that show the most opacified coronary artery. Second, a deep learning-based classification of stenosis on each keyframe is performed employing a pre-trained Inception-v3 on the ImageNet dataset. A single channel-wise and spatial-wise attention modules from CBAM are arranged in parallel at the bottom of the model to maximize the attention of the baseline network.

On the other hand, if only limited label images are available, a patch-based approach is suitable to solve the stenosis detection task. In this popular approach, the classification process is achieved at a patch level instead of classifying a complete image. As such, one full-size image generates n-patches of a predefined size (i.e., 32×32 pixels), augmenting the number of training images. Figure 8.14 shows in detail this process.

In such a context, Antczak and Liberadzki made publicly available a dataset for patch-based stenosis detection [4]. Moreover, a shallow patch-based CNN, only five-layer deep, was employed in this work. A pre-trained step was conducted to improve the network detection rates. Thus, a generative model creates a synthetic dataset that assumes that a vessel can be modeled as a Bezier curve.

Ovalle-Magallanes et al. introduced a network-cut approach to reduce the number of layers needed to be transferred and fine-tuned from a source model pre-pre-trained on a large dataset, i.e., transfer learning [37]. An exhaustive search selected the optimal cut and trainable layers for three different state-of-the-art architectures: VGG16, ResNet50, and Inception-v3. The Inception-v3 showed the best detection result, keeping and fine-tuning only the first three inception blocks.

New hybrid models combining classical CNNs elements and quantum circuits are recently investigated to accomplish and improve different classification tasks. In this wise, Ovalle-Magallanes et al. solve a patch-based coronary stenosis detection in X-ray angiography images proposing a classical-quantum CNN within a distributed-quantum layer splitting the quantum processing workload into multiple variational quantum circuits [38]. Moreover, an L_2-tanh activation function was presented to avoid the vanishing gradient problem and improve the quantum layer performance. Table 8.2 summarizes the deep-learning approaches to solve the stenosis detection task.

Table 8.2 Summary of the CNN employed for stenosis detection

Author	Year	Backbone network	Dataset
Antczak and Liberadzki [4]	2018	5-layer CNN	- 250 patches of size 32×32 pixels
Cong et al. [13]	2019	Inception-v3	• 194 XCA sequences, each with 60 to 120 images of 512×512 or 1024×1024 pixels
Wu et al. [60]	2020	VGG19	• 148 XCA sequences, each with 40 to 70 images of 512×512 pixels
Ovalle-Magallanes et al. [37]	2020	Inception-v3*	• 250 patches of 32×32 pixels
Pang et al. [39]	2021	ResNet50	• 1260 images of 512×512 pixels
Moon et al. [34]	2021	Inception-v3	• 312 XCA sequences, each at 15 fps with an image size of 512×512
Danilov et al. [16]	2021	ResNet101*	• 8325 images of 512×512 pixels
Ovalle-Magallanes et al. [38]	2022	ResNet18	• 250 patches of 32×32 pixels

The symbol ⋆ highlights the best model concerning multiple networks evaluation

8.7   Illustrative Study Cases

Object-based stenosis classification outcome is a set of bounding boxes surrounding the positive cases detected by the network. Figure 8.15 presents an example of this approach type obtained by different state-of-the-art methods. Hence, the patch-based or image-based stenosis classification is used to obtain the class-discriminative localization map. In such a case, the Gradient-weighted Class Activation Mapping (Grad-CAM) uses the gradient information flowing into the last convolutional layer [48]. The precedent process retains high-level semantics and detailed spatial information of the CNN architectures.

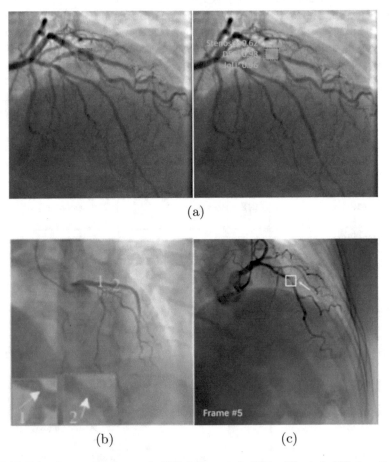

Fig. 8.15 Taken from: **a** Danilov et al. [16], **b** Pang et al. [39], **c** Wu et al. [60]. In **a** the left image with the red box shows the ground truth for the stenosis case, and the right figure with the green box shows the detection outcome. The ground truth is not provided in the (**b**) and (**c**) cases. The green boxes in (**b**) display the true positive detection while in (**c**) are given in yellow boxes

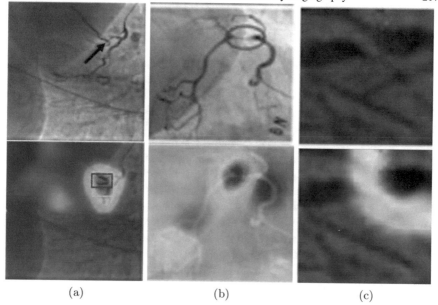

(a)   (b)   (c)

Fig. 8.16 Taken from: **a** Cong et al. [13], **b** Moon et al. [34], **c** Ovalle-Magallanes et al. [38]. The images in the top id the raw image, showing the stenosis case. Notice that (**c**) is a patch-based classification. Therefore, the patch represents a stenosis case. The red tones reflect the high-interest regions in each image, while blue/purple tones the lower importance regions

This method is widely employed to visualize discriminative regions with different contribution weights for the classification decision. Taking a particular class c, the Grad-CAM is obtained as follows,

$$L^c_{\text{Grad-CAM}} = \delta \left(\sum_k \alpha^c_k A^k \right),$$ (8.43)

where δ is the ReLU activation function, A^k is the feature map k, and α^c_k is the neuron importance weights defined as

$$\alpha^c_k = \frac{1}{Z} \sum_i \sum_j \frac{\partial y^c}{\partial A^k_{i,j}}.$$ (8.44)

Notice that the score gradient y^c for class c, concerning A^k is first computed (before the softmax). Then, these gradients are back-propagated and global-average-pooled. Hence, α^c_k captures the importance of their respective feature map k for a target class c.

Figure 8.16 shows some illustrative cases taken from the state-of-the-art DL-based methods where the Grad-CAM was applied to give a first stenosis detection positioning.

8.8   Challenges and Future Work

Nowadays, CADx systems play a crucial role in supporting the medical diagnosis. One of the significant CADx applications is the differentiation of stenosis and non-stenosis in XCA images. CADx system based on deep learning extract, select, and classify features within the optimization process of the same deep architecture. In such a way, they confirm the feasibility of XCA stenosis detection using deep learning methods. Nevertheless, these methods manifest the main drawback: they cannot give a stenosis degree quantification, which is also required in clinical diagnosis.

Moreover, stenosis tends to occur in curved or bifurcation regions in the vascular tree [32, 43]. However, there is a lack of detailed analysis of this specific vessel characterization, particularly in a deep learning context employing XCA images [5, 11, 12, 25]. Thus, some strategies can be developed to improve stenosis detection by identifying coronary bifurcations regions. Another limitation of the existing methods, particularly those that took the complete XCA sequence as input, is that they need a vast amount of annotated data to train and validate the model performance, i.e., keyframe validation and the segmented image ground truth.

These methods also show the potential of transfer learning, taking the ImageNet pre-trained network instead of training from scratch as a starting point. By doing so, the classification performance is drastically boosted.

Moreover, attention mechanisms start to be studied for medical image segmentation (lung and skin), where a Spatial and Channel Attention Module (SCAM) adaptively highlights interdependent channel maps and focuses on more discriminant regions by selecting useful channel features [18]. Also, a triple attention network (A^3Net) learns channel-wise, element-wise, and scale-wise attention simultaneously to cope with thoracic disease diagnosis on chest X-ray [55]. The abnormal cervical cell detection task was also improved by combining channel attention and spatial attention with an Attention Feature Pyramid Network (AttFPN) [10]. However, the application of attention modules remains unexplored regarding stenosis classification in XCA images.

Recently, vision transformers have been applied to medical image analysis despite limited data availability. For instance, MIL-VT used in the retinal disease classification task included the Multiple Instance Learning (MIL) heading to improve the backbone transformer [61]. Besides, a 3D Medical image Transformer based on MRI images was used for knee cartilage defect assessment [57]. Also, the TransMed system combines the advantages of CNN and *Transformers* to efficiently extract low-level features of images for parotid gland tumors classification and knee injury classification [15]. The ViT approach has not been widely studied in XCA image analysis. It is also important to notice that ViT requires a full-size image (i.e., 512×512 pixels) as input to encode spatial position.

The new hybrid model has been proposed to improve deep learning algorithms based on quantum computing. As such, two new variants of hybrid models have emerged: Quantum to Classical (QC) and Classical to Quantum (CQ). In the first case, Henderson et al. introduce a new type of layer, so-called a quantum convolution layer [21]. The quantum convolution transforms classical data using a predefined number of random quantum circuits analogously to a classical convolutional layer. Such a layer is placed at the bottom of the network to process the input image.

The quantum convolution layer approach has been explored to perform COVID-19 detection in X-ray in Computed Tomography (CT) scans [3] and in fundus retinal images for blood vessel segmentation [2].

Contrarily, the classical to the quantum network plug a quantum layer at the top of the network to only process and enhance the feature vector representation (i.e., after a global pooling layer). In this wise, Mari et al. introduced a quantum layer jointly trained along the classical sub-module [31]. This layer interacts as a classical fully-connected layer but learns the variational quantum circuit weights. COVID-19 detection from CT images [1, 52] and diabetic retinopathy detection in fundus images have been improved by employing this hybrid model, where the top features of a classical network feed a 4-qubit variational quantum circuit [33]. In this direction, Ovalle-Magallanes et al. introduce a quantum circuit within a parallel variational quantum circuit to reduce computation time to improve a patch-based classical-quantum CNN for stenosis detection in XCA images [38].

Although the previous methods present hybrid methods to improve the performance of convolutional networks, they do not consider the bottleneck of the encoding and decoding process from classical to quantum data and vice versa. Nowadays, quantum computers dispose of a limited amount of qubits and QRAM [26, 42]. However, quantum simulators are available for working with quantum algorithms in a classical local or cloud platform [7, 40].

8.9 Conclusions

Stenosis detection is challenging because of the limited availability and complex image conditions. This work showed an overview of the state-of-the-art deep-learning-based methods to handle this task. The existing methods used object detection and patch-based approaches exploiting either the availability of a full-length XCA test or the transfer learning paradigm to improve accuracy.

Thereby, the fundamentals of attention mechanisms, ViT, and quantum computing were presented, and how they have begun to explore the medical image domain. Quantum computing exhibits performance improvements over classical machine learning and deep learning algorithms. As quantum computers expand in the next decade in terms of qubits and fault tolerance, research in this field will grow. This limited hardware availability was experienced in deep learning when GPUs were not yet widespread. Once trained deep learning and hybrid models, the computational costs associated with model inference are low enough to run on a standard modern CPU in real-time.

Identifying future trends can help researchers in the stenosis detection task guide their efforts to overcome the main challenges for more robust and optimal systems employed in medical practice. Nevertheless, many challenges remain that need to be addressed in future studies.

Acknowledgements This work was supported in part by the University of Guanajuato Grant NUA 147347, and in part by the Mexican Council of Science and Technology CONACyT under Grant No. 626154/755609 and 626155/719327, and by the Mexican National Council of Science and Technology under project Cátedras-CONACyT No. 3150-3097.

Conflict of Interest The authors declare that they have no conflict of interest. The funders had no role in the design of the study; in the collection, analyses, or interpretation of data; in the writing of the manuscript, or in the decision to publish the results.

References

1. Acar, E., Yilmaz, I.: COVID-19 detection on IBM quantum computer with classical-quantum transfer learning. Turk. J. of Electr. Eng. Comput. Sci. **29**(1), 46–61 (2021)
2. Alvarado-Carrillo, D.E., Ovalle-Magallanes, E., Dalmau-Cedeño, O.S.: D-GaussianNet: adaptive distorted Gaussian matched filter with convolutional neural network for retinal vessel segmentation. Geom. Vis. **1386**, 378 (2021)
3. Amin, J., Sharif, M., Gul, N., Kadry, S., Chakraborty, C.: Quantum machine learning architecture for COVID-19 classification based on synthetic data generation using conditional adversarial neural network. Cogn. Comput. 1–12 (2021)
4. Antczak, K., Liberadzki, Ł.: Stenosis detection with deep convolutional neural networks. In: MATEC Web of Conferences, vol. 210, p. 04001. EDP Sciences (2018)
5. Antoniadis, A.P., Mortier, P., Kassab, G., Dubini, G., Foin, N., Murasato, Y., Giannopoulos, A.A., Tu, S., Iwasaki, K., Hikichi, Y., et al.: Biomechanical modeling to improve coronary artery bifurcation stenting: expert review document on techniques and clinical implementation. Cardiovasc. Interv. **8**(10), 1281–1296 (2015)
6. Athanasiou, L.S., Fotiadis, D.I., Michalis, L.K.: Atherosclerotic Plaque Characterization Methods Based on Coronary Imaging, 1 edn. Academic Press (2017)
7. Bergholm, V., Izaac, J., Schuld, M., Gogolin, C., Alam, M.S., Ahmed, S., Arrazola, J.M., Blank, C., Delgado, A., Jahangiri, S., et al.: Pennylane: Automatic differentiation of hybrid quantum-classical computations. arXiv preprint arXiv:1811.04968 (2018)
8. Biamonte, J., Wittek, P., Pancotti, N., Rebentrost, P., Wiebe, N., Lloyd, S.: Quantum machine learning. Nature **549**(7671), 195–202 (2017)
9. Britannica, The Editors of Encyclopaedia: Coronary Heart Disease (2021, October). https://www.britannica.com/science/coronary-heart-disease
10. Cao, L., Yang, J., Rong, Z., Li, L., Xia, B., You, C., Lou, G., Jiang, L., Du, C., Meng, H., Wang, W., Wang, M., Li, K., Hou, Y.: A novel attention-guided convolutional network for the detection of abnormal cervical cells in cervical cancer screening. Med. Image Anal. **73**, 102197 (2021)
11. Chang, C.F., Chang, K.H., Lai, C.H., Lin, T.H., Liu, T.J., Lee, W.L., Su, C.S.: Clinical outcomes of coronary artery bifurcation disease patients underwent Culotte two-stent technique: a single center experience. BMC Cardiovasc. Disord. **19**(1), 1–8 (2019)
12. Chiastra, C., Iannaccone, F., Grundeken, M.J., Gijsen, F.J., Segers, P., De Beule, M., Serruys, P.W., Wykrzykowska, J.J., van der Steen, A.F., Wentzel, J.J.: Coronary fractional flow reserve measurements of a stenosed side branch: a computational study investigating the influence of the bifurcation angle. Biomed. Eng. **15**(1), 1–16 (2016). (online)

13. Cong, C., Kato, Y., Vasconcellos, H.D., Lima, J., Venkatesh, B.: Automated stenosis detection and classification in X-ray angiography using deep neural network. In: International Conference on Bioinformatics and Biomedicine (BIBM). pp. 1301–1308. IEEE, San Diego, CA, USA (Nov 2019)
14. Dai, J., Li, Y., He, K., Sun, J.: R-FCN: object detection via region-based fully convolutional networks. In: Advances in Neural Information Processing Systems, pp. 379–387. Curran Associates Inc., Red Hook, NY, USA (2016)
15. Dai, Y., Gao, Y., Liu, F.: Transmed: transformers advance multi-modal medical image classification. Diagnostics 11(8), 1384 (2021)
16. Danilov, V.V., Klyshnikov, K.Y., Gerget, O.M., Kutikhin, A.G., Ganyukov, V.I., Frangi, A.F., Ovcharenko, E.A.: Real-time coronary artery stenosis detection based on modern neural networks. Sci. Rep. 11(1), 1–13 (2021)
17. Dosovitskiy, A., Beyer, L., Kolesnikov, A., Weissenborn, D., Zhai, X., Unterthiner, T., Dehghani, M., Minderer, M., Heigold, G., Gelly, S., Uszkoreit, J., Houlsby, N.: An Image is worth 16×16 words: transformers for image recognition at scale. In: International Conference on Learning Representations (2021)
18. Fang, W., Han, X.H.: Spatial and channel attention modulated network for medical image segmentation. In: Computer Vision—ACCV 2020 Workshops, pp. 3–17. Springer International Publishing, Kyoto, Japan (2020, December)
19. Fard, E.R., Aghayar, K., Amniat-Talab, M.: Quantum pattern recognition with multi-neuron interactions. Quant. Inf. Process. 17(3), 42 (2018)
20. He, K., Zhang, X., Ren, S., Sun, J.: Deep residual learning for image recognition. In: 2016 IEEE Conference on Computer Vision and Pattern Recognition, CVPR 2016, Las Vegas, NV, USA, June 27–30, 2016, pp. 770–778. IEEE Computer Society (2016)
21. Henderson, M., Shakya, S., Pradhan, S., Cook, T.: Quanvolutional neural networks: powering image recognition with quantum circuits. Quantum Mach. Intell. 2(1), 1–9 (2020)
22. Hu, J., Shen, L., Albanie, S., Sun, G., Vedaldi, A.: Gather-excite: exploiting feature context in convolutional neural networks. In: Advances in Neural Information Processing Systems, pp. 9423–9433. Curran Associates, Inc., Montréal, Canada (Dec 2018). https://proceedings.neurips.cc/paper/2018/hash/dc363817786ff182b7bc59565d864523-Abstract.html
23. Hu, J., Shen, L., Sun, G.: Squeeze-and-excitation networks. In: Proceedings of the IEEE Conference on Computer Vision and Pattern Recognition, pp. 7132–7141. Salt Lake City, UT, USA (Jun 2018)
24. Huang, G., Liu, Z., Maaten, L.V.D., Weinberger, K.Q.: Densely connected convolutional networks. In: 2017 IEEE Conference on Computer Vision and Pattern Recognition (CVPR), pp. 2261–2269. IEEE Computer Society, Los Alamitos, CA, USA (2017, July)
25. Iakovou, I., Foin, N., Andreou, A., Viceconte, N., Di Mario, C.: New strategies in the treatment of coronary bifurcations. Herz 36(3), 198–213 (2011)
26. IBM, Q.: IBM Quantum. Retrieved from https://quantum-computing.ibm.com/. Accessed 25 June 2021 (2021, June)
27. Johal, G.S., Goel, S., Kini, A.: Coronary anatomy and angiography. In: Practical Manual of Interventional Cardiology, pp. 35–49. Springer, Berlin (2021)
28. Kishore, A.N., Jayanthi, V.: Automatic stenosis grading system for diagnosing coronary artery disease using coronary angiogram. Int. J. Biomed. Eng. Technol. 31(3), 260–277 (2019)
29. Li, X., Lei, L., Sun, Y., Li, M., Kuang, G.: Multimodal bilinear fusion network with second-order attention-based channel selection for land cover classification. IEEE J. Sel. Top. Appl. Earth Obs. Remote Sens. 13, 1011–1026 (2020)
30. Liu, W., Anguelov, D., Erhan, D., Szegedy, C., Reed, S., Fu, C.Y., Berg, A.C.: SSD: single shot multibox detector. In: European Conference on Computer Vision, pp. 21–37. Springer, Berlin (2016)
31. Mari, A., Bromley, T.R., Izaac, J., Schuld, M., Killoran, N.: Transfer learning in hybrid classical-quantum neural networks. Quantum 4, 340 (2020)
32. Markl, M., Wegent, F., Zech, T., Bauer, S., Strecker, C., Schumacher, M., Weiller, C., Hennig, J., Harloff, A.: In vivo wall shear stress distribution in the carotid artery: effect of bifurcation

geometry, internal carotid artery stenosis, and recanalization therapy. Circ. Cardiovasc. Imaging **3**(6), 647–655 (2010)
33. Mir, A., Yasin, U., Khan, S.N., Athar, A., Jabeen, R., Aslam, S.: Diabetic retinopathy detection using classical-quantum transfer learning approach and probability model. Comput. Mater. Continua **71**(2), 3733–3746 (2022)
34. Moon, J.H., Lee, D.Y., Cha, W.C., Chung, M.J., Lee, K.S., Cho, B.H., Choi, J.H.: Automatic stenosis recognition from coronary angiography using convolutional neural networks. Comput. Methods Programs Biomed. **198**, 105819 (2021)
35. National Heart, Lung, and Blood Institute: Atherosclerosis (2021, October). https://www.nhlbi.nih.gov
36. Nielsen, M.A., Chuang, I.L.: Quantum computation and quantum information. Am. J. Phys. **70**(5), 558 (2002)
37. Ovalle-Magallanes, E., Avina-Cervantes, J.G., Cruz-Aceves, I., Ruiz-Pinales, J.: Transfer learning for stenosis detection in X-ray coronary angiography. Mathematics **8**(9), 1510 (2020)
38. Ovalle-Magallanes, E., Avina-Cervantes, J.G., Cruz-Aceves, I., Ruiz-Pinales, J.: Hybrid classical-quantum convolutional neural network for stenosis detection in X-ray coronary angiography. Expert Syst. Appl. 116112 (2021)
39. Pang, K., Ai, D., Fang, H., Fan, J., Song, H., Yang, J.: Stenosis-DetNet: sequence consistency-based stenosis detection for X-ray coronary angiography. Comput. Med. Imaging Graph. **89**, 101900 (2021)
40. Qiskit: Qiskit. Retrieved from https://qiskit.org/. Accessed March 10, 2022 (March 2022)
41. Ren, S., He, K., Girshick, R., Sun, J.: Faster R-CNN: towards real-time object detection with region proposal networks. Adv. Neural Inf. Process. Syst. **28**, 91–99 (2015)
42. Rigetti: Think quantum. Retrieved from https://www.rigetti.com/. Accessed 25 June 2021 (2021, June)
43. Rodriguez-Granillo, G.A., García-García, H.M., Wentzel, J., Valgimigli, M., Tsuchida, K., van der Giessen, W., de Jaegere, P., Regar, E., de Feyter, P.J., Serruys, P.W.: Plaque composition and its relationship with acknowledged shear stress patterns in coronary arteries. J. Am. Coll. Cardiol. **47**(4), 884–885 (2006)
44. Ronneberger, O., Fischer, P., Brox, T.: U-Net: Convolutional networks for biomedical image segmentation. In: International Conference on Medical Image Computing and Computer-Assisted Intervention, pp. 234–241. Springer, Berlin (2015)
45. Roy, A.G., Navab, N., Wachinger, C.: Recalibrating fully convolutional networks with spatial and channel squeeze and excitation blocks. IEEE Trans. Med. Imaging **38**(2), 540–549 (2019)
46. Sameh, S., Azim, M.A., AbdelRaouf, A.: Narrowed coronary artery detection and classification using angiographic scans. In: 2017 12th International Conference on Computer Engineering and Systems (ICCES). pp. 73–79. IEEE, Cairo, Egypt (Dec 2017)
47. Sandler, M., Howard, A., Zhu, M., Zhmoginov, A., Chen, L.C.: Mobilenetv2: inverted residuals and linear bottlenecks. In: IEEE Conference on Computer Vision and Pattern Recognition, pp. 4510–4520 (2018)
48. Selvaraju, R.R., Cogswell, M., Das, A., Vedantam, R., Parikh, D., Batra, D.: Grad-CAM: visual explanations from deep networks via gradient-based localization. In: IEEE International Conference on Computer Vision (ICCV), 2017, pp. 618–626. IEEE Computer Society, Venecia, Italia (2017, October)
49. Simonyan, K., Zisserman, A.: Very deep convolutional networks for large-scale image recognition. In: Bengio, Y., LeCun, Y. (eds.) 3rd International Conference on Learning Representations, ICLR 2015, San Diego, CA, USA, May 7-9, 2015, Conference Track Proceedings, pp. 1–14 (2015). http://arxiv.org/abs/1409.1556
50. Szegedy, C., Ioffe, S., Vanhoucke, V., Alemi, A.A.: Inception-v4, inception-ResNet and the impact of residual connections on learning. In: Thirty-first AAAI Conference on Artificial Intelligence (2017)
51. Szegedy, C., Liu, W., Jia, Y., Sermanet, P., Reed, S.E., Anguelov, D., Erhan, D., Vanhoucke, V., Rabinovich, A.: Going deeper with convolutions. In: IEEE Conference on Computer Vision and Pattern Recognition, CVPR 2015, Boston, MA, USA, June 7–12, 2015. pp. 1–9. IEEE Computer Society (2015)

52. Umer, M.J., Amin, J., Sharif, M., Anjum, M.A., Azam, F., Shah, J.H.: An integrated framework for COVID-19 classification based on classical and quantum transfer learning from a chest radiograph. Concurrency Comput. Prac. Experience e6434 (2021)
53. Vaswani, A., Shazeer, N., Parmar, N., Uszkoreit, J., Jones, L., Gomez, A.N., Kaiser, Ł., Polosukhin, I.: Attention is all you need. In: Advances in Neural Information Processing Systems, pp. 5998–6008. Curran Associates, Inc. (2017)
54. Wan, T., Feng, H., Tong, C., Li, D., Qin, Z.: Automated identification and grading of coronary artery stenoses with X-ray angiography. Comput. Methods Programs Biomed. **167**, 13–22 (2018)
55. Wang, H., Wang, S., Qin, Z., Zhang, Y., Li, R., Xia, Y.: Triple attention learning for classification of 14 thoracic diseases using chest radiography. Med. Image Anal. **67**, 101846 (2021)
56. Wang, Q., Wu, B., Zhu, P., Li, P., Zuo, W., Hu, Q.: ECA-Net: efficient channel attention for deep convolutional neural networks. In: Proceedings of the IEEE Conference on Computer Vision and Pattern Recognition, pp. 11531–11539. Seattle, WA, USA (Jun 2020)
57. Wang, S., Zhuang, Z., Xuan, K., Qian, D., Xue, Z., Xu, J., Liu, Y., Chai, Y., Zhang, L., Wang, Q., Shen, D.: 3DMeT: 3D medical image transformer for Knee Cartilage defect assessment. In: Lian, C., Cao, X., Rekik, I., Xu, X., Yan, P. (eds.) Machine Learning in Medical Imaging, pp. 347–355. Springer International Publishing, Cham (2021)
58. Woo, S., Park, J., Lee, J., Kweon, I.S.: CBAM: convolutional block attention module. In: Proceedings of the European Conference on Computer Vision. pp. 3–19. Munich, Germany (2018, September)
59. World Health Organization: Cardiovascular Diseases (CVDs) (Oct 2021). https://www.who.int/news-room/fact-sheets/detail/cardiovascular-diseases-(cvds)
60. Wu, W., Zhang, J., Xie, H., Zhao, Y., Zhang, S., Gu, L.: Automatic detection of coronary artery stenosis by convolutional neural network with temporal constraint. Comput. Biol. Med. **118**, 103657 (2020)
61. Yu, S., Ma, K., Bi, Q., Bian, C., Ning, M., He, N., Li, Y., Liu, H., Zheng, Y.: Mil-vt: multiple instance learning enhanced vision transformer for fundus image classification. In: de Bruijne, M., Cattin, P.C., Cotin, S., Padoy, N., Speidel, S., Zheng, Y., Essert, C. (eds.) Medical Image Computing and Computer Assisted Intervention (MICCAI), pp. 45–54. Springer International Publishing, Cham (2021)
62. Zoph, B., Vasudevan, V., Shlens, J., Le, Q.V.: Learning Transferable Architectures for Scalable Image Recognition. arXiv preprint http://arxiv.org/abs/1707.07012. arXiv:1707.07012 (2017)

Chapter 9
Potential Benefits of Artificial Intelligence in Healthcare

Nathalie Hoppe, Ralf-Christian Härting, and Anke Rahmel

Abstract Healthcare systems worldwide are confronted with numerous challenges such as an aging population, an increasing number of chronically ill patients, innovations as cost drivers and growing cost pressure. The COVID-19 pandemic causes additional burden for healthcare systems. In order to overcome these challenges, digital technologies are increasingly used. Especially the past decade witnessed a tremendous boom of artificial intelligence (AI) within the healthcare sector. AI has the potential to revolutionize healthcare and to mitigate the challenges healthcare systems are confronted with. The existing literature has frequently examined specific benefits of AI within the healthcare sector. However, there are still research gaps according to different application areas in healthcare. For this reason, an empirical study design has been conducted to investigate the potentials of AI in healthcare and to consequently identify its role. Based on a Systematic Literature Review (SLR), the following application areas for key determinants in healthcare have been identified: *management tasks, medical diagnostics, medical treatment* and *drug discovery*. By means of structural equation modeling (SEM), the study confirmed *medical diagnostics* and *drug discovery* as positive and significant influencing factors on the potential benefits of AI in healthcare. The other determinants didn't prove a significant influence. Based on the findings of the study, various recommendations have been derived to further exploit the potentials of AI in healthcare.

Keywords Artificial intelligence · AI · Healthcare · Potential benefits · Digitalization · Systematic literature review · Structural equation modeling

N. Hoppe · R.-C. Härting (✉) · A. Rahmel
Aalen University of Applied Sciences, Aalen, Germany
e-mail: ralf.haerting@hs-aalen.de

N. Hoppe
e-mail: nathalie_vanessa.hoppe@kmu-aalen.de

A. Rahmel
e-mail: anke.rahmel@hs-aalen.de

© The Author(s), under exclusive license to Springer Nature Switzerland AG 2023
C. P. Lim et al. (eds.), *Artificial Intelligence and Machine Learning for Healthcare*,
Intelligent Systems Reference Library 229,
https://doi.org/10.1007/978-3-031-11170-9_9

9.1   Introduction

Artificial Intelligence (AI) is considered to be "the new electricity" [1] and thus the foundation for numerous applications. AI can be briefly defined as "intelligence demonstrated by machines" [2] and is increasingly applied in various industries such as retail, finance, manufacturing and also in healthcare [3]. It is attributed by many experts to create a new era of healthcare [4–6]. The growing availability of patient data and advances in analytics have contributed to this development [4].

Healthcare systems worldwide have to face numerous challenges such as aging populations, staff shortages and a rise of chronic diseases [7]. The COVID-19 pandemic has exacerbated these challenges by substantially increasing the demand for protective equipment, medications and medical devices [8]. To mitigate or even eliminate these challenges, new solutions have to be identified. According to the opening statement by Andrew Ng, AI can be harnessed as the "new electricity" [1] for addressing healthcare challenges. At the same time, the question arises of what concrete role AI will play in this regard.

Researchers and computer scientists have examined how various AI approaches, especially Machine Learning (ML) and Deep Learning (DL) models, can be used for specific tasks or problems [9, 10]. One research focus is the application of AI-based systems in intensive care units [11, 12]. Moreover, AI is considered to support healthcare personnel in administrative tasks [13]. Additionally, numerous scientific papers can be identified that examine the role of AI and its approaches in relation to the COVID-19 pandemic [14, 15]. Suri et al. (*in 2020*) investigate how AI and medical imaging can contribute to the severity classification of COVID-19 infections [15].

The existing literature comprises AI algorithms, models and experimental studies that predominantly address specific problems or targets within medicine and healthcare [16, 17]. A study examining the potential benefits of AI according to various application areas in healthcare has not yet been conducted. Apart from medical application areas, an additional focus is on the area of management within the healthcare sector. Due to various factors like cost and competitive pressure, a tremendous focus is on efficiency and productivity within healthcare organizations [18]. Therefore, management tasks could also be subject for improvements thanks to AI [19].

The research project is based on an empirical investigation, more precisely a quantitative study among AI experts in healthcare. Based on the findings, recommended actions for different stakeholders such as physicians, AI developers, managers and researchers will be derived.

First, the authors provide theoretical insights into AI in healthcare by addressing the beginnings of AI as well as current developments (see Sect. 9.1.2). The subsequent section represents the main part as it comprises the individual components of the research design. A systematic literature review (SLR) represents the basis for the generation of hypotheses and the creation of a conceptual model (see Sect. 9.1.3.2). The model is built as a structural equation model (SEM) which is a type of multivariate analysis, i.e. multiple variables can be analyzed simultaneously [20]. For the purpose of generating primary data and deriving statements on the hypotheses, an online survey among AI experts with focus on the healthcare sector in Germany was conducted. Within Sect. 9.1.3.3, the process of data collection is explained in detail including information on the acquisition of participants. The following section presents the results and contains the characteristics of the expert group, the examination of different quality criteria and the evaluation of the SEM. The interpretation of the results in Sect. 9.1.5 is followed by different recommended actions to fully exploit the potential benefits of AI. Finally, the authors summarize the results and give an outlook on the further development of AI in the healthcare sector (see Sect. 9.1.7).

9.2 Artificial Intelligence in Healthcare

The beginnings of AI in healthcare and medicine can already be traced back to the 1950s. At this time, physicians conducted first trials to support diagnostics by means of computer-aided programs [21]. One famous example is the diagnosis of abdominal pain by Gunn [22]. Nowadays, both the availability of healthcare data and various methods of big data analytics are supposed to transform healthcare sectors worldwide [4].

At the same time, the almost exploding availability of patient data from a huge variety of electronic sources represents a major challenge to healthcare professionals. Gathering this data and transforming it into a suitable decision is hardly feasible for them [6]. Over the past years, there has been an enormous rise of electronic health records (EHR). Considering the availability of medical knowledge, it is estimated that a physician would have an effort of 29 h per day assimilating new medical knowledge [6]. This is where AI plays an increasing role. Especially the past decade is characterized by a tremendous boom of AI technologies and applications. The improvements in computer processing speed, the availability of a larger amount of data and the pool of talented AI engineers have contributed to it [23].

The idea of using AI to detect and treat diseases such as cancer at an early stage is already an inspiration for many researchers and developers. Cosma et al. (*in 2017*) examine different approaches of computational intelligence for predictive modeling in prostate cancer [24]. Additionally, Carter et al. (*in 2020*) examine the effects of AI applied to breast cancer care [25].

The essential core of AI-based systems is that they require training based on data. These data are derived from numerous clinical sources like diagnosis, screening or treatment. The overall goal is to identify patterns, associations between features and relevant outcomes within the data [4]. The support of AI-based systems can cover many clinical and administrative areas such as diagnostics, therapy or documentation [23]. In order to give an insight into the present and future role of AI in healthcare, there is an introduction to current numbers and figures.

The rise of AI technologies in healthcare is emphasized by the growth of the global market revenue. The market revenue is supposed to increase from 6.9 U.S. dollars in 2021 to 67.4 billion U.S. dollars in 2027 [26]. Additionally, the revenue for the market of *diagnostics and medical imaging* is estimated at 2.5 billion U.S. dollars and the one of *drug discovery* is estimated at 4 billion U.S. dollars by 2024 [27]. The increasing and rapid development of AI technologies in healthcare also results in a growing number of AI startups [28]. Compared to the share of AI startups worldwide, AI startups in healthcare and biotech have a share of 9% [29].

9.3 Research Design

The empirical study is based on a quantitative research design. In general, a distinction can be made between qualitative and quantitative research designs. Whereas qualitative research focuses on exploratory and small data sets, quantitative research comprises structured data collection with a large number of datasets [30]. In a first step of the research design, relevant questions have been identified from a systematic literature review (SLR). The derived conceptual model and hypotheses build the foundation for the data collection and further findings through an online survey.

Figure 9.1 illustrates the main elements of the research design. Based on the aim to identify the potential benefits of AI according to different application areas in healthcare, a SLR was conducted. The findings from the SLR are used to derive hypotheses and create a conceptual model that can subsequently be used for the data collection and the evaluation of the results. The data collection was carried out through an online survey and is based on a questionnaire which reflects the theoretically gained insights through the SLR. Subsequently, the data was analyzed by means of the statistical software SmartPLS [31]. The results are interpreted based on the findings from the literature and ultimately lead to answering the research question.

In the following sections, each step of the research design is explained in detail, starting with the strategy of the SLR.

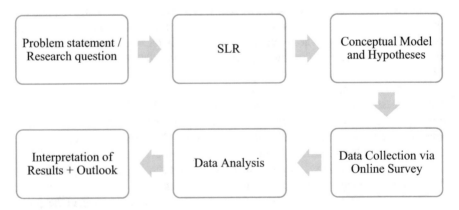

Fig. 9.1 Research design

9.3.1 Systematic Literature Review (SLR)

SLRs can be, inter alia, traced back to the field of medicine. Nowadays, they are increasingly applied to other sciences like management and international development [32]. The development of a hypothesis framework is necessary for the subsequent study and consequently for answering the research question. In order to develop hypotheses, a SLR was conducted. The search strategy comprises the keywords that were used for the search, scientific databases and the quality assessment of the articles.

According to the main research question, the following keywords were used for the literature review:

"Artificial Intelligence", "Artificial Intelligence in Healthcare", "AI in Healthcare", "Artificial Intelligence in Medicine", "Machine Learning in Healthcare", "Deep Learning in Healthcare", "Potentials of Artificial Intelligence in Healthcare", "Benefits of Precision Medicine", "Economic benefits of AI in healthcare", "Medical Artificial Intelligence", "ANN in healthcare", "Impact of Artificial Intelligence in Healthcare OR Medicine".

As the research question covers the areas of business studies, computer science and medicine/healthcare, a wide range of databases were accessed: ScienceDirect, AIS eLibrary, JSTOR, SAGE Journals, INFORMS PubsOnLine, Google Scholar, Wiley Online Library, IEEE Xplore, Springer Link, EconBiz, Taylor & Francis Online, PubMed.

In order to evaluate the scientific quality of journals and conferences, different rankings can be used. The literature review is based on two ranking portals: VHB-Jourqual3 [33] and CORE Rankings Portal [34]. The "Verband der Hochschullehrer für Betriebswirtschaft e.V. (VHB)" deals with scientific topics related to business science [35]. VHB-JOURQUAL3 is a rating of business relevant journals based on judgements of VHB members [33]. Only journals with a rating from A+ to C have been used for the literature research to ensure a good quality of the articles. The CORE (Computing Research and Education) Rankings Portal assesses especially conferences but also journals of the computing disciplines [34]. Conferences and journals ranked between A+ and B were considered to ensure a good quality of the articles.

9.3.2 Generation of Hypotheses and Conceptual Model

Four hypotheses were generated based on the findings of the SLR:

H1: Management tasks positively influence the potential benefits of AI in healthcare.
H2: Medical diagnostics positively influences the potential benefits of AI in healthcare.

H3: Medical treatment positively influences the potential benefits of AI in healthcare.
H4: Drug discovery positively influences the potential benefits of AI in healthcare.

These hypotheses are part of the conceptual model that was developed based on *Structural Equation Modeling (SEM)*. SEM is a multivariate analysis method that enables the evaluation of multiple variables which are not directly observable. In order to describe and measure these variables, indicators have to be identified. A specific method of SEM is called *Partial Least Squares SEM (PLS-SEM)* which can be used for the development of theories [36].

Within SEM, hypotheses and the relation of variables are illustrated as *path models* [36]. A distinction is made between independent (exogenous) and dependent (endogenous) variables. Independent variables can be considered as causes that have effects on the dependent variable [36]. Each PLS path model consists of a *structural model,* also known as *inner model*, and a *measurement model,* known as *outer model*. The structural model specifies the relationship between the latent variables whereas the measurement model illustrates the relationship between the latent variables and indicators [36]. *Latent variables* are not directly observable and require suitable measurement models whereas *manifest variables* can be directly observed [37].

Figure 9.2 depicts the hypothesis model that was created based on the findings of the SLR.

According to the hypotheses, the model consists of four latent variables and 18 indicators. It considers medical application areas as well as the area of management as influences on the potential benefits of AI in healthcare. The measurement model is designed as a *reflective measurement model*. Thus, the reflective indicators can be

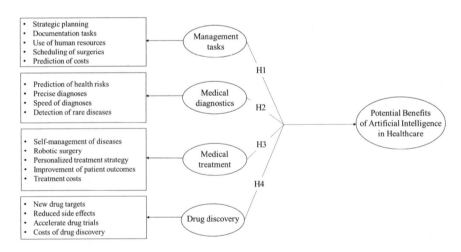

Fig. 9.2 Conceptual model

considered as representative examples within the definition of the construct and are interchangeable [38].

The results of the SLR, and thus the evidence for the development of the hypotheses and related indicators, are outlined below. Additionally, the authors provide an overview of articles including ranking, resulting items and the assignment to different constructs (see [39]).

Hypothesis 1—Management Tasks

Due to various factors like cost and competitive pressure, there is a tremendous focus on efficiency and productivity within healthcare organizations [18]. Therefore, management tasks can also be subject for improvements due to AI.

H1: Management tasks positively influence the potential benefits of AI in healthcare.

Krämer et al. (*in 2019*) developed a ML model for the classification of hospital admissions into elective and emergency care. This approach can support case mix planning which is a key component of *strategic planning* [40]. Additionally, Akter et al. (*in 2022*) conclude that ML is able to increase hospital bedding efficiency which can lead to an improved long-term strategic planning in hospitals [9]. In doing so, they refer to Turgeman et al. (*in 2017*) who developed a ML model for predicting patients' length of stay in a hospital [41].

Kocaballi et al. [13] and Doraiswamy et al. [42] confirm with their study that AI-based systems can support *documentation tasks* like writing referrals or medical records of patients. Fairley et al. (*in 2019*) introduce an optimization and ML model to improve the efficiency of operating rooms. The authors assume that their approach can support schedulers in *calculating staffing needs* and ultimately reduce staffing requirements [17]. In addition, an *efficient use of human resources* can arise due to the ability of ML to predict how long a patient will stay in hospital [9].

Onukwugha et al. (*in 2016*) show that their survival grouping algorithm can improve the *prediction of 5-year costs* [43]. Additionally, Thesmar et al. (*in 2019*) expect AI to be able to predict upcoming health costs [44].

Hypothesis 2—Medical Diagnostics

The decision-making process in diagnostics can be divided into two phases, namely differential diagnosis and final or provisional diagnosis [45]. Within the first phase, the medical history of the patients, specific symptoms and laboratory tests like blood testing are considered as input data. The final/provisional diagnosis is provided by means of the medical knowledge of physicians [45]. The following results of the SLR show that AI can have the potential to improve medical diagnostics.

H2: Medical diagnostics positively influences the potential benefits of AI in healthcare.

Kaplan and Haenlein (*in 2020*) mention the capability of AI to "predict serious health risks such as skin cancer and strokes" [46] by even better operating than humans. Thereby, the authors allude to the third evolutionary stage, the AI super-intelligence [47]. Additionally, Garbuio and Lin (*in 2019*) refer to the medical DL company Enlitic and see AI's potential to *identify patients with risk factors* for a specific disease [28].

The ability of AI to enable more *precise diagnoses* is subject of a large number of scientific papers. Pee et al. (*in 2019*) state that medical imaging systems based on AI have the ability to review computed tomography images and can diagnose diseases with an increased accuracy [48]. Fan et al. (*in 2020*) examine the impact factors for healthcare professionals to adopt an AI-based medical diagnosis support system (AIMDSS). The authors present AIMDSS like those of Enlitic and Freenome which are able to provide more precise diagnoses than radiologists [49]. Additional evidence can be found in the paper of Yuan et al. [50]. The researchers show that their AI-based system can achieve sepsis diagnoses with an accuracy of more than 80%. It is thus outperforming the traditional SOFA score used for sepsis diagnosis [50].

Garbuio and Lin (*in 2019*) see potential in AI to enable a *faster detection* of small variations within data [28]. Especially the combination of AI with medical imaging can lead to faster diagnoses [15]. Within their case study, Pee et al. (*in 2019*) introduce a robot that is able to recommend diagnoses even faster than a human due to the large amount of data he is able to process [48].

One main benefit of AI is the ability to examine large and multidimensional datasets by determining important variables. Through the identification of (complex) patterns in patients' data the *detection of rare diseases* can be supported [44].

Hypothesis 3—Medical Treatment

The treatment of patients is an essential component of healthcare provision. The trend is increasingly moving towards personalized medicine to be able to take the needs of the individual patient into account [19].

H3: Medical treatment positively influences the potential benefits of AI in healthcare.

Bardhan et al. (*in 2020*) see the potential of AI in wearables or mobile applications to *support the management of chronic conditions* and promote healthy lifestyles. According to the authors, possible applications would be health monitoring or virtual coaching for managing diabetes [5].

Shin et al. (*in 2019*) implement two different learning algorithms in a *surgical robot* for tissue manipulation. As a result, both algorithms implemented in the surgical robot could fulfill the task and thus improve this sub-process of the surgery [51]. Moreover, AI-based systems can support surgeons by automatically guiding surgical instruments [52].

Paranjape et al. (*in 2020*) show the potential of ML algorithms by means of two medical application areas: Lung cancer and sepsis. ML can provide personalized radiation therapy and a *treatment strategy tailored to the patient* [6]. Further evidence that AI can support personalized treatment can be found in the study of Bertsimas et al. [16]. The authors developed different data-driven models for personalized coronary artery disease management as well as supervised ML algorithms for regression models. Overall, the authors see ML's potential of identifying an optimal treatment strategy for patients [16].

Schinkel et al. (*in 2019*) demonstrate that the early diagnosis of diseases and early initiation of treatment by means of AI-based systems can ultimately lead to an *improvement of patient outcomes* [53]. Additionally, Garbuio and Lin (*in 2019*) indicate that AI-based systems have been improving health outcomes [28].

Within the scope of their analysis, Vemulapalli et al. (*in 2016*) examine the use of AI-based methods like Bayesian networks for chronic disease management. As a result, the researchers are able to demonstrate the ability of Bayesian networks to reveal non-obvious correlations in the data. The use of these algorithms can lead to the *reduction of treatment costs* [54]. Additionally, the AI algorithm of Yuan et al. (*in 2020*) not only leads to more precise sepsis diagnoses but can also lead to cost reduction due to early treatment [50].

Hypothesis 4—Drug Discovery

Drug discovery is a decisive factor for healthcare provision and can be divided into different phases. It mainly includes target selection and validation, compound screening and lead optimization, preclinical studies and clinical trials. After the selection of targets appropriate for a specific disease, various molecular components are identified. Various preclinical and clinical studies follow [55]. AI is supposed to support drug discovery in various task which are presented below.

H4: Drug discovery positively influences the potential benefits of AI in healthcare.

Davenport and Ronanki (*in 2018*) refer to Pfizer using IBM Watson to support drug discovery in immuno-oncology. The system is based on the combination of an extended literature review and Pfizer's data. Finding hidden patterns can accelerate the *identification of new drug targets* [56]. Akter et al. (*in 2022*) introduce the cooperation of Novartis and Intel on the development of deep neural networks to accelerate drug discovery [9]. Additionally, Dezső and Ceccarelli (*in 2020*) show that their ML approach can predict and identify new drug targets in oncology. With this method, they offer a *cost-effective* and efficient solution for drug discovery [57].

Akay and Hess (*in 2019*) examine the potentials as well as needs of ML and DL applications in medicine and technology. Accordingly, DL combined with predictive analysis and patient database meta-searches can support drug design and prevent serious side-effects during the drug regimen [10]. The study of Doraiswamy et al. (*in 2020*) among psychiatrists additionally discovered that AI/ML is able to provide personalized drug targets with *reduced side effects* [42].

Garbuio and Lin (*in 2019*) introduce Enlitic, a medical deep learning company based in San Francisco that offers clinical decision support products. By analyzing health data, the system can *accelerate drug trials* [28].

9.3.3 Data Collection

Subsequent to the presentation of the conceptual model and the hypotheses, the procedure of data collection is explained in detail. Figure 9.3 depicts the different steps of the data collection.

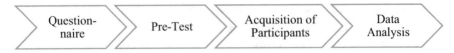

Fig. 9.3 Main steps of the data collection

The questionnaire was created based on the conceptual model (see Sect. 9.1.3.2) and includes 19 questions. The questions on the conceptual model correspond to section B.

Additionally, three further sections were included:

(A)   Experience with AI in Healthcare
(B)   Assessment of the Potential Benefits of AI in Healthcare
(C)   Enterprise-specific Questions
(D)   Socio-demographic Questions.

The results are presented in detail within Sect. 9.1.4.

LimeSurvey was selected as tool for data collection. It is an online survey tool that allows the integration of different question types into the survey [58]. A pre-test was carried out to review the comprehensibility of the questions, eliminate content overlaps and test the usability of the survey. The pre-test proved to be an essential part of the preliminary work and considerations.

The target group of the online survey includes experts on AI in healthcare. In detail, it comprises employees in the areas of management, consulting, computer science, engineering, medicine, health sciences and pharmacy. The main focus has been on the German healthcare sector. To gain comprehensive insights, users, developers and manufacturers as well as researchers have been included. Section 9.1.4.1 presents the main characteristics of the expert group.

9.4   Results

This section presents the results of the expert survey. First of all, the process of data analysis is introduced, followed by the sample characteristics including the experience with AI in healthcare as well as socio-demographic and enterprise-specific questions. Section 9.1.4.2 examines the quality criteria of the model, followed by the results of the SEM in Sect. 9.1.4.3.

9.4.1   Data Analysis and Sample Characteristics

A total of 127 complete responses were indicated via the survey tool LimeSurvey [58]. This number also included participants who selected "No" when asked about their experience with AI in healthcare. Due to the implemented "exit scenario", people without experience with AI in healthcare were excluded. This results in 105 complete responses used for the subsequent evaluation.

There are various software tools to evaluate models based on SEM. As the conceptual model presented in Sect. 9.1.3.2 is based on PLS-SEM, the most suitable software is SmartPLS [31]. It has a high level of usability and extended reporting features [59] and is thus used for the evaluation of the results.

The participants who indicated having no experience with AI in healthcare were asked if they plan to address the topic in the future. 77% indicate that they will address AI within healthcare in the future. 18% may want to engage with it while 5% of the participants do not want to deal with AI in healthcare.

91 participants indicated that their enterprise is located in Germany. Additionally, 6 participants stated that their organization is operating globally. Two experts are from the United States, respectively one expert is from Brazil and Israel. 4 experts did not provide an answer in which country their enterprise is located.

Examining the gender of the participants, 85.7% are male. 11.4% are female and 2.9% of the experts did not indicate an answer.

In order to more precisely assess the experience of the participants, they were asked on how many years of experience they have with AI in healthcare. Most of the experts have 1–2 years of experience with AI in healthcare, followed by 30 respondents who have 3–4 years of experience. 27 participants have even more than 6 years of experience with AI in healthcare. The experience of 9 participants amounts to 5–6 years while 7 respondents have less than one year of experience with AI in healthcare. The results show that the experience of the experts varies considerably in terms of years.

In addition, the experts were asked which application areas in healthcare their experience refers to (see Fig. 9.4). The participants had the option to indicate multiple responses. 35.3% of the participants have experience with AI related to diagnostics. 16.4% refer their experience to treatment, followed by health prevention (11.8%). 10.1% of the participants relate their experience to the manufacturing of medical devices. Further application areas are drug discovery / drug manufacturing and administration with respectively 8%. The participants had the opportunity to add further application areas. This results in the following additional application areas: Patient monitoring, translation of AI to the clinical setting, guidance to care, clinical evaluation, speech recognition, structuring of medical data, performance analysis of medical devices, research, supply chain monitoring, standardization and benchmarking of AI in healthcare, sales effectiveness and AI-based suggestion in healthcare.

The question on AI approaches (see Fig. 9.5) shows that most of the experience refers to ML, followed by DL with 23.1%. The participants had again the opportunity to provide multiple responses. 21.9% of the experts indicate that their experience refers to Artificial Neural Networks (ANN) which can also be assigned to ML/DL [60]. While 14% are experienced in predictive analytics, 6.1% of the participants are experienced in Natural Language Processing (NLP). 3.2% of the experts have experience with robotics. In addition, the experts indicated the following AI approaches: medical image analysis and image processing, surgical data science, probabilistic

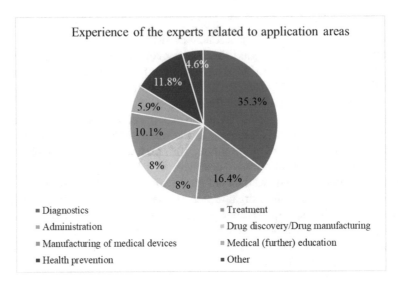

Fig. 9.4 Experience of the experts related to application areas

reasoning, cognitive modeling as well as fuzzy logic. Cognitive modeling contains theories describing the reasoning in people [61]. Fuzzy logic is based on the fuzzy set theory which comprises linguistic variables, fuzzy if–then rules and more [61].

According to their function in the enterprise, 42.9% of the experts can be attributed to the field of *management and administrative staff*. 28.6% of the participants are computer/data scientists while 14.3% are (AI) engineers. Additionally, 8 research

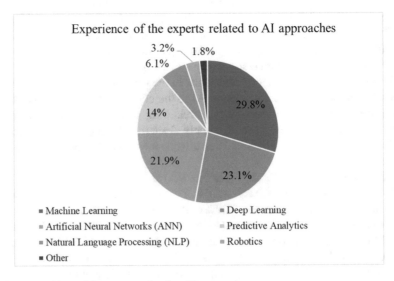

Fig. 9.5 Experience of the experts related to AI approaches

scientists took part in the survey. 5 experts are physicians and 2 participants did not indicate an answer. In order to assess the size of the enterprise, the number of employees and the amount of turnover were queried. 52 enterprises have more than 250 employees whereas 35 have less than 50 employees. 10.5% of the companies employ 50–250 people and 7 participants did not indicate an answer on the number of employees in their enterprise.

Considering the amount of turnover in 2019, 34 enterprises record a turnover of more than 50 million euros. In contrast, 21.9% of the enterprises have a turnover of less than 10 million euros. Three enterprises record a turnover of 10–50 million euros. It has to be noted that the majority did not indicate the amount of turnover. According to the recommendation of the European Commission, enterprises with less than 250 employees and an annual turnover below 50 million euros can be attributed to the category of micro, small and medium-sized enterprises (SMEs) [62]. Accordingly, about one third of the enterprises can be considered to be SMEs.

The experts were also asked to which category their enterprise can be assigned. 30 enterprises can be attributed to the area of software and IT. 22 enterprises can be assigned to medical technology. 14 participants work in a hospital while 12.4% of the experts assign themselves to research institutes or universities. Additionally, nine pharmaceutical enterprises are represented. Respectively one expert works in a nursing home, non-profit organization or has no current enterprise.

The COVID-19 pandemic is affecting all sectors and especially the healthcare sector, which is facing an increasing number of patients [8]. In order to investigate whether the pandemic also has an impact on the use, development or general engagement with AI in healthcare, the following statement was included into the questionnaire (see Fig. 9.6).

20 experts completely agree with the statement whereas 30 participants rather agree. 31 experts responded neutrally. 14.3% rather disagree and 9 participants completely disagree that the COVID-19 pandemic has led to an increased focus on

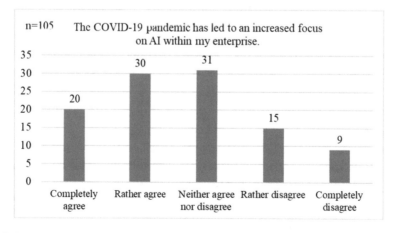

Fig. 9.6 Impact of the COVID-19 pandemic on the focus of AI

AI within the enterprise. The responses show that nearly half of the experts perceive an increased focus on AI within their enterprise.

9.4.2 Examination of Quality Criteria

Section 9.1.4.3 focuses on the evaluation of the hypothesis model using SEM. In order to assess the quality of the model, various quality criteria are initially considered within this section.

The main quality criteria to assess the quality of a measurement are *objectivity*, *reliability* and *validity*. *Objectivity* can be assumed when different investigators obtain the same results. In addition, participants should not be influenced and the same results should lead to the same conclusions. *Reliability* reflects the stability of the measuring instrument. The third criterion *validity* indicates the accuracy of the measuring instrument and its fit to the measurement target [37].

To examine the *reliability,* two criteria can be used. The quality criterium *Composite Reliability (CR)* determines the reliability of internal consistency by taking into account different indicator loadings. In order to confirm the reliability of the indicators, values of at least 0.6 are acceptable [37]. *Cronbach's Alpha (CA)* additionally makes statements on the reliability of internal consistency. In contrast to CR, it assumes equal indicator loadings [37]. To confirm an *acceptable* reliability, CA values should be at least 0.7 in constructs with four or more indicators [38].

Convergence validity is the extent to which a measurement correlates positively with an alternative measurement of the same construct. The items belonging to a construct should share a large amount of variance. The convergence validity can either be examined by considering the loadings of the indicators or by means of *average variance extracted (AVE)* [37]. The focus of the following section is on AVE. Outer loadings are especially considered in reflective measurement models and determine the contribution of an indicator toward the construct it is assigned to [37]. The target value of the AVE to be able to confirm a variance has to exceed the threshold of 0.5 [63]. The *coefficient of determination* R^2 describes the proportion of the variance explained by a linear regression [64]. Values of 0.67 can be considered "substantial" whereas results of 0.33 are "moderate" and values up to 0.19 are considered "weak" [63].

The higher the R^2 value, the better is the explanation of the dependent variable by the latent variables in the structural model [37].

Table 9.1 provides an overview of the quality criteria.

First, the CR values are being considered. All values clearly exceed the threshold of 0.6. *Drug discovery* has the highest value of 0.893, followed by *medical diagnostics* with a value of 0.855 and *medical treatment* with 0.826. The construct *management tasks* shows a CR value of 0.808. Additionally, all CA values exceed the threshold of 0.7 and thus represent an acceptable internal consistency.

The examination of *AVE* shows that the values of *drug discovery* and *medical diagnostics* are above the threshold of 0.5. Consequently, the constructs explain

Table 9.1 Quality criteria

	Composite reliability (CR)	Cronbach's Alpha (CA)	Average variance extracted (AVE)
Management tasks	0.808	0.711	0.459
Medical diagnostics	0.855	0.770	0.599
Medical treatment	0.826	0.738	0.489
Drug discovery	0.893	0.846	0.676

more than half of the variance of their indicators [37]. In contrast, the values of *medical treatment* and *management tasks* are below the target value. However, they are only slightly below the threshold.

To examine how adequately the dependent variable "Potential benefits of AI in healthcare" is explained by the four independent variables, R^2 was examined. The R^2 value of 0.261 represents a result considered as "weak" to "moderate" [63].

9.4.3   Evaluation of the SEM

After examining the quality criteria, the model based on SEM is being evaluated. Figure 9.7 shows the structural model with the t-statistics and significance levels of the respective paths.

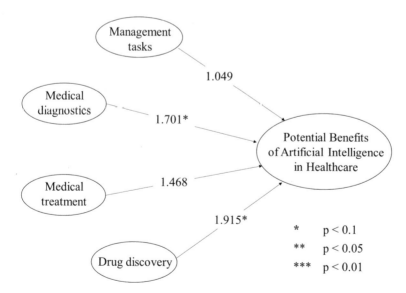

Fig. 9.7 T-statistics of the path model

Table 9.2 Results of the SEM

	Original sample (O)	Sample mean (M)	Standard deviation	T-statistics	P-value
Management tasks	0.095	0.115	0.090	1.049	0.295
Medical diagnostics	0.205	0.198	0.120	1.701	0.089
Medical treatment	0.175	0.178	0.119	1.468	0.142
Drug discovery	0.162	0.167	0.084	1.915	0.056

In the following section, the results are discussed in more detail in order to be able to derive statements relating to the hypotheses. Table 9.2 illustrates the individual values.

A two-sided test with a significance level of 10% was conducted. Considering the original sample, values of at least 0.2 are considered "meaningful" [65]. Additionally, the t-value is used as a decisive criterion. T-statistics are used to determine the significance of a parameter estimator. For a two-sided test with a significance level of 10%, the critical t-value is 1.65. If the measured t-value exceeds the critical t-value, the null hypothesis can be rejected [59]. In order to confirm the significance, the p-value has to be below 0.1 [37].

H1: *Management tasks positively influence the potential benefits of AI in healthcare.*

Considering the *t-statistics,* the value is below the critical t-value of 1.65. Additionally, the p-value of 0.295 exceeds the threshold value of 0.1. Consequently, the hypothesis has to be rejected. A slightly positive but no significant influence on the potential benefits of AI in healthcare can be assumed.

H2: *Medical diagnostics positively influences the potential benefits of AI in healthcare.*

The t-value of 1.701 exceeds the critical t-value while the p-value is below the threshold of 0.1. Additionally, the value of the original sample exceeds the desired threshold of 0.2. A positive and significant influence can be assumed. Consequently, *hypothesis 2 can be accepted*. Medical diagnostics positively influences the potential benefits of AI in healthcare.

H3: *Medical treatment positively influences the potential benefits of AI in healthcare.*

The t-value of 1.468 is below the critical t-value and the p-value exceeds the mark of 0.1. With an o-value of 0.175, the construct shows a positive but no statistically significant influence. Therefore, *the hypothesis has to be rejected*.

H4: *Drug discovery positively influences the potential benefits of AI in healthcare.*

The t-value of 1.915 exceeds the threshold. Additionally, the p-value is below 0.1 whereby a significant influence can be assumed. As the o-value is below 0.2, a weak positive influence is implied. Nevertheless, based on the confirmed p-values and t-values, hypothesis 4 can be accepted. With a p-value of 0.056, the construct shows the most significant influence on the potential benefits of AI in healthcare.

In summary, the experts consider AI to offer significant potential benefits within the application areas *medical diagnostics* and *drug discovery*.

9.5 Interpretation

The COVID-19 pandemic represents a massive and global challenge. It has caused more than 6 million deaths worldwide [66], overwhelmed healthcare systems as well as the economy [14]. As the empirical investigation shows, nearly half of the experts perceive an increased focus on AI within their enterprise due to the COVID-19 pandemic. It can be assumed that the pandemic has increased the need for assistive technologies like AI. The literature additionally shows that new AI approaches emerged since the COVID-19 pandemic. Researchers investigate how AI can support drug discovery and vaccine development [14] or how image-based AI can contribute to tissue characterization and classification of COVID-19 patients [15].

Considering the results of the SEM, the determinants *medical diagnostics* and *drug discovery* respectively show a positive and significant influence on the potential benefits of AI in the healthcare sector. Whereas *medical diagnostics* shows the most positive influence, *drug discovery* has the most significant influence. In the following, the construct *medical diagnostics* is examined more closely.

According to the findings from the literature, *medical diagnostics* has been confirmed by the experts to be a beneficial application area of AI. For example, AI-based systems can support the prediction of health risks like strokes [28, 46]. The prediction of health risks is essential for the prevention and early treatment of diseases [50]. AI can therefore be a decisive contribution. AI-based systems can further increase the precision of diagnoses [48] and could ultimately reduce false diagnoses. Furthermore, the speed of diagnoses can be enhanced by means of AI [28, 48]. This can lead to *increased efficiency* and more time for physicians to care for patients. It could ultimately improve the interaction between patients and physicians [48].

Additionally, the literature shows that AI is already widely used for diagnostics [15, 49, 50] which is also reflected by the results of the study. More than 35% of the experts indicated that their experience with AI refers to diagnostics. Considering the construct *drug discovery*, a positive significant influence can be assumed. However, the construct *drug discovery* presumably has only a weak influence, as the original sample value is below the desired threshold of 0.2 [65]. AI is able to support the development of drugs with reduced side effects. It has the potential to enhance optical drug design and reduce side effects during the drug regimen [10]. Through the use of AI and the increased efficiency, the costs of drug discovery can be reduced [57]. The results show that AI is also able to accelerate drug trials, as stated by Garbuio and Lin (*in 2019*) [28]. Additionally, AI-based systems can accelerate the identification of new drug targets [9, 57] which can also have a positive influence on the development of vaccine and medication against COVID-19 [14].

The construct *medical treatment* could not be confirmed as significant influencing factor on the potential benefits of AI in healthcare. However, the assumption that AI can lead to the *improvement of patient outcomes* shows the best indicator loading. AI technologies such as ML algorithms can contribute to the improvement of patient outcomes [16, 53]. The non-significant results might be due to the fact that medical treatment usually requires direct contact to physicians and caregivers. Kocaballi et al. [13] identified within their study that empathy still represents a main task of physicians. AI-based systems can hardly replace this contact.

Whereas in the area of diagnostics procedures could be more standardized, the individual treatment of patients is very important [19].

The application area *management tasks* is also not considered by the experts to have a significant influence on the potential benefits of AI in healthcare. The results could be caused by the fact that management tasks usually require a high level of sense-making and judgmental competence in order to derive comprehensible decisions [67]. According to the results, AI-based systems may be rather considered as assistants to managers allowing them to focus on complex and meaningful tasks [67]. Consequently, AI can lead to *an efficient use of human resources* within healthcare [17], thereby facilitating staffing [9]. The results could also stem from the circumstance that AI has not yet been widely applied to management tasks.

According to the literature, there is also a challenge in creating *transparency*. This is especially emphasized by the "black box problem" referring to the difficulty for healthcare professionals and patients to understand the decisions made by AI systems [68, 69]. Another challenge is how to determine who is responsible or even legally liable for medical errors. The more stakeholders are involved in the development or use of AI, the more difficult it is to define those responsibilities [70].

Through the survey and the literature review, various challenges of AI in healthcare emerged. To mitigate the challenges, recommended activities are provided in the following section.

9.6 Recommended Activities: Cooperation and Exchange Between Different Stakeholders

The stakeholders considered here correspond to the professions indicated by the experts. The professions of the experts cover management/administrative staff, engineers, data/computer scientists, research scientists and physicians. As patients are a key group of stakeholders within the healthcare sector and should also benefit from AI, they are also integrated in the recommendation.

Factors such as perceived performance anxiety and communication barriers decrease the intention to use AI [3]. Some studies indicate that health professionals could be afraid of being replaced by AI-based systems [13, 46]. As the study shows, AI does not (yet) demonstrate significant potential benefits in all areas that were examined. Empathy and human connection can only hardly be provided by AI [13].

Developers and manufacturers, like data scientists and AI engineers, can play a central role in increasing the willingness to use AI-based systems among healthcare professionals. Specific workshops and continuous support by developers and manufacturers could help healthcare professionals to deal with AI-based systems well and safely. This requires time investments in the first step. The fact that AI-based systems can lead to time savings (e.g. by accelerating diagnostics) would make this investment worthwhile. A basic understanding of AI could help healthcare professionals to create transparency regarding the functionality of AI. The developers and manufacturers should therefore support the implementation process at different levels within the healthcare facility.

Through a continuous exchange between users and manufacturers, support can be provided in case of problems and users can give feedback to developers. Through the practical experience of the users, the developers can obtain suggestions for improvement or align the systems according to the needs in the healthcare sector. As health professionals are directly involved into clinical processes, the insights can be more specified than the ones of developers and manufacturers. This process could support the continuous development of AI-based systems.

In order to provide a functioning and reliable human-AI collaboration, not only healthcare professionals but also patients should be integrated into the use of AI [3]. One of the most important goals in healthcare is to maintain and regain patients' health through the provision of optimal healthcare [8]. Patients should be made aware of the benefits and limitations of AI-based systems. As suggested by Esmaeilzadeh (*in 2020*), patients' concerns about AI-based systems should be addressed before the implementation of such systems [3]. However, generating transparency is hindered by the "black box problem" [68]. Consequently, decisions made by AI-based systems are not always transparent. Physicians should therefore explain to their patients both the role that human caregivers play and the role of AI-based systems in a diagnostic or treatment process. Additionally, physicians should communicate the potential benefits of AI compared to other methods, thereby also referring to potential risks. Thus, possible misperceptions of AI by patients can be reduced or even eliminated [70]. In return, patients could share their experiences of AI-based systems with physicians so they can in turn provide feedback to AI developers.

Digital transformation in healthcare organizations is confronted with regulation and statutory requirements [71]. When AI is going to be implemented, it should be holistically integrated into the (digital) infrastructure and organizational culture [72]. Managers should take the role of a "guiding light" in order to exploit the potentials of AI. Another important task is to increase the employees' awareness of what AI can achieve and what not [70]. The systems should be designed to meet the needs of both patients and employees. In order to ensure this requirement, the management should maintain a continuous exchange with the developers. Tasks of the upper management would be to understand the capabilities of AI-based systems and to decide whether existing capabilities should be improved or whether there is a need for new capabilities [72]. As there is the risk of organizational resistance [73], AI acceptance should already be realized during the implementation process [72]. According to Lee et al. (*in 2019*), possible measures that could increase acceptance are pilot projects and AI training [73]. Another main task for managers would be to develop an AI strategy [73] in order to holistically integrate AI into organizational processes.

While researchers and consultants provide theoretically founded insights, health professionals and developers can in turn provide researchers with practical insights. Accordingly, there should be a continuous exchange between researchers, developers/manufacturers and healthcare professionals.

9.7 Conclusion and Outlook

The empirical investigation confirmed *medical diagnostics* and *drug discovery* as positive and significant influencing factors on the potential benefits of AI in healthcare. In contrast, *management tasks* and *medical treatment* could not be confirmed as significant influencing factors. AI can increase the precision [48, 49], the speed of diagnoses [15] and predict health risks [46]. In drug discovery, there is potential for the development of drugs with reduced side effects [42]. Drug trials can be accelerated [28] and costs for drug discovery can be reduced [57].

The feedback from the experts revealed that the intention to use AI-based systems plays a decisive role. Accordingly, physicians could feel that their decision-making authority is impaired by the use of AI. Some even express the fear of being replaced by AI. As the study shows, AI-based systems cannot completely replace physicians and nurses at the current state of development. Especially in medical treatment, human intervention and providing empathy towards patients are important aspects AI can only hardly fulfill. However, AI could contribute to increased efficiency, thereby reducing the workload of healthcare personnel [74]. This could ultimately allow more time for physicians to provide empathetic care and to focus on complex cases. AI can play a critical role in improving healthcare processes as an assistant to healthcare professionals.

The mixed results of the investigation might be partly caused by the fact that AI is still rarely used within the German healthcare sector. This also illustrates that the study is subject to some limitations. First of all, the study could be extended by including more experts from other countries. This would provide a more generalized view on the potential benefits of AI in healthcare. Additionally, the sample size of 105 is rather small. Increasing the sample size could help to derive more general statements. Another approach could be to conduct the empirical investigation solely among users or exclusively among developers. This would allow to attribute the results to a more specific target group. Future research could focus on how to eliminate or mitigate the challenges associated with AI in healthcare.

The potential benefits of AI in healthcare are promising. However, there are hurdles such as data privacy, ethical concerns and missing transparency that impede the full exploitation of the potential benefits. The future challenge will be to generate the balance between necessary regulation, especially with regard to data protection, and the necessary "design freedom" for AI developers [75].

To pursue the developments of AI in the healthcare sector, the research areas "Management for Small and Medium-sized Enterprises" and "Healthcare Management" at Aalen University are continuing their research in this field. Currently, the barriers of AI in the healthcare sector are empirically investigated in order to be able to derive suggestions for improvement for the application and development of AI-based systems.

Returning to the opening quote "AI is the new electricity" by Andrew Ng [1], parallels can certainly be drawn between the beginnings of electricity and AI. Just a few hundred years ago, the subject on electricity was associated with numerous myths. The invention of electric light and widespread power supplies finally led to a tremendous boom at the turn of the nineteenth century [76]. Despite the current boom of AI, it still does not seem to be truly tangible for some people and is associated with some myths. Taking electricity as an example, continuous developments and appropriate responses and actions to failures can contribute decisively to a long-term and beneficial establishment of AI. This can ultimately lead to an increased acceptance of AI among people. Reliable and ethically oriented AI-based systems are especially important in the healthcare sector, where uncertainty, medical errors and additional risks can have serious consequences. The idea of AI revolutionizing healthcare by reducing the workload of health professionals, improving patient outcomes and add benefit to many other areas within healthcare sectors is definitely worth holding on to AI.

References

1. Ng, A.: cited by C. Jewell, Artificial Intelligence: The New Electricity (2019), Available online at https://www.wipo.int/wipo_magazine/en/2019/03/article_0001.html. Accessed 20 March 2022
2. Obschonka, M., Audretsch, D.B.: Artificial intelligence and big data in entrepreneurship: a new era has begun. Small Bus. Econ. 55(3), 529–539 (2020). https://doi.org/10.1007/s11187-019-00202-4
3. Esmaeilzadeh, P.: Use of AI-based tools for healthcare purposes: a survey study from consumers' perspectives. BMC Med. Inform. Decis. Mak. 20, 170 (2020). https://doi.org/10.1186/s12911-020-01191-1
4. Jiang, F., et al.: Artificial intelligence in healthcare: past, present and future. Stroke Vasc. Neurol. 2, 1–14 (2017). https://doi.org/10.1136/svn-2017-000101
5. Bardhan, I., et al.: Connecting systems, data, and people: a multidisciplinary research roadmap for chronic disease management. MISQ 44(1), 185–200 (2020). https://doi.org/10.25300/MISQ/2020/14644
6. Paranjape, K., et al.: Short keynote paper: mainstreaming personalized healthcare-transforming healthcare through new era of artificial intelligence. IEEE J. Biomed. Health Inf. 24(7), 1860–1863 (2020). https://doi.org/10.1109/JBHI.2020.2970807

7. Meskó, B., et al.: Will artificial intelligence solve the human resource crisis in healthcare? BMC Health Serv. Res. **18**, 545 (2018). https://doi.org/10.1186/s12913-018-3359-4

8. Bundesministerium für Gesundheit: The German healthcare system: Strong. Reliable. Proven. (2020)

9. Akter, S., et al.: Transforming business using digital innovations: the application of AI, blockchain, cloud and data analytics. Ann. Oper. Res. **308**, 7–39 (2022). https://doi.org/10.1007/s10479-020-03620-w

10. Akay, A., Hess, H.: Deep learning: current and emerging applications in medicine and technology. IEEE J. Biomed. Health Inf. **23**(3), 906–920 (2019). https://doi.org/10.1109/JBHI.2019.2894713

11. Barda, A.J., et al.: A qualitative research framework for the design of user-centered displays of explanations for machine learning model predictions in healthcare. BMC Med Inform Decis. Mak. **20**, 257 (2020). https://doi.org/10.1186/s12911-020-01276-x

12. Hagan, R., et al.: Comparing regression and neural network techniques for personalized predictive analytics to promote lung protective ventilation in intensive care units. Comput. Biol. Med. **126**, 104030 (2020). https://doi.org/10.1016/j.compbiomed.2020.104030

13. Kocaballi, A.B., et al.: Envisioning an artificial intelligence documentation assistant for future primary care consultations: a co-design study with general practitioners. JAMIA **27**(11), 1695–1704 (2020). https://doi.org/10.1093/jamia/ocaa131

14. Keshavarzi Arshadi, A., et al.: Artificial intelligence for COVID-19 drug discovery and vaccine development. Front. Artif. Intell. **3**, 65 (2020). https://doi.org/10.3389/frai.2020.00065

15. Suri, J.S., et al.: COVID-19 pathways for brain and heart injury in comorbidity patients: a role of medical imaging and artificial intelligence-based COVID severity classification: a review. Comput. Biol. Med. **124**, 103960 (2020). https://doi.org/10.1016/j.compbiomed.2020.103960

16. Bertsimas, D., et al.: Personalized treatment for coronary artery disease patients: a machine learning approach. Health Care Manag. Sci. **23**, 482–506 (2020). https://doi.org/10.1007/s10729-020-09522-4

17. Fairley, M., et al.: Improving the efficiency of the operating room environment with an optimization and machine learning model. Health Care Manag. Sci. **22**, 756–767 (2019). https://doi.org/10.1007/s10729-018-9457-3

18. Reinhardt, R., Oliver, W.J.: The cost problem in health care. In: Gurtner, S., Soyez, K. (eds.) Challenges and Opportunities in Health Care Management, pp. 3–13. Springer International Publishing, Cham (2015). https://doi.org/10.1007/978-3-319-12178-9_1

19. Denicolai, S., Previtali, P.: Precision Medicine: implications for value chains and business models in life sciences. Technol. Forecast Soc. Chang. **151**, 119767 (2020). https://doi.org/10.1016/j.techfore.2019.119767

20. Latan, H., Noonan R. (eds.): Editor's preface. In: Partial Least Squares Path Modeling. Cham, Springer International Publishing (2017). https://doi.org/10.1007/978-3-319-64069-3

21. Tran, B.X., et al.: Global evolution of research in artificial intelligence in health and medicine: a bibliometric study. J. Clin. Med. **8**(3), 360 (2019). https://doi.org/10.3390/jcm8030360

22. Gunn, A.A.: The diagnosis of acute abdominal pain with computer analysis. J. R. Coll. Surg. Edinb. **21**(3), 170–172 (1976)

23. Bohr, A., Memarzadeh, K.: The rise of artificial intelligence in healthcare applications. Artif. Intell. Healthc. 25–60 (2020). https://doi.org/10.1016/B978-0-12-818438-7.00002-2

24. Cosma, G., et al.: A survey on computational intelligence approaches for predictive modeling in prostate cancer. Expert Syst. Appl. **70**, 1–19 (2017). https://doi.org/10.1016/j.eswa.2016.11.006

25. Carter, S.M., et al.: The ethical, legal and social implications of using artificial intelligence systems in breast cancer care. Breast **49**, 25–32 (2020). https://doi.org/10.1016/j.breast.2019.10.001

26. MarketsandMarkets: Artificial Intelligence in Healthcare Market by Offering. (Hardware, Software, Services), Technology (Machine Learning, NLP, Context-aware Computing, Computer Vision), Application, End User and Geography—Global Forecast to 2027 (2022). https://www.marketsandmarkets.com/Market-Reports/artificial-intelligence-healthcare-market-54679303.html. Accessed 15 Jan 2022

27. IP PRAGMATICS: Artificial Intelligence in the Life Sciences & Patent Analytics: Market Developments and Intellectual Property Landscape (2018)
28. Garbuio, M., Lin, N.: Artificial intelligence as a growth engine for health care startups: emerging business models. Calif. Manag. Rev. **61**(2), 59–83 (2019). https://doi.org/10.1177/000812561 8811931
29. Roland Berger: Artificial Intelligence—A Strategy for European Startups (2018)
30. Slevitch, L.: Qualitative and quantitative methodologies compared: ontological and epistemological perspectives. J. Qual. Assur. Hosp. Tour. (2011). https://doi.org/10.1080/1528008X. 2011.541810
31. Ringle, C.M., et al.: SmartPLS 3 (2015). Available online at http://www.smartpls.com. Accessed 20 March 2022
32. Durach, C.F., et al.: A new paradigm for systematic literature reviews in supply chain management. J. Supply Chain Manag. **53**(4), 67–85 (2017). https://doi.org/10.1111/jscm.12145
33. VHB e.V., VHB-JOURQUAL 3 (2019). https://vhbonline.org/vhb4you/vhb-jourqual/vhb-jou rqual-3. Accessed 20 March 2022
34. Computing Research & Education, CORE Rankings Portal (2016). https://www.core.edu.au/conference-portal. Accessed 20 March 2022
35. VHB e.V., Über den Verband (2019). https://vhbonline.org/ueber-uns. Accessed 20 March 2022
36. Sarstedt, M., et al.: Partial least squares structural equation modeling. In: Homburg, C. et al. (ed.) Handbook of Market Research. Springer, Cham (2017), pp 1–40. https://doi.org/10.1007/978-3-319-05542-8_15-1
37. Chin, W.W.: How to write up and report PLS analyses. In: Esposito Vinzi, V. et al. (ed.) Handbook of Partial Least Squares. Springer, Berlin, Heidelberg (2010), pp. 655–690. https://doi.org/10.1007/978-3-540-32827-8_29
38. Henseler, J., et al.: Partial least squares path modeling: updated guidelines. In Latan, H., Noonan, R. (eds.) Partial Least Squares Path Modeling, pp. 19–39. Springer, Cham (2017). https://doi.org/10.1007/978-3-319-64069-3_2
39. Hoppe, N.: Benefits of artificial intelligence in healthcare—a systematic literature review (2021). http://www.kmu-aalen.de/kmu-aalen/forschung/publikationen/. Accessed 19 March 2022
40. Krämer, J., et al.: Classification of hospital admissions into emergency and elective care: a machine learning approach. Health Care Manag. Sci. **22**(1), 85–105 (2019). https://doi.org/10.1007/s10729-017-9423-5
41. Turgeman, L., et al.: Insights from a machine learning model for predicting the hospital length of stay (LOS) at the time of admission. Expert Syst. Appl. **78**, 376–385 (2017). https://doi.org/10.1016/j.eswa.2017.02.023
42. Doraiswamy, P.M., et al.: Artificial intelligence and the future of psychiatry: Insights from a global physician survey. Artif. Intell. Med. **102**, 101753 (2020). https://doi.org/10.1016/j.artmed.2019.101753
43. Onukwugha, E., et al.: Cost prediction using a survival grouping algorithm: an application to incident prostate cancer cases. Pharmacoeconomics **34**(2), 207–216 (2016). https://doi.org/10.1007/s40273-015-0368-6
44. Thesmar, D., et al.: Combining the power of artificial intelligence with the richness of healthcare claims data: opportunities and challenges. Pharmacoeconomics **37**, 745–752 (2019). https://doi.org/10.1007/s40273-019-00777-6
45. Azzi, S., et al.: Healthcare applications of artificial intelligence and analytics: a review and proposed framework. Appl. Sci. **10**(18), 6553 (2020). https://doi.org/10.3390/app10186553
46. Kaplan, A., Haenlein, M.: Rulers of the world, unite! The challenges and opportunities of artificial intelligence. Bus. Horiz. **63**(1), 37–50 (2020). https://doi.org/10.1016/j.bushor.2019.09.003
47. Bostrom, N.: Superintelligence. Oxford University Press, Oxford, England (2014)
48. Pee, L.G., et al.: Artificial intelligence in healthcare robots: a social informatics study of knowledge embodiment. JASIST **70**(4), 351–369 (2019). https://doi.org/10.1002/asi.24145

49. Fan, W., et al.: Investigating the impacting factors for the healthcare professionals to adopt artificial intelligence-based medical diagnosis support system (AIMDSS). Ann. Oper. Res. **294**, 567–592 (2020). https://doi.org/10.1007/s10479-018-2818-y
50. Yuan, K.-C., et al.: The development an artificial intelligence algorithm for early sepsis diagnosis in the intensive care unit. Int. J. Med. Inform. **141**, 104176 (2020). https://doi.org/10.1016/j.ijmedinf.2020.104176
51. Shin, C., et al.: Autonomous tissue manipulation via surgical robot using learning based model predictive control. In: 2019 International Conference on Robotics, pp. 3875–3881 (2019). https://doi.org/10.1109/ICRA.2019.8794159
52. Kalis, B., et al.: 10 promising AI applications in health care. Harv. Bus. Rev. REPRINT H04BM0, 1–5 (2018)
53. Schinkel, M., et al.: Clinical applications of artificial intelligence in sepsis: a narrative review. Comput. Biol. Med. **115**, 103488 (2019). https://doi.org/10.1016/j.compbiomed.2019.103488
54. Vemulapalli, V., et al.: Non-obvious correlations to disease management unraveled by Bayesian artificial intelligence analyses of CMS data. Artif. Intell. Med. **74**, 1–8 (2016). https://doi.org/10.1016/j.artmed.2016.11.001
55. Chan, H.C.S.: Advancing drug discovery via artificial intelligence. Trends Pharmacol. Sci. **40**(8), 592–604 (2019). https://doi.org/10.1016/j.tips.2019.06.004
56. Davenport, T.H., Ronanki, R.: Artificial intelligence for the real world. Don't start with moon shots. Harv. Bus. Rev. 1–10 (2018)
57. Dezső, Z., Ceccarelli, M.: Machine learning prediction of oncology drug targets based on protein and network properties. BMC Bioinform. **21**, 104 (2020). https://doi.org/10.1186/s12859-020-3442-9
58. LimeSurvey: Turn questions into answers. (2021). https://www.limesurvey.org/. Accessed 20 March 2022
59. Wong, K.K.-K.: Partial least squares structural equation modeling (PLS-SEM) techniques using SmartPLS. Market. Bull. (24, Technical Note 1), 1–32 (2013)
60. Kose, U., et al.: Deep Learning for Medical Decision Support Systems. Springer Singapore, Singapore (2021). https://doi.org/10.1007/978-981-15-6325-6
61. Chowdhary, K.R. (ed.): Fundamentals of Artificial Intelligence. Springer India, New Delhi (2020). https://doi.org/10.1007/978-81-322-3972-7
62. European Commission: Commission Recommendation of 6 May 2003 Concerning the Definition of Micro, Small and Medium-Sized Enterprises. L 124/36 (2003)
63. Chin, W.W.: The partial least squares approach for structural equation modeling. In: Marcoulides, G.A. (ed.) Modern Methods for Business Research (Quantitative Methodology Series), pp. 295–336. Psychology Press, New York, NY (1998)
64. Schuberth, F., Cantaluppi, G.: Ordinal consistent partial least squares. In: Latan, H., Noonan, R. (eds.) Partial Least Squares Path Modeling, pp. 109–150. Springer, Cham (2017). https://doi.org/10.1007/978-3-319-64069-3_6
65. Chin, W.W.: Issues and opinion on structural equation modeling. MIS Q. vii–xvi (1998)
66. Center for Systems Science and Engineering (CSSE): Johns Hopkins University (JHU), COVID-19 Dashboard (2022). https://gisanddata.maps.arcgis.com/apps/opsdashboard/index.html#/bda7594740fd40299423467b48e9ecf6. Accessed 19 March 2022
67. Keding, C.: Understanding the interplay of artificial intelligence and strategic management: four decades of research in review. Manag. Rev. Q. **71**, 91–134 (2020). https://doi.org/10.1007/s11301-020-00181-x
68. Astromskė, K., et al.: Ethical and legal challenges of informed consent applying artificial intelligence in medical diagnostic consultations. AI Soc. **36**, 509–520 (2021). https://doi.org/10.1007/s00146-020-01008-9
69. Rai, A.: Explainable AI: from black box to glass box. J. Acad. Mark. Sci. **48**(1), 137–141 (2020). https://doi.org/10.1007/s11747-019-00710-5
70. Schiff, D., Borenstein, J.: How should clinicians communicate with patients about the roles of artificially intelligent team members? AMA J. Ethics **21**(2), E138-145 (2019). https://doi.org/10.1001/amajethics.2019.138

71. Kraus, S., et al.: Digital transformation in healthcare: analyzing the current state-of-research. J. Bus. Res. **123**, 557–567 (2021). https://doi.org/10.1016/j.jbusres.2020.10.030
72. Reim, W., et al.: Implementation of artificial intelligence (AI): a roadmap for business model innovation. AI **1**(2), 180–191 (2020). https://doi.org/10.3390/ai1020011
73. Lee, J., et al.: Emerging technology and business model innovation: the case of artificial intelligence. JOItmC **5**(3), 44 (2019). https://doi.org/10.3390/joitmc5030044
74. Gombolay, M., et al.: Robotic assistance in the coordination of patient care. Int. J. Robot. Res. **37**(10), 1300–1316 (2018). https://doi.org/10.1177/0278364918778344
75. Laï, M.-C., et al.: Perceptions of artificial intelligence in healthcare: findings from a qualitative survey study among actors in France. J. Transl. Med. **18**(1), 14 (2020). https://doi.org/10.1186/s12967-019-02204-y
76. Brox, J.: Brilliant: The Evolution of Artificial Light. Houghton Mifflin Harcourt, Boston (2010). ISBN: 978-0-547-48715-1

Chapter 10
Barriers of Artificial Intelligence in the Health Sector

Laura Beltempo, Jasmin Zerrer, Ralf-Christian Härting, and Nathalie Hoppe

Abstract Demographic change, shortage of qualified employees and increasing cost pressure—the healthcare sector has to deal with various challenges. Coping with the current COVID-19 pandemic is an additional issue. All these barriers contribute to the fact that digitalization in the healthcare sector is moving forward more and more. Without the application of advanced technologies, healthcare organizations would reach their limits. In this context, the use of AI is becoming increasingly important. The potentials are wide-ranging and include applications in diagnostics and therapy, as well as the development of pharmaceuticals. But what challenges are associated with the use of AI in healthcare? Within the framework of a qualitative empirical study according to Mayring, this question has been investigated. Based on a systematic literature review, the following barriers of AI in healthcare have been identified and examined: Disagreement in data protection, lack of compatibility with ethical aspects, quality of training data, knowledge, and trust of physicians in AI-supported systems. The next step in the research design have been expert interviews among medical staff as well as AI developers with focus on AI in the healthcare sector mainly in Germany. According to these interviews, the data are analyzed and evaluated. Based on the results of the study, potential activities have been derived in order to be able to successfully overcome the barriers of AI in the healthcare sector in the future. Finally, the opinions of physicians and developers on the identified barriers are compared and discussed.

L. Beltempo · J. Zerrer · R.-C. Härting (✉) · N. Hoppe
Aalen University of Applied Sciences, Aalen, Germany
e-mail: ralf.haerting@hs-aalen.de

L. Beltempo
e-mail: laura.beltempo@kmu-aalen.de

J. Zerrer
e-mail: jasmin.zerrer@kmu-aalen.de

N. Hoppe
e-mail: nathalie_vanessa.hoppe@kmu-aalen.de

© The Author(s), under exclusive license to Springer Nature Switzerland AG 2023
C. P. Lim et al. (eds.), *Artificial Intelligence and Machine Learning for Healthcare*,
Intelligent Systems Reference Library 229,
https://doi.org/10.1007/978-3-031-11170-9_10

Keywords Artificial intelligence · AI · Healthcare · Barriers · Digitalization ·
Trust · Data privacy · Expert interviews · Systematic literature review · Qualitative
study

10.1   Introduction

Digitalization became one of the most important economic topics of the future [1]. Big
Data technologies have the potential to process large amounts of data from different
origins and various source structures with high speed [2]. This capability is also
used by artificial intelligence systems to generate far-reaching changes in treatment
methods [3]. Machine Learning, Deep Learning, Natural Language Processing, Big
Data Analytics, and a lot more, are terms that are summarized as artificial intelligence
(AI). But what exactly is meant by the term AI? Since there is currently no general
accepted definition, AI can be defined as an empirical discipline of computer science
that explores the mechanisms of intelligent human behavior [4]. With the help of
computer program simulations, algorithms are programmed that resemble the functionality of a human brain. In this way, artificial neurons are used to form networks
that enable machine learning. The two main requirements that an AI system must
fulfill are the ability to learn and the ability to deal with uncertainty and probabilities
[2].

In order to strengthen Germany's position in the development, research and application of AI in international competitions, the German government adopted the
"Artificial Intelligence" strategy in November 2018. The goal is to promote the
trademark "AI Made in Europe" to further establish and expand responsible and
public welfare-oriented application and development of AI systems in Germany and
Europe. The funding is aimed to advance the application areas of AI in all parts of
society, including medicine [5].

Automating human or manual decision-making behaviors using AI makes it
possible to improve patient care while reducing costs and long waiting times. In
some medical fields, AI is even better than humans. Currently, the most prominent
field of application of AI-based technologies is radiology, followed by oncology
and pathology [6]. However, despite many opportunities, the use of AI also creates
some hurdles. Besides trust and privacy issues, ethics is a controversial subject,
especially autonomous decision-making [7]. Particularly in times of COVID-19, the
need for immediate ethical consideration of medical actions become the focus of
current debates [8]. The main ethical implications are negative consequences, such
as damaging things or, in the worst case, harming people. Since an algorithm is not
a legal entity, the question of who can be liable for an AI-based failure in general
needs to be clarified [7]. Unfortunately, so far, there are no specific liability rules for
any damage resulting from AI application. Therefore, human and machine actions
must not be directly equated [9].

Digitalization and the use of AI in healthcare is an inevitable process that many
people cannot fully grasp and appreciate [7]. Therefore, this study uses a qualitative

research approach to explore the impact of AI, focusing on barriers in the healthcare sector.

10.2   Empirical Investigation

This section describes the applied strategy step by step and presents the results of the systematic literature review. The literature-based hypotheses build the foundation for the data collection using expert interviews. The process of data collection and the data analysis are also explained in detail.

10.2.1   Research Design

The empirical investigation is based on a qualitative research design. Due to the fact that the research subject is very current and that there is plenty of literature on the topic, a deductive-inductive method according to Philipp Mayring was used.

Figure 10.1 provides an overview of the applied research design. The aim of the research is to investigate the barriers of AI in the health sector. For this purpose, a systematic literature review was conducted in the first step. Several challenges were identified, which were subsequently formulated as a hypothesis. In order to substantiate the generated hypotheses, semi-structured expert interviews have been con ducted for the data collection. Afterwards, the interviews were transcribed and coded with the software MAXQDA. The results from the analysis of the interviews are interpreted together with the findings from the literature research and finally lead to answer the research question. The original hypotheses were extended by new hypotheses, which resulted from the analysis of the interviews. Based on that, a conceptual model was developed, which can be used as a basis for a quantitative research work in the future.

The individual steps of the empirical investigation are described more detailed in the following sections.

10.2.2   Systematic Literature Review and Generation of Hypotheses

The development of a hypothesis framework provides the basis for a deductive investigation according to Mayring, with the aim of answering the research question. For the literature review, the following databases were accessed: ScienceDirect, Google Scholar, Springer and IEEE Xplore. Because the topic AI in healthcare is a current

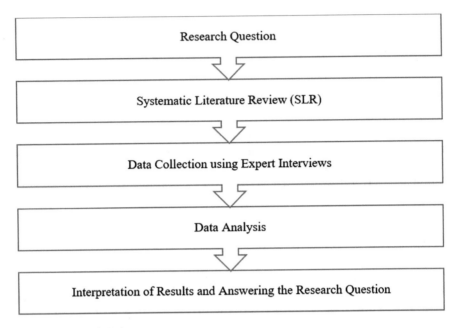

Fig. 10.1 Research design

issue, the selection of journals focused on the most recent ones available. In addition, only journals with a rating of A and B were used to ensure a good quality of the articles. The two ranking portals CORE Rankings Portal [10] and VHB-Jourqual3 [11] were used to check and evaluate the scientific quality. The following section presents the results of the SLR and the hypotheses that were derived based on these findings. A total of six hypotheses were formulated in order to identify barriers for the application of AI in healthcare.

Quinn et al. (*in 2021*) mention that the recommendations and actions of AI systems cannot be explained for proprietary or technical reasons. In this context, the "Black Box" phenomenon is often discussed. The lack of transparency can diminish autonomy and affect trust in the recommendations of an AI mechanism [12].

Cheng et al. (*in 2021*) describe explainability and interpretability as a key for transparent AI algorithms. They distinguish between local and global transparency. While local transparency focuses on explaining decisions in a specific context, global transparency aims to understand the entire AI System. At the same time, total transparency can also create potential risks. For example, disclosing additional data and information can make AI more vulnerable to hacker attacks. Therefore, a balance needs to be found between necessary transparency and the associated risks [13]. As a lack of transparency is assumed to influence the use of AI in healthcare, the following hypothesis is derived:

H1: Lack of transparency impairs the use of AI.

Kokciyan et al. (*in 2021*) describe that the misbehavior of AI technologies is not always clear or statistically detectable. For this reason, regulatory structures are needed to constrain these behaviors without compromising autonomy [14]. The focus is placed on decision algorithms such as classification or evaluation to minimize undesired misbehavior and to achieve fairness. Another cause emerges as a result of failures in measuring algorithm performance. When scientists present their research results, they usually argue that algorithms have a certain level of accuracy. However, this assumption depends on whether the training and testing samples are representative of the target group and whether their distributions are similar enough. In practice, it has been demonstrated that the learned AI algorithm achieves zero training bias for unrepresentative samples in the beginning phase. Due to the fact that new added data increases the probability of AI-misbehavior [13], the following hypothesis is generated:

H2: Misbehavior of systems complicates the use of AI.

Khullar et al. (*in 2021*) focus their study on the issue of liability when using AI in healthcare. This includes the question of who should be responsible for medical failures resulting from joint treatment between physicians and algorithms. In their study, they concluded that the public is significantly inclined to believe that physicians should be liable. However, physicians believe that healthcare providers and organizations should be responsible for AI-related medical failures. Because the use of AI in healthcare is new, there is currently not much established jurisprudence on how liability issues should be decided. So far, it is also unclear how these issues will be resolved in the future, because no major cases involving the use of AI in medicine have been decided by the courts. It is imaginable that physicians will take responsibility in situations where AI is recommended, instead of the machine or its AI algorithm. In addition, the liability issue may depend on who developed the used algorithm. If a physician uses an AI system developed by their own healthcare organization, the organization may be assigned a higher liability risk due to "Enterprise liability." In this case, hospitals and medical groups are blamed for failures rather than individual physicians [15]. This leads to the following hypothesis:

H3: Liability issues complicate the use of AI.

Bartoletti et al. (*in 2019*) mention data privacy as a challenging factor for the use of AI in healthcare. In this study on ethical and data protection aspects, it was clearly shown that data protection laws are a hurdle to achieving medical innovations. Privacy is tied to cultural norms and evolves over time. Therefore, it is also conceivable that data protection will change along with technological progress. However, this is always dependent on the respective country and generation. Data can also be quickly misused by hackers and thus increase distrust in the release of data to collection points. In addition, many people are insecure about the lack of transparency in data protection. This is because data protection notices are often too long and incomprehensible to the layperson. When it comes to health data, this is the most private information a person has, so there must be a high level of trust. On the one hand, health data is very sensitive and requires special protection. On the other hand, the use of such data in a research context can improve health conditions enormously. Therefore, finding a good balance is a major challenge, especially in the development of AI algorithms in healthcare [16]. Due to the challenging factors on data privacy, the following hypothesis is generated:

H4: Uncertainty in data privacy hampers the use of AI.

Straw (*in 2020*) describes that bias in health care can lead to data-driven, algorithmic, and human errors. Prejudices in AI data can bring terrible consequences in healthcare. This can put certain groups of people at a disadvantage when it comes to medical care. The reason for this usually lies in deep-rooted inequalities between ethnicities and genders, which are now reflected in the underrepresented datasets. Accordingly, AI systems can reinforce discrimination based on the trained dataset. Therefore, the challenge of choosing the right dataset should be countered by using standardized training specifications and continuous development of datasets. However, there is still a risk that unconscious bias may appear in the data, putting certain groups of people at a disadvantage through the use of AI [17, 18]. This leads to the following hypothesis:

H5: Discrimination has a negative impact on the use of AI.

Boddington et al. (*in 2017*) focus their study on answering ethical questions in relation to AI. In society, artificial intelligence can scare people through various levels of unpredictability. This lack of knowledge about the degree of autonomy of systems makes the public skeptical and distrustful. Machines are often ascribed the same kind of autonomy as humans and consequently there is concern about how to control them [19]. Today, AI systems are used in hospitals, law enforcement, and other sensitive areas. Therefore, it is highly desirable that AI behaves correctly in these areas. Doctors, therefore, do not find it easy to rely on AI systems and perhaps transfer their decision-making authority to the machine in the future. In most cases, physicians are not properly informed about how such an AI algorithm works and about its strengths and weaknesses. The lack of knowledge among physicians leads to a negative attitude toward the use of AI systems [20]. Due to the misunderstanding in society that AI is at risk of taking over the world the following hypothesis was formulated:

H6: Decision-making authority impairs the use of AI.

10.2.3 Data Collection

The data collection includes sixteen semi-structured interviews with nine physicians, who have experience with AI in the healthcare sector, as well as seven AI-researchers and AI-developers. The interviews were conducted between December 2021 and February 2022 and the main focus has been on the German healthcare sector. Only one expert was from Austria. Participants from different functional areas were interviewed to gain a broad understanding of the situation and minimize individual bias.

Table 10.1 Interviewee overview

Number	Gender	Professional field	Position
1	Female	Surgery	Senior dental radiologist
2	Male	Cardiology	Specialist for cardiac surgery
3	Male	Radiology	Radiologist
4	Male	Researcher	Manager digital health & innovation
5	Male	Researcher/developer	Research assistant/Ph.D. student
6	Male	Radiology	Radiologist
7	Female	Researcher/developer	Senior AI and FEM Expert
8	Male	Researcher	Research group leader
9	Female	Surgery	Dentist
10	Male	Researcher/developer	Research group leader
11	Male	Researcher/developer	Developer and project manager
12	Male	Researcher/developer	Research assistant
13	Male	Surgery	Hand surgeon
14	Male	Radiology	Radiologist
15	Male	Radiology	Radiologist
16	Male	Internal medicine	Doctor, program director telemedicine, E-health and artificial intelligence

The interviewees in this study are between 25 and 64 years old and have an average of 8.3 years of experience with AI in healthcare, so a high level of expertise in this research topic is assumed. Table 10.1 gives an overview about all participants.

The questionnaire was created based on the hypothesis model and includes eighteen questions. The questionnaire consists of six parts. Part A includes socio-demographic questions, such as age, gender, or academic background. Part B includes questions about the experience with AI in the healthcare sector and part C to F contain one or two questions about each hypothesis. The questionnaire was distributed a few days before the interview, so that the experts had the opportunity to prepare the topics. The interviews were conducted and digitally recorded via the platform Zoom with a duration of 30–60 min. Afterwards, the answers were transcribed in the original German language, coded, and subsequently analyzed. The results are presented in detail within Sect. 10.3.

After the preparation of the questionnaire, a pre-test was carried out together with a physician in order to check the comprehensibility of the questions and to eliminate overlaps in content.

10.3   Results

This section presents the results of the expert interviews. First, the process of data analysis is presented. Then the conceptual model is introduced by the results from the expert interviews, followed by the derived hypotheses.

10.3.1   Data Analysis

After the semi-structured interviews were completely transcribed, the data analysis process started. The data was analyzed by using the Philipp Mayring coding guideline. For this process, the software MAXQDA was used. In the first step, individual categories were created by generating inductive and deductive codes. The inductive codes consist of keywords that can be derived from the structured literature research and were searched in the interviews. Deductive codes emerged from the analysis of the interviews and were generated for topics that were mentioned by many experts. At the end, a combination of inductive and deductive codes was formed. The individual categories were substantiated during the analysis with the help of anchor examples, so that the assignment of codes was transparent and comprehensible.

In this way, subcategories of related categories could be formed in the next step. For example, the codes "Black Box", "Misbehavior/wrong decisions" and "Lack of Empathy" build the third-order category, which is combined into the second-order category "Trust of Physicians". The second order categories are divided into "Data Privacy", "Ethical Principles", "Knowledge of Physicians", "Training Data" and "Trust". In this study, the core category represents the barriers of AI in the health sector.

A total of 623 codes were generated from all 16 interviews. These were subcategorized and grouped into 22 categories. To decide which of the codes would ultimately be included in the conceptual model, it was determined which codes were most frequently addressed by the experts. The remaining codes were not included in the analysis because they were only mentioned by a few experts. In this way, it was possible to identify the most important aspects that have a negative influence on AI in healthcare.

10.3.2   Empirical Findings and Model Conceptualization

To understand the method, a conceptual model was developed, which is presented in Fig. 10.2. It is based on the coded expert interviews and the previous SLR. A total of five main hypotheses and seventeen sub-hypotheses were identified, which were explained in detail in the following.

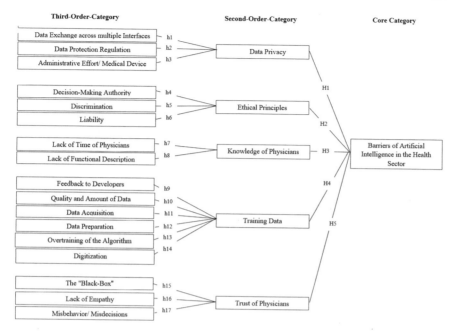

Fig. 10.2 Conceptual model

10.3.2.1 Data Privacy

To minimize the risk of hacking, hospitals avoid exchanging data between multiple interfaces. Each hospital has its own data center that is completely isolated from the outside. Because of sensitive data in medicine, the IT security level is very high. Therefore, the use of medical data is associated with a lot of effort for AI developers. To guarantee a secure transmission of the data, the encryption and anonymization of the data is essential. In this context, the permission of the patients is required for the use of data in the research framework.

[…] Clearly, if data is exchanged with other university hospitals via interfaces or even uploaded to some cloud, there is a huge risk. […]

On the one hand, IT security is a hurdle, because data collection is made more difficult. On the other hand, personal data are particularly worth protecting.

[…] In other words, this is not something that is thought up for fun; it is about handling data sensibly. And that is why it is good that something like this exists. And it has to be balanced somehow. […]

In Germany, there are doubts about data being exchanged between interfaces. In other countries, this is seen as an opportunity to provide better and faster medical care in emergencies. Therefore, data transfer between hospitals should be made possible in general. The framework of encryption and anonymization of the data must be observed at all costs. Sometimes it can be difficult to anonymize data when they are needed from a specific application area, e.g., from the head area. It should not be possible to draw conclusions about individuals.

[...] But I think if the data is all anonymized and encrypted, it should actually already be possible to transfer it with a relatively high level of security. [...]

h1: Data exchange across multiple interfaces has a significant impact on data privacy.

The data in Germany must be processed in a DSGVO-compliant manner. Patients and participants in studies should be informed immediately about what happens to their data and that the data can be withdrawn at any time. This should be followed without exception in order to avoid uncertainties and complications with data protection. A way should be found that supports the publication of knowledge and not the privatization of knowledge or algorithms.

[...] A European path that is linked to the data protection regulation. I think this is really important, even if it's tiresome, even if it slows down. [...]

For many researchers and developers, the effort to follow the requirements of the DSGVO and other ethics committees is too high. Therefore, they have less motivation to research AI-innovations in connection with patients. To sum it up, data protection is a major barrier to the use of AI because developers don't get enough data. In addition, ethics committees are becoming stricter, leading to even higher hurdles for physicians in acquiring data.

[...] Sorry, but I don't feel like doing that. It's probably incredibly difficult to find a balance between the need for data and the need to protect data. [...]

Compared to other countries, such as the USA, Germany is already lagging in terms of data collection and computing power. It can be seen as a risk but also as an opportunity to say that if we can't centralize the data, then we can develop methods to achieve good quality without centralizing the data. This would be a locational advantage, to build AI in Europe that is compliant with data protection. The reason why other countries are more advanced in AI development is because of less regulation in terms of data protection, less complicated paperwork, and more freedoms. This leads to the risk that qualified specialists will prefer to deploy their expertise abroad. However, the management of the Corona pandemic in Germany shows how damaging strict data protection laws are for an efficient IT infrastructure in healthcare. It can be concluded that if Germany fails to catch up with other countries by adapting the data protection regulation, the country runs the risk of buying expensive AI algorithms from abroad instead of selling themselves.

[...] We are good at basic AI research, but we are losing a lot of ground in developing products because it is really difficult in Germany at the moment. [...]

Another problem is that politicians in Germany are making demands that contradict each other. They would prefer all data to be centrally available and visible to every-one, but totally privacy-compliant and totally private. These goals are not easy to combine. In addition, the German healthcare system is one of the most complex in the world. Because of this great interaction between and against each other of the most diverse institutions, it is extremely inhibiting to innovation. This does not just affect AI; it affects the entire digitalization and innovation readiness in healthcare. In this context, the difficult structures but also the convenience of doctors, who do not want to change anything in their paper documentation, are major inhibiting factors.

[...] And that is also the biggest barrier, that this structure of the health care system is reorganized a bit, so that it becomes a bit more fluid. [...]

h2: Data protection regulation has a significant impact on data privacy.

Practically, AI systems have a supportive role in medical treatments. Therefore, there is an increasing development towards structured reporting, especially in radiology. Currently, AI is implemented to support faster decision-making and minimize risks. Physicians report that this makes their daily work easier.

[...] To facilitate administrative activities, so that time is again made possible for the encounters between people, doctors, and patients on both sides. [...]

You need standardized data to train an AI. The problem is that the documentation must be personalized. So, standards are actually not correct from a legal point of view.

h3: Administrative effort has a significant impact on data privacy.

In summary, it was found that physicians and developers see a major hurdle to the use of AI in data privacy laws. Compared to other countries, the many administrative requirements imposed by ethics committees and approval applications slow down technological progress in healthcare.

H1: Uncertainty in data privacy hampers the use of AI.

10.3.2.2   Ethical Principles

Doctors can quickly be offended in their position as physicians if you want to replace their work with AI. However, this often depends on the gender, age, area of application and perception of the person. In this context, today's AI systems are purely for support, and they are an aid to decision-making. Nevertheless, there is a high level of skepticism on the part of physicians about the replacement of medical decisions through AI systems. However, some experts have the opinion that these concerns will become less pronounced in the future or will be ignored. Interviewee 4 mentioned in this regard:

[...] The question is merely how quickly and to what extent will certain physicians and areas of application be replaced. Perhaps not 100 percent, but I can very well imagine that in the medium to long term a 90 percent replacement rate could prevail. [...]

The majority of respondents believe that complete replacement by AI will never be possible. Medicine is too complex and multi-layered for that. There are always special cases. In addition, talking to patients is an important part of medical treatment. There are ethical questions that cannot be taken over by artificial intelligence. The living is just one example where the human being must make the decision.

[...] And in the end, it is always very important that the human factor does not disappear completely, because computers can calculate well and calculate quickly, but they can't replace the human factor. [...]

On the other hand, standardized treatment decisions can be replaced by AI soon. Ultimately, this transfer tends to give doctors more time for each patient rather than replacing them. It is also possible that staff will be eliminated by assistance systems, thereby somewhat countering the shortage of personnel in the healthcare sector. This always depends on the situation and the area of application. For example, radiology with its imaging processes is already very advanced with the use of AI. Interviewee 6 explained:

[…] So we do individual CT examinations in radiology today. We have 3000 images for one examination. And that is of course time-consuming to look at. People are not always one hundred percent concentrated. We get tired, and of course these systems can help us. […]

In the end, doctors will see AI systems as an aid, but they would never allow them to replace them. Interviewee 1 said the following statement:

[…] We have different roles and different stakeholders. And I don't think they're going to be able to replace that because we're probably not going to allow it to happen in the first place, which is to be replaceable. After all, we want to be loved. […]

In summary, taking over medical decisions is going to take a long time, if AI ever catches on. This will be difficult, as the use of AI is contrary to the preservation instinct of physicians. However, it is to be expected, that in the future the demographic change and the shortage of staff will continue to come to a head and at some point, there will be no other option for the widespread use of AI systems in healthcare.

h4: Decision-making authority has a significant impact on ethical principles.

When AI is used, certain groups of people may be favored. This is not intentional but happens unintentionally and depends on the data set used. Researchers often exercise a training set in good faith and do not detect bias that may occur. If the data set contains more information about men than about women, the AI will work well with men and worse with women. To prevent this, attention must be paid to the quality of the data. If it is a specific disease, then discrimination would make sense. There is a chronic disease that is more prevalent in dark-skinned people. If the disease is detected early, deadly consequences can be prevented. That means, in this case, you want a discriminatory model that is specifically positive for dark-skinned people. In healthcare, AI applications must pass a high study setting before they are allowed to use. The bottom line is that it must be defined in advance where and for which group of people the system is to be used. From this point of view, data should be categorized so that a qualitative evaluation in medicine is possible.

[…] AI systems show discriminatory behavior, but they are not proactive agents. It is a tool. It is not an autonomous system in its own right. […]

Often, incorrect data sets are discovered only when the AI is used. Then it is important to report the mistakes to a central location and to reprogram the AI. The patient makes a contract with the doctor. Therefore, the doctor will always remain responsible for his actions. In this context, physicians need to be informed about the training data so that they do not exceed the target group. In addition, AI can be used for social scoring systems, especially in other countries. Social scoring would be used to decide whether a person is preferred for medical treatment or not. That would be very discriminatory and could be abused by AI.

[…] And that just shows that there is definitely, […], a big risk of discrimination. Also, scientifically, so not only social discrimination. […]

On the one hand, AI is more objective and neutralizes certain prejudices that people can have. On the other hand, AI generates a new form of discrimination that is not caused by emotions, but by errors in the input of basic data. Often this happens un-consciously and should be closely examined by ethics committees before AI is introduced in healthcare.

h5: Discrimination has a significant impact on ethical principles.

Experts have different opinions on the liability situation regarding AI. Who is liable in the context of damage caused by faulty measurement of AI? Five interviewees can imagine that the developer can also be held liable in the future. If AI should make decisions on its own at some point and a guarantee for safe results is given by the developer, he will be liable. If no guarantee is given, the hospital must expect possible errors and learn to deal with them. In general, it is also fact that developers or the company are always responsible for a defect in the product.

[…] And that would also be difficult in the development of such products if the user were then held liable, for a product problem. […]

Other 7 interviewees see the liability rather with the physicians. If the medical device is not defective, the user is responsible. In the case of assistance systems, it is difficult not to hold the physician liable because the developer only offers a recommendation with the AI. In the end, the physician must make the final decision and is therefore responsible. The risk for medical technology manufacturers to spend a lot of money on liability cases is too high. That is why the companies will not be liable. From this point of view, the liability will probably remain with the physicians, because they are expected to check the results of the AI system with their expertise and then make a decision. The opinion of interviewee 1 was:

[…] The physician performing the action is the one who makes the decisions and the one who is liable for them. […]

Another option would be to have the liability run through insurance companies in the future. In principle, customers would then pay part of the insurance when they purchase the product, and this would be balanced out somehow. This is how malpractice is handled in hospitals. If it can be proven that the doctor was in fault, the hospital is liable for the doctor via an insurance policy.

[…] I could imagine that a hospital would then also be liable via *insurance for an error by the AI system. […]*

In addition, it is very important for the development of AI algorithms that the liability does not belong to the producers. Otherwise, no scientist would take the risk and develop an AI. To sum it up, an AI software ends up being a medical device and has to go through a very strict approval process. So, when the software comes onto the market, it can be considered that the quality is of a very high standard, especially in Europe. Since AI has no identity, it cannot be considered a legal entity. Therefore, the solution to the liability issue via insurance should be the closest.

h6: Liability has a significant impact on ethical principles.

To conclude, all mentioned aspects, decision-making authority, discrimination and liability issues complicate the use of AI in healthcare. This leads to the following hypothesis:

H2: Ethical principles hampers the use of AI.

10.3.2.3 Knowledge of Physicians

For doctors, lack of time is always present. That is why AI systems that make a pre-selection are a time-saving help. In this way, the workload can be minimized, and output can be increased at the same time. In addition, AI helps to make decisions faster and reduce errors in medical treatments.

[…] It was actually a great relief to have this kind of AI support, so that you didn't have to do the paperwork 20 times again but could check it off quickly with this kind of AI support. […]

The time problem also means that physicians don't even find the time to inform about AI and to implement AI systems in their practices. This is because they have to ensure patient care and are thereby focused on medical care. It is a dilemma because in the end, AI would save them time again. So, a big challenge is to even realize AI in the first place and then implement it despite the lack of time and complex insurance policies.

[…] but it, just makes life difficult for doctors because they have to decide between two things. But their main job is to care for patients, so that's the main hurdle. […]

h7: Lack of time of physicians has a significant impact on the knowledge of physicians.

There is the problem that we use AI systems in practice that have theoretical errors that we do not even know about. This means that if doctors use such an assistance system, it should only work in the background and provide suggestions. No decisions should be imposed on the physician. An experienced physician should still be able to estimate the results and determine the level of confidence. A broad knowledge transfer of AI will not take place due to time constraints. There is always an explanation of possible risks when using a device, but there is no time or desire for more in most cases. Nevertheless, doctors should be made aware of AI tools. It is important that developers communicate exactly what AI can and cannot do, so that doctors can interpret the results of AI correctly.

[…] I mean doctors specialize in a thousand things, have to learn so much, have such a hard job. I don't think they want to deal with the theory of deep learning. […]

For most physicians, AI is incomprehensible, especially if they are not familiar with machine learning. As an external user, decisions made by AI systems are difficult to understand. In this context, it would be useful to provide appropriate and easy-to-understand instructions for the use by the developer or via user manual. Depending on the requirements, instructions may not be sufficient in some cases. Therefore, good training by the developer and information about the risks should not be neglected in any case.

[…] I don't think you just have to specify that in a user manual, but you also have to clearly train the doctor. […]

h8: Lack of functional description has a significant impact on the knowledge of physicians.

Mainly, the time limitation and the recording capacity of physicians prevent the flow of knowledge about AI. In addition, in many cases, there is insufficient training on how to operate AI systems. Physicians should be made more aware of the benefits of AI implementation, and sensitization to the topic should be promoted.

H3: Lack of Knowledge of Physicians hampers the use of AI.

10.3.2.4   Training Data

AI is a learning system. In practice, learning ends at a certain point and the system is integrated into practice. However, learning is actually not completely finished, because the same learning data can be used again and improved if necessary. This continuous learning process is very important for an AI system to improve its quality in the long-term. The interaction between physicians and developers plays a major role in this process because developers and manufacturers depend on feedback from physicians so that they can optimize the algorithm. After all, the accuracy of the AI results must still be determined with a specialist in the end, and this determination can minimize undesirable misbehavior. It is also conceivable to develop a feedback system that directly informs the AI system of the failure. In this way, the algorithm in the AI system would be trained further by telling it:

[…] Hey, here is another example of a situation where there is actually no tumor. But you said there is one, just take a look at it again. Try to update your model again. Hoping that if the same picture or a similar picture comes in, this failure will not happen again. […]

The challenge is that once a system is approved, it can't be changed. In this case, the AI system would have to go through the approval process again due to the strict regulatory requirements, which involves a lot of time and effort.

h9: Feedback to developers has a significant impact on training data.

A large amount of data that has simultaneously a high quality is important for an effective and specific training of AI. This is the only way to ensure that AI algorithms are provided with one hundred percent quality to the users. Interviewee 6 mentions in this regard:

[…] one of the main problems is the lack of well-adopted datasets. We require them to train the AI systems, so that they all perform a super learning. We need large amounts of annotated, and qualitatively well-annotated datasets! […]

h10: Quality and amount of data has a significant impact on training data.

In medicine, a lot of data is generally available and well documented, but the challenge is to gain access to the data. Interviewee 1 commanded:

[…] My hurdle right now is getting data out of these thousands of x-rays from the hospital. So, I wish that we could get better access to research data. […]

Because we are dealing with sensitive patient data, it is usually stored on local servers in hospitals and doctors' offices. The data pool is highly protected, so it is not possible to simply pull out and merge the data needed to train the algorithm. Currently, there is no suitable tool in Germany to exchange and merge data, that is why interviewee 5 said:

[…] It would be a dream if there is a cloud or something like that, where all data is stored completely anonymized, with the same prerequisites as I just described. And that all research institutes would have access to the data, possibly also German companies, if they pay a bit of money for it. […]

h11: Data acquisition has a significant impact on training data.

Data need to be specially prepared for the training of AI, because they are not always structured in the same way. A typical example of this is marking a tumor in a CT scan. Some physicians mark the tumor with a cross, encircle it, or mark nothing. As every doctor has his or her own procedure, it is very time-consuming for the developer of an AI algorithm to prepare the dataset in such a way that it can be used for training. Interviewee 8 explains that:

[…] the heterogeneity of the data, i.e., how the data look, is another problem. You have to prepare it so that you can use them, for example for machine learning or other AI methods. […]

In most cases, a physician must be consulted to explain the data in detail to the developer. This is very time-consuming for both parties, so standardized documentation criteria in Germany can help to minimize the effort involved in data preparation.

h12: Data preparation has a significant impact on training data.

AI systems are trained with plenty of data before they are approved. During this process, it is important to ensure that the system is not overtrained. This means that a part of the available data must always keep aside, which will be used for the final validation. In this way, it is possible to check whether the AI only performs well based on training data or also based on validation data. If it comes to the realization at this point that there are certain misfitting during the training, it is probably an over fitting.

[…] If you have over-fitted the AI on training data, then you have to either increase the amount of data or just adjust the targeting of the data even more to match the target population. […]

Overtraining can also result because AI algorithms need to be adjusted and revised based on the feedback from the physicians. The training process is triggered again and, ideally, the algorithm learns this special case. However, a challenge is also, that retraining can lead to the AI forgetting what it has already learned. This means that whenever the AI system is extended, the complete validation process must be repeated to ensure that the AI can still do what it has already learned. This means it must be guaranteed by the developer that the algorithm is at least as good as before, so that no undesirable overtraining effects occur.

h13: Overtraining of the algorithm has a significant impact on training data.

Digitization plays a major role for the application of AI, because only where digitization is well-advanced, AI can be applied. Compared to other countries, like China or the USA, Germany is far behind in the healthcare sector. The entire digital areas are comparatively weak in the German healthcare system. Interviewee 10 mentions the Corona pandemic as an example for this:

[…] that fax machines are still used in Germany today, even in clinics or in administration. This is a shame. We are lagging in terms of digitization in general. The processes should be digital with reasonable interfaces that reach the target quickly […]

The complication that emerges especially for developers is that it is hard for them to get the data they need for the AI training. This is because one physician stores the data online, while another physician still writes the reports with a pen and a paper. To successfully integrate AI into the German healthcare system, according to interviewee 7.

[…] Germany really first requires the data as a digital document. That is the biggest hurdle. […]

h14: Digitization has a significant impact on training data.

AI systems are only as good as the training data they have used to learn specific functions. Raw data or test data are crucial to ensure that the system knows exactly what it is supposed to find during the application. If only an insufficient, perhaps unrepresentative, selection of training data is used, there is a risk that maybe wrong diagnoses may occur.

[…] Very important is that you have to know what kind of goal you have with AI, because if you do not define this goal exactly, then you are off the track! […]

Therefore, the developers of AI algorithms must pay close attention during training to guarantee that the system is trained on the correct data, which are relevant to the topic. The experience and expertise that a developer contributes also plays a major role, because not everyone can recognize patterns, for example in the field of imaging. If people with limited knowledge are hired in advance for AI training, the probability is high that the programmed algorithm will have weaknesses in the end.

H4: Training Data has a significant influence on AI.

10.3.2.5 Trust of Physicians

The term "Black Box" is a big problem for users, as described earlier in the SLR. For the experts, the challenge is to understand where the AI results come from. Only if the physician was directly involved in the technical development, there is a chance to understand the system better. Especially in the medical context, algorithms are comprehensible to the user from a certain perspective, or not at all. The lack of transparency naturally also has a negative impact on the trust of users. In the initial phase, every physician will only trust an AI system if it is possible to understand the decisions. Interviewee 3 has the following opinion:

[…] I think that it is still a issue, that people are very skeptical, also because the decisions or the results of the AI systems are often not completely comprehensible. And that creates a bit of a lack of trust. […]

To reduce this skepticism, the research area "Explainable AI" is currently working on making AI algorithms more transparent. For example, there are methods that are being used in the field of imaging. With some of these, an attempt is finally made to visualize which areas were relevant for the result and where the algorithm gained the most information. After all, when users trust in AI, patients' confidence will probably increase as well.

h15: The "Black Box" has a significant influence on the trust of physicians.

One challenge of using AI is the lack of empathy towards patients. This affects the trust of physicians, because they have to show empathy to their patients in certain situations. AI will probably never be able to replace empathy from a doctor. Interviewee 6 comments on this aspect:

[...] I do not think that AI will be able to replace the doctor or other medical professionals with all the humanity, with the attention as well as with the empathy. That is an important function. [...]

As an example, serves a patient with a malignant tumor. There is the possibility of an operation, which is not promising. In this case, the situation may arise that it is not useful or that the patient does not want the surgery. Since a human being is capable of empathy, it can better assess the situation. An AI would most probably try to save the patient's life, regardless of the patient's individual wishes. This contributes to the fact that a lack of empathy currently affects the confidence of users.

h16: Lack of empathy has a significant influence on the trust of physicians.

AI-based misbehavior or wrong decisions will probably always happen, the same way as human misbehavior exists. Because the current state of development in Germany is not yet advanced enough to use AI as an autonomously acting system in medicine, the term wrong decision is used more frequently. This is because misbehavior would imply that AI has a will of its own, which is currently not the case. Basically, it can be said that AI systems that make serious mistakes are not used in medicine at all. However, to give the physician more confidence and safety, the AI developer can indicate the probability that a mistake may occur. Then the users can decide for themselves whether it is acceptable to utilize the AI system or not. Interviewee 11 says:

[...] I don't want to go to a hospital where the algorithm might be able to detect a disease with 80 percent accuracy. That would be a disaster. That is why it is good that there is a regulatory framework for this. [...]

This means that trust in AI can be increased if the reliability of detection is more exactly defined.

[...] the good thing is that when a wrong decision is made, the algorithms are supposed to learn from it. In the context of technical development, it is something very good, this trial-and-error of learning AI systems [...]

Since AI is currently only used as a support system in Germany, a specialist always takes a final look at the AI results. In this way, the physician always has the final responsibility and can minimize possible errors.

h17: Misbehavior/ wrong decisions have a significant influence on the trust of physicians.

Humans are usually reluctant and skeptical towards new technologies at the beginning. But once they have been implemented for a period of time, they are accepted. Trust towards AI may not yet be completely established, for example, because physicians are afraid of being unconsciously influenced by AI. Interviewee 4 thinks:

[…] in reality, a person is influenced by these unconscious decision-making aids. And I think there is currently still a huge skepticism, if you directly confront someone as a medical professional. [...]

One way to eliminate skepticism and build more trust is to convince physicians, for example, through valid certifications and high-quality results and studies. Only in this way, AI can gradually build trust. But of course, trust can also be quickly destroyed if mistakes happen. Creating more transparency plays a crucial role in this regard, because the user will only trust such a system, especially in the initial phase, if it can understand the decision.

[…]What creates trust is when everything that happens is very transparent and the highest security standards are really maintained, so that there are no data scandals in this area. And people should be educated about what possibilities there are through the application of AI [...]

H5: Trust of physicians has a significant influence on AI.

10.4 Discussion

The barriers identified in this study are data privacy and ethical aspects such as the physicians' decision-making authority. In addition, it was figured out that the knowledge level of physicians has a significant impact on the use of AI in healthcare. Moreover, the quality and amount of training data as well as the trust of physicians turned out to be moderating factors. This study shows which influencing factors slow down the use and development of AI systems in healthcare. If this conceptual model will be considered, these issues can be targeted to drive forward the implementation of AI in Germany. One of the biggest barriers in this context is that Germany has stricter legislation and more requirements to meet than other countries. It is important to protect personal data, but there should be a balance between sharing data for research and data protection. Otherwise, the gap in technological progress will grow and may lead to a competitive disadvantage in the future. In addition, the influence of the various ethical aspects for the use of AI should be considered. A significant hurdle in decision-making authority is that the use of AI is contrary to the preservation instinct of physicians. It is to be expected, that in the future the demographic change and the shortage of medical staff will increase the need for AI in healthcare. Subsequently, attention must be directed to the selection of training data and the area of application to prevent discriminatory results of AI. In addition, uncertainty regarding the liability situation poses another challenge to the use of AI. Different opinions hold that in the case of AI errors, either the physicians, the developers or an insurance company is liable. The third option is most likely because the physician would not want to be liable for the use of a defective product and the developers would not take the risk of developing something for which they could be held liable. Therefore, impartial insurance companies are the best way to overcome this barrier. Moreover, the lack of knowledge of physicians about AI is an additional hurdle. This is mainly connected to the time limitation and the recording capacity of physicians. Nevertheless, physicians should receive extensive training before using AI systems and be made aware of potential risks. The topic of digitization and AI systems should be promoted more for physicians. Another influence on the research question is the quality and quantity of training data. In addition, the selected data must be relevant to the topic being researched. Therefore, people with good knowledge of AI systems are highly required. Otherwise, it could lead to weaknesses in the algorithm. The last major impact on the use of AI is the trust of physicians. To overcome physicians' skepticism and build more trust, it takes valid certifications and high-quality results and studies. More transparency also leads to greater acceptance and understanding for the decision of an AI. Even in the experience of errors, trust is not immediately lost if the AI is comprehensible to physicians.

Subsequently, the statements of the physicians and developers are contrasted and compared with each other. On the subject of data protection, a clear difference can be seen between the opinions of engineers and physicians. From the point of view of developers, data protection is a major hurdle. They also agree that data protection is holding back the development process and research into AI, particularly in Germany. Compared to the U.S., developers see a significant competitive disadvantage and fear that if regulations do not adapt, technology will have to be acquired from abroad in the future. The physicians' side mainly does not see the progress of AI threatened by data protection laws, since only anonymized data sets are used.

On the topic of decision-making authority, physicians and developers also differ in their opinions. On the one hand, the doctors see AI as a purely supportive activity whose task is to simplify the doctor's daily work. In addition, due to its lack of emotional and empathic capacity, AI does not have the potential to consider a treatment decision holistically and to place it in the overall context of the patient. In addition, doctors would never let technology get this far because they do not want to have the feeling of being replaceable. On the other hand, for some physicians it is conceivable that in the future AI will automate certain treatment decisions and the physician will merely act as confirmation of the measure. In individual cases, this could be feasible in the future, especially in the fields of radiology, pathology, and ophthalmology.

The ethical aspects also include discrimination. The majority of doctors agree with the hypothesis that discrimination has a negative impact on the use of AI. But there are also three participants who said that the AI system is only as discriminating as the data set on which the algorithms are based and trained. The developers are determined that AI, on the one hand, neutralizes certain prejudices that humans may have, on the other hand, new forms of discrimination can be generated. In general, discrimination already exists to some extent in the testing of drugs. These are often tested only on men. However, it is known that drugs frequently have a different effect on women. Discrimination in healthcare is therefore a general problem that should be combated.

Compared to the uncertainty in liability, the most doctors and developers think doctors are responsible when AI makes a wrong decision. The executing physician is the one who makes the decisions and the one who is liable for them. It would make the development of an AI much more difficult and not allow any further development if the one who offers the software is responsible for it. Because the claims for damages are so high that no manufacturer will take over. Therefore, it may be likely in the future that insurance companies will pay for such damage. Compared to the study mentioned in Sect. 10.2.2, the liability issue may also depend on who developed the used algorithm. In this case, hospitals and medical groups are blamed for failures rather than individual physicians.

On the subject of doctors' lack of knowledge and training data, the experts are agreed, regardless of whether they are doctors or developers. The time limitation and the recording capacity of physicians prevent the flow of knowledge about AI. In connection with insufficient training on how to operate these systems, this hampers the use of AI. Moreover, the continuous learning process is very important for an AI system to improve its quality in the long term. The interaction between the physician and the developer plays a major role, because the developers depend on feedback from the physicians so that they can optimize the algorithm. After all, the accuracy of the AI results must still be determined with a specialist in the end, and this determination can minimize undesirable misbehavior. It is also conceivable to develop a feedback system that directly informs the AI system of the error.

Regarding the last hypothesis about trust, the most physician's experts referred to AI as a black box. AI systems cannot be understood at the moment of decision because they are very complex. But, since they are based on algorithms, any decision can be decoded or unlocked in retrospect. Also, it's a support for the physicians, they always have a final look over it anyway. So, the physicians can understand decisions to a certain extent, but not always. If physicians were involved in the development and know how the algorithm is structured, then they can understand relatively well what it has done. In this context, physicians then also have more confidence in AI systems. In contrast, the developers are of the opinion that AI is a black box for the physician. AI is only used as a support and the doctors always have to look over it themselves. That is why it is not so bad if not everything is comprehensible for doctors. There is a field of research called "Explainable AI" that is trying to make AI algorithms a bit more comprehensible to increase the level of trust.

10.5 Limitations and Further Research

As a result of the qualitative study, expert interviews were used to investigate the barriers of AI in the healthcare sector. Five influencing factors were identified with their associated indicators, and possible coping strategies were presented. A conceptual model was created for a further quantitative research. Future research should quantitatively verify or refute the established hypotheses of this qualitative approach. The study provides added theoretical value by providing initial insights into a very current area of research in medicine.

It must be considered that this study has limitations. It focuses exclusively on the aspects mentioned in the qualitative expert interviews. The sample represents the knowledge of physicians, researchers, and developers. By interviewing a targeted group, the respective barriers in the individual medical fields can be addressed more precisely. Radiology appears to be well suited for this purpose, because AI is most advanced in the field of imaging.

A total of 16 experts were interviewed. This means that the sample size was higher than expected, which is why the validity of this study can be classified as good. Furthermore, the sample was relatively homogeneous. Out of the sixteen experts, four worked in radiology and seven have a background in research and/or development. Since 13 of the sample were male, an interview with female experts could therefore lead to discrepancies or possibly different results. Furthermore, a heterogeneous group should be interviewed to achieve higher validity and representativeness.

Additionally, it seems promising to conduct an international study, e.g., with physicians and AI developers from the U.S., to get a different perspective on the topic. During the interviews, it became obvious that many countries are already more advanced in the area of AI. It would also be interesting to compare the AI challenges or potentials between Germany and other countries.

Since digitalization and the new technologies that come along with it are advancing faster and faster, it can be expected that the topic AI will play an increasingly important role in the healthcare sector in the next years. When using well-functioning AI algorithms, there is the chance to support doctors and medical professionals considerably and to relieve them of time. In that context, the shortage of specialists can possibly be compensated in the future and doctors can focus more on the individual patient.

Acknowledgements We thank Professor Lakhmi C. Jain and all reviewers for supporting our research. Thank you for your valuable and helpful comments.

References

1. Härting, R.-C., et al.: The Potential Value of Digitization for Business: Insights from German-speaking Experts (2017) https://doi.org/10.18420/IN2017_pp.165
2. Dai, D., Boroomand, S.: A review of artificial intelligence to enhance the security of Big Data systems: state-of-art, methodologies, applications, and challenges. Arch. Computat. Methods Eng. **29**, 1291–1309 (2022). https://doi.org/10.1007/s11831-021-09628-0
3. Gjellebaek, C., et al.: Management challenges for future digitalization of healthcare services (2020). https://doi.org/10.1016/j.futures.2020.102636
4. Helm, J.M., et al.: Machine learning and artificial intelligence: definitions. Appl., Future Dir. (2020). https://doi.org/10.1007/s12178-020-09600-8

5. Federal Ministry for Economic Affairs and Climate Action: Digital Summit Event: Strengthening AI and Trust in Digital Technologies (2021). https://www.bmwi.de/Redaktion/EN/Pre ssemitteilungen/2021/05/20210518-digital-summit-event-strengthening-aI-and-trust-in-dig ital-technologies.html (accessed on 04/03/2022).
6. Mintz, Y., Brodie, R.: Introduction to artificial intelligence in medicine. Minim. Invasive Ther. Allied Technol. **28**, 73–81 (2019). https://doi.org/10.1080/13645706.2019.1575882
7. Siau, K., Wang, W.: Artificial intelligence (AI) ethics: ethics of AI and ethical AI. J. Database Manag. 14 (2020). https://doi.org/10.4018/JDM.2020040105
8. Saxena, S.: Evolving uncertainty in healthcare service interactions during COVID-19: artificial intelligence—a threat or support to value cocreation? Cyber-Phys. Syst. (2022). https://doi.org/10.1016/B978-0-12-824557-6.00014-5
9. Ludvigsen, K.R., Nagaraja, S.: Dissecting liabilities in adversarial surgical robot failures: a national (Danish) and EU law perspective. Comput. Law Secur. Rev. **44** (2022). https://doi.org/10.1016/j.clsr.2022.105656
10. Core: http://portal.core.edu.au/jnl-ranks/. Accessed on 02/07/2022
11. VHBonline (2022) https://vhbonline.org/vhb4you/vhb-jourqual/vhb-jourqual-3/gesamtliste. Accessed on 02/07/2022
12. Quinn, T.P., et al.: Trust and medical AI: the challenges we face, and the expertise needed to overcome them. J. Am. Med. Inform. Assoc. **28**(4), 890–894 (2021). https://doi.org/10.1093/jamia/ocaa268
13. Cheng, L., et al.: Socially responsible AI algorithms: issues, purposes, and challenges (2022). http://arxiv.org/abs/2101.02032
14. Kokciyan, N., et al.: Sociotechnical perspectives on AI ethics and accountability, IEEE Internet Comput. **25**(06), 5–6 (2021). https://doi.org/10.1109/MIC.2021.3117611
15. Khullar, D., et al.: Public versus physician views of liability for artificial intelligence in health care. J. Am. Med. Inform. Assoc. **28**(7), 1574–1577 (2021). https://doi.org/10.1093/jamia/oca b055
16. Riaño, D., et al.: Artificial Intelligence in Medicine: 17th Conference on Artificial Intelligence in Medicine, AIME 2019, Poznan, Poland, Proceedings, vol. 11526. Springer International Publishing, Cham (2019). https://doi.org/10.1007/978-3-030-21642-9
17. Straw, I.: The automation of bias in medical artificial intelligence: de-coding the past to create a better future. Artif. Intell. Med. (2020). https://www.sciencedirect.com/science/article/pii/S09 33365720312306
18. Norori, N., et al.: Addressing bias in big data and AI for health care: a call for open science. J. Patterns Cell Press. 1–9 (2021). https://doi.org/10.1016/j.patter.2021.100347
19. Boddington, P., et al.: Minds and machines special issue: ethics and artificial intelligence. Minds Mach. **27**(4), 569–574 (2017). https://doi.org/10.1007/s11023-017-9449-y
20. Lokhorst, G.-J.C.: Computational meta-ethics Minds Mach. (2011). https://doi.org/10.1007/s11023-011-9229-z

Printed in the United States
by Baker & Taylor Publisher Services